QUALITY MANAGEMENT
IN THE IMAGING SCIENCES

QUALITY MANAGEMENT
IN THE IMAGING SCIENCES

FIFTH EDITION

JEFFREY PAPP, PhD, RT(R) (QM)
Professor of Physics and Diagnostic Imaging
College of DuPage
Glen Ellyn, Illinois

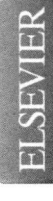
ELSEVIER

ELSEVIER
MOSBY

3251 Riverport Lane
St. Louis, Missouri 63043

QUALITY MANAGEMENT IN THE IMAGING SCIENCES,
FIFTH EDITION

ISBN: 978-0-323-26199-9

Copyright © 2015 by Mosby, an imprint of Elsevier Inc.
Copyright © 2011, 2006, 2002, 1998 by Mosby, Inc., an affiliate of Elsevier Inc.

All rights reserved. No part of this publication may be reproduced or transmitted in any form or by any means, electronic or mechanical, including photocopying, recording, or any information storage and retrieval system, without permission in writing from the publisher. Details on how to seek permission, further information about the Publisher's permissions policies and our arrangements with organizations such as the Copyright Clearance Center and the Copyright Licensing Agency, can be found at our website: www.elsevier.com/permissions.

This book and the individual contributions contained in it are protected under copyright by the Publisher (other than as may be noted herein).

Notices

Knowledge and best practice in this field are constantly changing. As new research and experience broaden our understanding, changes in research methods, professional practices, or medical treatment may become necessary.

Practitioners and researchers must always rely on their own experience and knowledge in evaluating and using any information, methods, compounds, or experiments described herein. In using such information or methods they should be mindful of their own safety and the safety of others, including parties for whom they have a professional responsibility.

With respect to any drug or pharmaceutical products identified, readers are advised to check the most current information provided (i) on procedures featured or (ii) by the manufacturer of each product to be administered, to verify the recommended dose or formula, the method and duration of administration, and contraindications. It is the responsibility of practitioners, relying on their own experience and knowledge of their patients, to make diagnoses, to determine dosages and the best treatment for each individual patient, and to take all appropriate safety precautions.

To the fullest extent of the law, neither the Publisher nor the authors, contributors, or editors, assume any liability for any injury and/or damage to persons or property as a matter of products liability, negligence or otherwise, or from any use or operation of any methods, products, instructions, or ideas contained in the material herein.

International Standard Book Number: 978-0-323-26199-9

Executive Content Strategist: Sonya Seigafuse
Content Development Manager: Laurie Gower
Content Development Specialist: Charlene Ketchum
Publishing Services Manager: Julie Eddy
Project Manager: Jan Waters
Design Direction: Paula Catalano

Printed in the United States of America

Last digit is the print number: 9 8 7 6 5 4 3 2 1

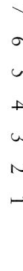

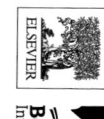

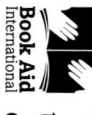

Working together
to grow libraries in
developing countries

www.elsevier.com • www.bookaid.org

To my daughter, Ashley Marie, and all of my students, past, present, and future.

CONTRIBUTORS

The author and publisher wish to acknowledge the following previous edition contributors.

Lorrie Kelley, MS, RT(R)(MR)(CT)
Associate Professor, Director, CT/MRI Programs
Boise State University
Boise, Idaho

James M. Kofler, Jr, PhD
Assistant Professor of Radiologic Physics, Mayo College of Medicine, Department of Diagnostic Radiology
Mayo Clinic
Rochester, Minnesota

Joanne M. Metler, MS, CNMT
Assistant Professor Emeritus, Nuclear Medicine Technology Program
College of DuPage
Glen Ellyn, Illinois

James A. Zagzebski, PhD
Professor, Departments of Medical Physics, Human Oncology, and Radiology
University of Wisconsin
Madison, Wisconsin

REVIEWERS

Angela Bland, MS, RT(R)
Online Instructor
Missouri College
Brentwood, Missouri

Sabrina M. Call, BS, RT(R)(CT)
Adjunct Faculty
Radiologic Sciences Department
Boise State University
Boise, Idaho
Lead CT/QA Technologist
Intermountain Medical Imaging
Boise, Idaho

Carolyn Cianciosa, MSRT(r)
Part-Time Faculty, Radiography Prior Learning Assessment
Empire State College, Niagara Frontier Center
Cheektowaga, New York

Cynthia M. Cobb, BS, RTRCT, CCRP
Manager, Imaging Quality and Safety
Lifespan; Rhode Island, Miriam, and Newport Hospitals
Providence, Rhode Island

Joe A. Garza, MS, RT(R)
Professor, Radiologic Science
Lone Star College – Montgomery
Conroe, Texas

Kerry Greene Donnelly, MBA, RT(R)(M)(CT)(QM)
Assistant Professor, Medical Imaging Sciences
College of Health Professions, Upstate Medical University
Syracuse, New York

Boyd Porowski, MDA, RT(R)
Instructor, Radiologic Technologist Program
Spencerian College
Louisville, Kentucky

Kathy McGarry, PhD, RT(R)(QM)
Learning Specialist
Cape Regional Medical Center
Cape May Court House, New Jersey

PREFACE

Quality management and its associated topics, quality assurance and quality control, are vitally important in modern diagnostic imaging departments. Government and accreditation agencies mandate procedures to ensure that equipment is functioning within accepted standards and that it is operated properly. Such procedures also must be appropriately documented. Because these responsibilities have been delegated to technologists, they need additional knowledge. The American Registry of Radiologic Technologists (ARRT) recognized this need by offering an advanced level examination in quality management in March 1997.

I have been teaching a course in quality assurance/quality management since 1983 and had never required a textbook because I could not find one single book that contained all of the necessary material. Instead, I had to reserve different books and government publications in our library for students to consult as reference sources or suggest that they consult individual chapters, research papers, and literature from various equipment manufacturers and suppliers. During discussions with other radiologic science educators, I discovered that most of them had the same problem in teaching this topic. I also had been besieged with requests from practicing technologists for study material for the Quality Management Advanced Level Examination. Previously, I could respond only by supplying a listing of several reference books.

From these many years of frustration came the impetus to write the first edition of *Quality Management in the Imaging Sciences*. The first four editions were very well received, so I am particularly pleased to offer this fifth edition, which will again fill several needs. Radiography educators find it to be a tailor-made text for instruction in quality management. It also serves as a practical reference for day-to-day consultation by practitioners responsible for implementing quality management programs in diagnostic imaging departments. Additionally, this comprehensive resource allows those practicing technologists studying for the Quality Management Advanced Level Examination to use a single reference book. The material contained in Chapters 13, 14, and 15 pertains to specialized areas of imaging (magnetic resonance imaging, sonography, and nuclear medicine) and is not covered on the Advanced Level Examination offered by the ARRT. Those readers preparing for the examination will find the material available in Evolve Resources particularly useful because it contains two sample tests based on the content outline developed by the ARRT for the Quality Management Examination.

Quality Management in the Imaging Sciences includes the most up-to-date information available on the quality management aspects of darkrooms, processing, equipment and accessories, fluoroscopic and advanced imaging equipment, artifacts, repeat analysis, and silver recovery. Quality assurance organizations and their web sites are listed in Appendix B, and full-page documentation forms are available in Evolve Resources.

The following special features are included, as in the first four editions:

- Federal regulations are set in boldface type in the text and the symbol appears beside them.
- Procedures are highlighted as separate elements with step-by-step guidelines.
- Key terms are identified at the beginnings of chapters, set in boldface type, and explained within chapters.
- Learning objectives, chapter outlines, and chapter review questions (with answers) are provided as study tools.
- Key term definitions are collected in a glossary.

NEW TO THE FIFTH EDITION

Additional updates continue to benefit the reader:

1. Revisions to the mammography chapter correspond with new digital mammographic systems that have received FDA approval.
2. The material on Evolve Resources that accompanies the text offers these features:
   a. Two 165-question mock examinations to encourage self-testing that are particularly convenient for those readers preparing for the updated ARRT Advanced Level Examination in Quality Management
   b. Full-size sample documentation forms that can be used "as is" or modified to meet the needs of a particular department
   c. Student experiments and analyses of them to correspond with appropriate chapters that have been modified for digital-only departments
   d. Questions for analysis and critical thinking that challenge the reader to prepare for real-life situations
3. Expanded material for digital imaging and quality control procedures for electronic image monitors is provided.
4. The latest changes in technology and current regulations have been updated throughout.

Quality Management in the Imaging Sciences continues to provide the wealth of information needed for instructors to guide students through quality management issues, for students and practitioners to prepare for the ARRT examination, and for technologists to succeed in the delivery of high-quality services.

INSTRUCTOR RESOURCES

Instructor ancillaries, including an ExamView Test Bank of over 400 questions; an electronic image collection of the images in the text; an instructor's manual of chapter outlines, teaching tips, and teaching strategies; and a new PowerPoint lecture presentation are all available at http://evolve.elsevier.com.

Jeffrey Papp, PhD, RT(R)(QM)

ACKNOWLEDGMENTS

Just as with the first four editions of this text, the production of this fifth edition has required the help and input of many people. I must start with my associates in the Diagnostic Medical Imaging program at the College of DuPage, namely, Pam Jankovsky and Shelli Thacker, for all of their support and understanding while I was preoccupied with writing this text. It is also important to include my Dean, Thomas Cameron, and my Associate Dean, Karen Solt. I also wish to thank Patty Holvey of Good Samaritan Hospital in Downers Grove, Illinois; Janet Petersen of Elmhurst Memorial Hospital, Elmhurst, Illinois; and Pam Verkuilen of Saint Alexius Medical Center in Hoffman Estates, Illinois, for all of their help in gathering information on digital imaging.

I am deeply indebted to my contributing authors, Lorrie Kelley, Program Director for CT/MRI at Boise State University; James M. Kofler, Assistant Professor, Department of Diagnostic Radiology, Mayo Clinic; Joanne M. Metler, Emeritus Coordinator for Nuclear Medicine at the College of DuPage; and James A. Zagzebski, Professor of Medical Physics at the University of Wisconsin, Madison.

I would also like to thank Charlene Ketchum, Andrea Hunolt, Sonya Seigafuse, and everyone at Elsevier for their help, support, and patience in the production of this text and the accompanying material found in the Evolve Resources.

Finally, I must thank Professor Gerard Lietz of DePaul University for giving me the knowledge, inspiration, and love of medical physics that allowed me to be successful in this profession.

Jeffrey Papp, PhD, RT(R)(QM)

CONTENTS

CHAPTERS

1. Introduction to Quality Management, 1
2. Quality Management Tools and Procedures, 19
3. Film/Screen Image Receptors, Darkrooms, and Viewing Conditions, 35
4. Film Processing, 52
5. Processor Quality Control, 69
6. Silver Recovery, 82
7. Quality Control of X-ray Generators and Ancillary Radiographic Equipment, 90
8. Quality Control of Fluoroscopic Equipment, 120
9. Digital and Advanced Imaging Equipment, 137
10. Outcomes Assessment of Radiographic Images, 177
11. Mammographic Quality Standards, 194
12. Quality Control in Computed Tomography, 267
13. Quality Control for Magnetic Resonance Imaging Equipment, 283
14. Ultrasound Equipment Quality Assurance, 301
15. Quality Assurance in Nuclear Medicine, 319

APPENDICES

A. Review of Radiographic Quality, 343
B. Agencies, Organizations, and Committees in Quality Assurance, 351

Bibliography, 352

Glossary, 353

CHAPTER 1 Introduction to Quality Management

TABLE 1-1 | Mandatory Reporting Requirements for User Facilities

Category	Report Form	To Whom	When
Death	FDA 3500 A	FDA and manufacturer	Within 10 working days
Serious injury	FDA 3500 A	Manufacturer; FDA only if manufacturer is unknown	Within 10 working days
Annual report of death and serious injury	FDA 3419	FDA	January 1

FDA, Food and Drug Administration.

assurance programs for all facilities that want to perform mammographic procedures to obtain FDA approval. Specific requirements were designed for dedicated equipment, physicians interpreting the images, medical physicists, and technologists. Most of these standards were formulated by or in conjunction with the American College of Radiology and were in use by many facilities before enactment of the MQSA. This law became effective October 1, 1994. The MQSA was replaced by the Mammography Quality Standards Reauthorization Act (MQSRA) of 1998, also known as Public Law 105-248. As part of the new law, final FDA regulations concerning mammographic procedures became effective April 28, 1999, replacing interim regulations that were used during the original law. The final regulations emphasize performance objectives rather than specify the behavior and manner of compliance. More specific information on the MQSA and MQSRA can be found in Chapter 11.

The **Health Insurance Portability and Accountability Act (HIPAA)** of 1996 (also known as the Kennedy-Kassebaum Act or Public Law 104-191) was enacted to simplify healthcare standards and save money for healthcare businesses by encouraging electronic transactions, but it also required new safeguards to protect patient security and confidentiality. HIPAA established national standards for healthcare e-commerce that include the following:

1. Electronic patient record system security requirements (security standard): This created a new national standard for the administrative, technical, and physical safety of protected health information (PHI).
2. Standard electronic formats for insurance transactions such as enrollment, encounters, and claims (transaction standard): This standard requires the implementation of a uniform set of codes and forms, such as the American National Standards Institute (ANSI) ASC X12N format for electronic healthcare transactions or professional and institutional claims.
3. Standard identifiers and codes for institutions, personnel, diagnoses, and treatments (national identifier standard): This created national numbers to identify employers (EIN), health plans (Payer ID) and healthcare providers (National Provider Identifiers or NPI). It also contains a set of codes that are used to encode all healthcare data. The four categories of these codes are (1) diseases (ICD-9); (2) injuries (ICD-10); (3) actions taken to prevent, diagnose, treat, or manage diseases (CPT-4); and (4) substances, equipment, and supplies (HCPCS).
4. Patient information, confidentiality, and privacy rules (privacy standard): This created a new national standard for privacy of protected health information.

The Department of Health and Human Services first issued proposed regulations for these standards in November 1999, with final rules approved in December 2000. They took effect April 14, 2001, and all healthcare organizations had to comply with and implement them by April 14, 2005. All medical records and patient information, whether electronic, on paper, or oral, are covered by these final rules.

Failure to comply with these standards resulted in significant penalties ranging from as little as $10 to $250,000 dollars and 10 years in prison. The **American Recovery and Reinvestment Act** of 2009 included the **Health Information Technology for Economic and Clinical Health Act** that amended HIPAA's enforcement regulations by adding several categories of violations and established ranges of penalty amounts for each category of violation. These regulations took effect on February 18, 2009, and include the following categories of violations and their respective penalty amounts available:

Violation Category—Section 1176 (a)(1)	Each Violation	All Such Violations of an Identical Provision in a Calendar Year
(A) Did not know	$100–$50,000	$1,500,000
(B) Reasonable cause	$1000–$50,000	$1,500,000
(C)(i) Willful neglect—corrected	$10,000–$50,000	$1,500,000
(C)(ii) Willful neglect—Not corrected	$50,000	$1,500,000

Further information can be found in the Federal Register/Vol. 74, No. 209/Friday, October 30, 2009/Rules and Regulations 56127.

This means that healthcare administrators must have policies and procedures including establishing a system of security and confidentiality, training all personnel in these policies, and appointing a staff member to act as a security officer to monitor compliance with these policies. This is discussed further in Chapter 2. Complete HIPAA guidelines can be found in the Federal Register under Title 45 of the Code of Federal Regulations Parts 160-164 (45 CFR 160-164).

The **Deficit Reduction Act** of 2005 (DRA), also known as Public Law 109-362, was enacted to help make $11 billion in cuts from 2007 (when the DRA went into effect) to 2015 in Medicare and Medicaid programs. One aspect of the program is to reduce payments for freestanding diagnostic imaging centers by capping some current procedural terminology (CPT) codes that were higher than hospital outpatient rates and freezing CPT codes already lower than hospital outpatient rates. Current procedural terminology codes were developed by the American Medical Association (AMA) and adopted by the federal government and private insurance providers to classify medical, surgical, and diagnostic services. The DRA also requires imaging centers to have quality control standards in place in order to receive reimbursement.

Having an effective quality management program also has become necessary as a condition of receiving reimbursement for services by the federal government. The United States Department of Health and Human Services, through its subbranch the CMS, emphasizes effective quality management procedures be documented in order for healthcare facilities to receive reimbursement for any healthcare service, and many private insurance companies have followed this practice.

The **Patient Protection and Affordable Care Act** of 2010, commonly known as "Obama Care" or Public Law 111-148, was enacted to increase health insurance coverage for Americans as well as reducing the overall cost of health care. There are far too many provisions of this bill to cover in a chapter of a book, so I will only mention the ones that should have a direct impact on diagnostic imaging departments. One provision (discussed earlier in this chapter) would change Medicare reimbursement from "fee for service" to a bundled payment for a "defined episode of care," which could lower the reimbursement rate to healthcare providers. Another provision adds a 2.3% excise tax on all medical devices (such as diagnostic imaging equipment) that is collected at the time of purchase. This could lead to more equipment being leased rather than purchased. It is also thought that having more people insured will increase the demand for healthcare services, thereby increasing the demand for imaging professionals in the workplace. Since many provisions are scheduled to become effective gradually between 2014 and 2018, it will take time to evaluate the impact of the law.

The Joint Commission

The Joint Commission (TJC), formerly known as the Joint Commission for the Accreditation of Healthcare Organizations or JCAHO) was founded in 1951, and is an independent, not-for-profit organization that accredits and certifies more than 20,000 healthcare organizations and programs in the United States. In the 1970s, TJC began requiring hospitals and other healthcare providers to perform and document specific quality assurance procedures in order for these facilities to obtain accreditation. Accreditation is voluntary, but hospitals and medical centers that do not have it may not possess Medicaid certification, hold certain licenses, have a residency program for training physicians, obtain reimbursements from insurance companies, or receive malpractice insurance. However, some hospitals may choose not to be accredited by TJC and instead have inspections by their state public health departments or other organizations such as DNV Healthcare (discussed later in this chapter). These hospitals include many rural hospitals that may be critical access hospitals and would still receive Medicaid and Medicare reimbursements. TJC accredits not only hospitals but also facilities for long-term care, ambulatory care, mental health, and chemical dependency. These quality management procedures are extensive and specific in nature. For example, any equipment that is inspected daily (Monday through Friday) also must be inspected on Saturday and Sunday if the opportunity exists that a patient would need that piece of equipment on the weekend. Second, refrigerators that contain medical supplies must have a thermometer, and a log of the daily recorded temperature (including weekends) must be kept. TJC also requires accredited institutions to have a process in place for correcting customer complaints (a process known as *service recovery*). This means that proper performance and documentation of quality management procedures are essential to pass TJC inspections. Standards set by TJC to receive accreditation require that healthcare organizations have a planned, systematic, and organization-wide approach for monitoring, evaluating, and improving the quality of care, as well as those of management, governance, and support activities. TJC standards also require that healthcare organizations must perform routine inspections of all equipment, devices, and supplies.

Before 1991, TJC used the concepts of quality assurance and quality control requiring systematic monitoring and evaluation, with the responsibility left to the medical director or department head. Because these concepts now have been incorporated into the newer quality management philosophy, an understanding of quality assurance and quality control is still important and is discussed in the following sections.

Det Norske Veritas Healthcare

DNV Healthcare, Inc. is part of Det Norske Veritas, a global foundation that was established in Oslo, Norway, in 1864 and has been operating in the United States since 1898. Their stated purpose is to safeguard life, property, and the environment. On September 26, 2008, DNV

Healthcare was granted authority to accredit hospitals by the CMS, and is therefore an alternative to The Joint Commission for hospitals to receive accreditation. Their philosophy is based on standards created by the International Organization for Standardization (ISO) based in Geneva, Switzerland (www.iso.org). These standards are based on very similar quality management principles as The Joint Commission standards, namely:

1. Customer focus
2. Leadership
3. Involvement of people
4. Process approach
5. System approach to management
6. Continual improvement
7. Factual approach to decision making
8. Mutually beneficial supplier relationships

Quality Assurance. Quality assurance (QA) is an all-encompassing management program used to ensure excellence in health care through the systematic collection and evaluation of data. The primary objective of a QA program is the enhancement of patient care; this includes patient selection parameters and scheduling, management techniques, departmental policies and procedures, technical effectiveness and efficiency, in-service education, and image interpretation with timeliness of reports. The main emphasis of the program is on the human factors that can lead to variations in quality care. Quality assurance should not be confused with **quality assessment**, which is the measurement of the level of quality at some point in time with no effort to change or improve the level of care.

Quality Control. Quality control (QC) is the part of the QA program that deals with techniques used in monitoring and maintaining the technical elements of the systems that affect the quality of the image. Therefore, quality control is the part of the QA program that deals with instrumentation and equipment. A quality control program includes the following three levels of testing:

Level I: Noninvasive and Simple. Noninvasive and simple evaluations can be performed by any technologist and include tests such as the wire mesh test for screen contact and the spinning top test for timer accuracy.

Level II: Noninvasive and Complex. Noninvasive and complex evaluations should be performed by a technologist who has been specifically trained in quality control procedures. This is because more sophisticated equipment, such as special test tools, meters, or the noninvasive evaluation of radiation output (NERO) computerized multiple function unit, is used. Many educational programs now include this level of competency for graduation, so the number of technologists with these skills is increasing. The American Society of Radiologic Technologists (ASRT) includes quality control and QA duties in its practice standards for radiographers, sonographers, nuclear medicine technologists, CT technologists, MRI technologists, mammographers, interventional radiographers, and bone densitometry technologists. The American Registry of Radiologic Technologists (ARRT) offers an advanced level certification exam for technologists wishing to document their knowledge of QA and quality control procedures and protocols. This can be used to verify qualification for a quality management technologist position.

Level III: Invasive and Complex. Invasive and complex evaluations involve some disassembly of the equipment and are normally performed by engineers or physicists. This textbook focuses on levels I and II of quality control testing. The following are the three types of quality control tests on various levels:

- Acceptance testing is performed on new equipment or equipment that has undergone major repair to demonstrate that it is performing within the manufacturer's specifications and criteria. It also can detect any defects that may exist in the equipment. The results obtained during acceptance testing are also used to establish the baseline performance of the equipment that is used as a reference point in future quality control testing.
- Routine performance evaluations are specific tests performed on the equipment in use after a certain amount of time has elapsed. These evaluations can verify that the equipment is performing within previously accepted standards and can be used to diagnose any changes in performance before becoming radiographically apparent.
- Error correction tests evaluate equipment that is malfunctioning or not performing at the manufacturer's specifications and are also used to verify the correct cause of the malfunction so that the proper repair can be made.

Continuous Quality Improvement. The older QA/QC program ensured that a certain level of quality was met; it required monitoring only periodically for maintenance. It was segmented in approach because each department in a facility monitored and evaluated its own structural outcomes, creating a tendency to view individual performances rather than the process or system in which that individual was functioning. In turn, the program was externally motivated because its emphasis was on demonstrating compliance with externally developed standards. As long as the standards were met, no further work was required to improve the system.

In 1991, TJC began incorporating the concepts of continuous quality improvement (CQI), which is defined as a structured organizational process for involving personnel in planning and executing a continuous flow of improvements to provide quality health care that meets or exceeds expectations, to replace the older QA/QC philosophy into their program of accreditation of healthcare organizations. CQI evolved from *total quality management* (TQM) concept in the manufacturing industry, also referred to as *total quality control* (TQC), *total quality leadership* (TQL), *total quality improvement* (TQI), and *statistical quality control* (SQC). This concept is based on the "14 Points for Management" developed by W. Edwards Deming (Box 1-1) and the Japanese management style.

The CQI concept does not replace the concept of quality assurance/quality control but incorporates it at a higher conceptual level. Instead of just ensuring and maintaining quality, it continually improves quality by focusing on improving the system or process in which individual workers function rather than on the individuals themselves. For these processes to improve, it is essential to focus on the organization as a whole, rather than on individual departments. It is important that each healthcare organization have a clear mission, values, and objectives that performance improvement processes are designed and implemented to support. It also promotes the need for objective data involving statistics to analyze and improve processes (known as data-driven or evidence-based analysis). Every employee should be actively involved in CQI (rather than just management or the quality control technologist) for the program to be successful. In this way, CQI can be internally motivating because employees will see that their involvement is tied to the success of the hospital, creating an atmosphere in which employees are motivated to do better because they are participating actively. Management must take the responsibility to promote this atmosphere, effectively allocate resources needed for improvement, treat employees as assets and not expenses, and work together toward shared goals. Managers/leaders should establish unity of purpose and direction of the organization. They should create and maintain the internal environment in which people can become fully involved in achieving the organization's objectives. For healthcare institutions, this should allow the ultimate focus to be on improving patient care, which should build a satisfied customer base and benefit the institution in the long term.

PROCESS IMPROVEMENT THROUGH CONTINUOUS QUALITY IMPROVEMENT

As mentioned earlier, CQI focuses on the process in which employees operate rather than on the employees themselves. The rationale is that problems and variability with the process are the main cause of poor quality. The concept of process improvement through CQI is based on the following premises:

- 85/15 Rule—the process or system in place is the cause of problems 85% of the time, and the people or personnel within the process are the cause of problems 15% of the time.
- 80/20 Rule—80% of the problems are the result of 20% of the causes.
- Workers who are closest to the problem probably know what is wrong with the process and are better able to fix it.
- Structured problem-solving processes that use statistical means to verify performance produce better long-term solutions than processes that are not structured.
- Improving quality is the responsibility of everyone within an organization because all are a part of the process. People at all levels are the essence of an organization, and their involvement enables their abilities to be used for the organization's benefit.

For healthcare organizations, most of the processes should be oriented toward the deliverance of high quality care and the achievement of customer satisfaction. A **process** is an ordered series of steps that help achieve a desired outcome or all the tasks directed at accomplishing one particular outcome grouped in a sequence. A **system** is a group of related processes. Identifying, understanding, and managing interrelated processes contributes to the healthcare organization's effectiveness and efficiency in achieving its objectives. The parts of any process include a supplier, input, action, output, and the customer.

- A **supplier** is an individual or entity that furnishes input to a process (e.g., person, department, organization) or one who provides the institution with goods or services. For diagnostic imaging departments, examples may include imaging equipment

---

BOX 1-1 Fourteen Points of Management

1. Create constancy of purpose toward improvement of product and service, with the aim to become competitive and stay in business and provide jobs.
2. Adopt a new philosophy.
3. Cease dependence on mass inspection to achieve quality. Build quality into the product in the first place.
4. End the practice of awarding business on the basis of price alone. Instead, minimize total cost. Move toward a single supplier for any one item because of a long-term relationship built on loyalty and trust.
5. Improve constantly and forever the system of production and service to improve quality and productivity and thus constantly reduce costs.
6. Institute on-the-job training.
7. Institute leadership to help people do the job better.
8. Drive out fear so everyone can work effectively for the good of the organization.
9. Break down barriers among departments.
10. Eliminate slogans, exhortations, and targets for the workforce.
11. Eliminate work quotas. Substitute leadership.
12. Eliminate merit rating systems.
13. Institute a vigorous program of education and self-improvement.
14. Involve everyone in the organization in the transformation of total quality improvement (TQI).

From Deming WE: *Out of the crisis*, Cambridge, Mass, 1986, Center for Advanced Educational Services, MIT Press.

vendors and referring physicians. An organization and its suppliers are interdependent, and a mutually beneficial relationship enhances the ability of both to create value for both parties.

- **Input** is information or knowledge necessary to achieve the desired outcome. For diagnostic imaging departments, examples may include patient information, examination requested, knowledge of procedures, and workload.
- **Action** is the means or activity used to achieve the desired outcome. Examples for diagnostic imaging departments may include computer entry and form completion and assignment of patients to appropriate rooms. The action steps are sometimes referred to as the *workflow*.

These first three steps are variable factors that influence the next portion of the process called the *output*.

- **Output** refers to the desired outcome, result, product, or characteristics that satisfy the customer. In diagnostic imaging departments, examples may include completed paperwork and completed diagnostic examination. A desired result is achieved more efficiently when activities and related resources are managed as a process.
- **Customer** refers to a person, department, or organization that needs or wants the desired outcome.

According to Deming, the customer determines what constitutes quality. This can be broken down into the following groups:

- *Internal customers:* Generally, these are individuals or groups from within the organization such as referring physicians, hospital employees, departments, and department employees.
- *External customers:* These are individuals or groups from outside the organization, such as patients and their families, third-party payers, and the community.

The satisfaction of the customer, both internal and external, is the driving force behind CQI because it focuses on the needs and expectations of customers and the continuous improvement of the product or service. By continually meeting or exceeding customer satisfaction, the process is considered to be successful. Both customer satisfaction and health outcomes should be used as performance measures to evaluate the success of a process in a healthcare environment. Organizations depend on their customers, and therefore should understand current and future customer needs, meet customer requirements, and strive to exceed customer expectations.

Key Quality Characteristics

Key quality characteristics are those qualities or aspects that have been identified as being most important to the customer. These characteristics must be constantly measured and improved in order for customer satisfaction to increase. Examples in diagnostic imaging departments would be availability of a procedure (e.g., MRI, PET), accurate report of image findings delivered promptly to the ordering physician, and minimal waiting time for patients.

Key Process Variables. Key process variables are the components of any process that may affect the final output of the process. Variability can have a negative impact on the quality of the final output, and systems must be developed to properly manage any variability that may arise. Unfortunately, patients, providers, and diagnostic categories found in health care are highly variable. There are five major categories of key process variables: manpower, machines, materials, environment, and policies.

- *Manpower* refers to the personnel involved in the process.
- *Machines* refers to the equipment used in the process.
- *Materials* refers to the type and quality of materials used in the process.
- *Environment* refers to the physical and psychological aspects on people involved in the process.
- *Policies* refers to the steps in the procedure or policy manual that have been used in the process.

Problem Identification and Analysis

Group Dynamics. For the continual improvement of the processes involved in customer satisfaction, several tools must be used to identify and analyze the data obtained. Groups or teams of individuals who are familiar with or are using the processes are generally the most successful in helping with problem identification in CQI. This is because a single individual may not have enough knowledge or experience, or both, with all of the aspects of a process. A team consists of at least two persons. For healthcare organizations, the ideal number for most teams or groups is 6–12 persons. To be effective, these teams should be goal oriented, share equal responsibility, and be empowered by management. By working together, team members not only can improve older processes and develop new and better ones but also develop a sense of ownership within the organization (and therefore be more productive workers). Group dynamic tools that can be used in quality management include brainstorming, focus groups, quality improvement teams, quality circles, multivoting, consensus, work teams, and problem-solving teams.

Brainstorming. Brainstorming is a group process used to develop a large collection of ideas without regard to their merit or validity. For example, a department meeting of all staff could be used to solicit ideas or suggestions for a particular topic. The leader of this session should encourage participation by everyone, not criticize any contribution made, and record all ideas for future assessment. It is also important to announce the topic to be discussed to all team members before the session.

It also may be more effective for the leader to review the particular subject at the beginning of the session and then phrase the topic that will be discussed in the form of a question. However, the discussion should be relevant to the topic being discussed, and the leader must direct members to adhere to this topic.

Focus Groups. A focus group is a small group that focuses on a particular problem and then hopefully derives a solution. Generally, the applicable ideas on a particular problem obtained from brainstorming are considered in this smaller group, which can come to a consensus. Focus groups also may be responsible for obtaining additional data such as the interviewing of customers and patient surveys. This may add to a higher implementation cost for focus groups as compared with other group dynamic tools. A focus group must have a skilled facilitator to be successful.

Quality Improvement Team. A quality improvement team is a group of individuals who implement the solutions that were derived by the focus group. This may or may not include members of the focus group. Ideally, quality improvement teams should have six or seven members who are key customers or suppliers, or both, of the steps in the process (i.e., the people who actually do the steps in the process). It is best to avoid teams of managers only because they usually do not have detailed knowledge of the process. Input from other customers and suppliers should be sought by the team.

Quality Circles. This type of group dynamic tool is normally composed of supervisors and workers who are from the same department or who may have the same function in a similar department. Quality circles should be scheduled to meet regularly and have the specific function to identify potential problems with departmental processes and then formulate solutions. Levels of productivity and quality of images produced within a department are possible issues that may be discussed by quality circles.

Multivoting. This method is normally used after a brainstorming session to dismiss nonessential or nonrealistic ideas and then concentrate on those that can realistically solve the problem. All members of the brainstorming session are given a list of all of the ideas that were formulated and then asked to vote on which one they consider the most important. The ideas with the fewest votes are discarded and the process repeated (thus the name, *multivoting*) until just one key idea remains. This method reduces a large number of ideas or options to a manageable few judged important by the participants.

Consensus. This is another method that can follow a successful brainstorming session. After the initial ideas are formulated during the brainstorming session, the group members, through discussion and teamwork, come to an agreement on the most important idea to be addressed. Total agreement within the group is unnecessary, but any decision should at least be acceptable to all group members.

Work Teams. These teams focus on solving a complete problem or completing an entire task, rather than focusing on any one particular step in a process. Some work teams, known as *self-managed teams (SMTs)* are composed of 6–18 persons and are empowered by management to take any corrective action necessary to solve the assigned problem or task. The SMT members should be highly trained in the particular area in which they are working. The teamwork created by these teams is highly successful in facilitating CQI and solving potential problems.

Problem-Solving Teams. These teams work on specific tasks and meet to solve particular problems, as well as *root cause analysis (RCA)*, which tries to identify the root causes of faults or problems within the process. They normally function to identify, analyze, and then solve both quality and productivity issues. Problem-solving teams must have a knowledgeable facilitator who is responsible for teaching team members the appropriate problem-solving tools for guiding them through the process. Two common problem-solving tools are *5 Why's* and the *Thought Process Map.*

5 Why's. This is a question-asking method developed by the Toyota Corporation that is used to explore the cause-and-effect relationships that may underlie a particular problem. Its ultimate goal is to determine the root cause of a problem. For example:

The department waiting time is excessive. (The problem)

1. Why?—One of the five X-ray rooms in the department is always malfunctioning.
2. Why?—The unit in the room is used 24 h/day 7 days/week.
3. Why?—The unit is 10 years old.
4. Why?—It is beyond its useful service life and has never been replaced.
5. Why?—Administration will not approve the purchase of a new unit.

Once the root cause is identified, a solution can then be devised to solve it. A fishbone diagram (discussed in Chapter 2) is most helpful in identifying multiple causes of problems during root cause analysis.

Thought Process Map. The thought process map (TPM) is one of the first tools that should be employed for a process improvement project. It presents thoughts, ideas, and questions at the beginning of a project to help a team or person identify all information and progress. There are five basic steps to create a TMP:

- Define the project's goal(s). The project improvement team needs to clearly define what needs to be accomplished or what problem needs to be solved. Brainstorming among the group is a good way to define the goal.
- List the knowns and unknowns. The team leader should use a large poster board or easel pad and make two columns—one for what the team knows

and one for what the team does not know. This can help identify the amount and type of data necessary to complete the project.
- Ask grouped questions or questions that define, measure, analyze, improve, or control (DMAIC). Focusing on the unknowns from step 2, create questions from the categorical perspectives of DMAIC. These perspectives are discussed in more detail later in this chapter.
- Sequence and link the questions. The questions in step 4 are now linked together using a flowchart (discussed in Chapter 2).
- Identify possible tools to be used. This step involves identifying potential tools that can be used to answer the questions posed In step 3. The most effective way to accomplish this step is to create a four-column matrix that assigns a column for the question, the tool or method, who is responsible, and the due date.

Specific Quality Management Quality Improvement Processes

TJC 10-Step Process. In 1985, TJC introduced the 10-step monitoring and evaluation process as the mechanism for satisfaction of accreditation. Although it is still in use today, the emphasis of some of its steps has changed from QA to CQI.

Step 1: Assign responsibility for the department's monitoring and evaluation activities. In QA, the medical director is ultimately responsible, but the task is usually delegated to a supervisor or QA technologist. With CQI, both intradepartmental and interdepartmental committees work together with hospital management participation. A separate quality management department is found in many healthcare facilities, while others use a unit or section within the diagnostic imaging area for QM responsibilities. Regardless, each department or committee is responsible for documenting the effectiveness of its quality management activities and for reporting such activities to the organization-wide program. Staff members who perform quality management responsibilities also should make sure that the overall organizational program is functional and effective.

Step 2: Delineate the scope of care and service provided by the department. With the QA model, the major services of a particular department are listed (e.g., imaging modalities offered, types of patients served, credentials of staff), whereas under CQI, the scope of care or service for the hospital as a whole is defined.

Step 3: Identify important aspects of care and service. Under QA, specific departmental tasks or functions are identified, with emphasis on high volume (chest radiography), high risk (mammography interpretations and angiography), and high risk/problem prone (and diagnostic imaging procedure requiring intravenous contrast media). With CQI, the entire hospital determines the key functions to be monitored. This should include important functions relating to patients, care of patients, leadership, use of medications, use of blood and blood components, and determination of the appropriateness of admissions and continued hospitalization.

Step 4: Identify indicators or performance measures. The Joint Commission defines an **indicator** as a valid and reliable quantitative process or outcome measure related to one or more dimensions of performance. There are two important types of indicators.

Adverse Event Indicator. An adverse event (or complication) is an untoward, undesirable, and usually unanticipated event that is caused by medical management rather than by the underlying disease or condition of the patient. In general, adverse events prolong the hospitalization, produce a disability at the time of discharge, or both. Examples might include perforation of a vessel during an angiographic or interventional procedure. Incidents such as patient falls or improper administration of medications are also considered adverse events, even if there is no permanent effect on the patient.

Sentinel Event Indicator. A sentinel event is an unexpected occurrence involving death or serious physical or psychological injury, or the risk thereof. Serious injury specifically includes loss of limb or function. The phrase "or the risk thereof" includes any process variation for which a recurrence would carry a significant chance of a serious adverse outcome. The events are called "sentinel" because they signal the need for immediate investigation and response. A **sentinel event indicator** identifies an individual event or phenomenon that is significant enough to trigger further review each time it occurs. These events are undesirable and occur infrequently, such as the death of a patient during a diagnostic examination as a result of contrast media reaction, suicide of a patient in a setting where the patient receives around-the-clock care, unanticipated death of a full-term infant, infant abduction or discharge to the wrong family, sexual assault of a patient, hemolytic transfusion reaction involving administration of blood or blood products having major blood group incompatibilities, and surgery on the wrong patient or wrong body part.

Aggregate Data Indicator. An **aggregate data indicator** quantifies a process or outcome related to many cases. It may occur frequently and may be desirable or undesirable. Examples include the number of cesarean sections, interventional procedures, and reported medication errors.

Using QA, each department identifies indicators, whereas under CQI, an interdisciplinary team identifies indicators that focus more on the process of care. The performance indicators that are most relevant to healthcare organizations would include the following:

- **Appropriateness of care** is whether the type of care (i.e., specific test, procedure, or service) that has been

requested is necessary. In other words, is it relevant to the patient's clinical needs, given the current state of knowledge (Are you doing the right thing?).
- **Continuity of care** is the degree to which the care/intervention for the patient is coordinated among practitioners or organizations, or both, over time.
- **Effectiveness of care** is the level of benefit when services are rendered under ordinary circumstances by average practitioners for typical patients, as defined by K.N. Lohr.* It also may be defined as the degree to which the care/intervention is provided in the correct manner, given the current state of knowledge, in order to achieve the desired/projected outcome for the patient.
- **Efficacy of care** is the level of benefit expected when healthcare services are applied under ideal conditions and the best possible circumstances or the degree to which the care/intervention has been shown to accomplish the desired outcome (i.e., Are you doing the right thing well?). Most healthcare systems deliver care that is somewhere between effectiveness and efficacy. QA attempts to bring effectiveness to efficacy, whereas CQI goes a step further in allowing for continued improvement once effectiveness has been reached.
- **Efficiency of care** refers to the outcome obtained when the highest quality of care is delivered in the shortest amount of time, with the least amount of expense, and with a positive outcome for the patient condition.

An aggregate data indicator involves the relationship between the outcomes (results of care) and the resources used to deliver patient care.

- **Respect and caring** is defined as the degree to which the patient or a designee is involved in his or her own care decisions and to which those providing services do so with sensitivity and respect for the patient's needs, expectations, and individual differences. Respect and caring refers to how well patients are treated during the delivery of healthcare service, what the patient's level of satisfaction is, and how well a patient's complaints are handled by staff and management.
- **Safety in the care environment.** This is the degree to which the risk of an intervention and the risk in the care environment are reduced for the patient and others, including the healthcare provider. Safety in the care environment includes equipment functioning and operation, application of universal precautions, and competency of staff.
- **Timeliness of care.** This is defined as the degree to which the care/intervention is provided to the patient at the most beneficial or necessary time. Timeliness of care refers to the delivery of health care within a reasonable amount of time, with minimal waiting time.

---
*From Lohr KN: Outcomes measurement: concepts and questions, *Inquiry* 25:37-50, 1988

- **Cost of care.** Cost of care refers to the delivery of health care that is reasonable for the current marketplace.
- **Availability of care.** This is defined as the degree to which appropriate care/intervention is available to meet the patient's needs. Availability of care refers to the availability at the clinical facility of the type of care or procedure required by the patient. A good example would be how early a patient who has a breast lump would be able to have a mammogram.

Step 5: Establish a Means to Trigger Evaluation. Under QA, a level of expectation is to be identified for each indicator. TJC identifies a level of expectation (formerly known as a *threshold*) as a preestablished level of performance applied to a specific indicator. The levels can be determined internally (on the basis of past performance of the facility) or externally (on the basis of federal and state regulations or professional guidelines such as those of TJC). As long as the indicator is below the expectation level in a negative event or condition, no further action or evaluation is required. For a highly desirable condition or event, the level of expectation is set at 100%. Under CQI, interdisciplinary teams use statistical methods to determine levels or patterns that trigger evaluation.

Step 6: Collect and Organize Data. Under QA, the department determines the protocol for data collection. First, the method of collection is determined. These data must be collected systematically and on important processes and outcomes that are related to the care of the patient or the functions of the healthcare organization. Options for collection include the following: *Patient surveys and questionnaires.* These should be sent to patients 3–7 days after discharge or on service dates for outpatients. These are the simplest mechanisms for obtaining customer/patient information. These should be brief (completed in 15 min or less, to generate a high response rate), have responses that can be measured quantitatively (such as multiple choice or Likert scale—a response that ranges from strongly disagree to strongly agree), and be clearly worded so that patients understand what is being asked of them.

- *Patient records.* Information such as sentinel events or other data is easily obtained.
- *Staff reports.* These include patient care logs, diaries, drug reaction reports, medication variance reports, and so on.
- *Focus groups.* As previously discussed, these small groups collect data that focus on finding a solution to a specific problem.
- *Computer database.* Considerable patient information and relevant data from across the country may be available in some computer databases. However, privacy concerns such as those addressed in the HIPAA (previously discussed) may limit access to database information.

CHAPTER 1 Introduction to Quality Management

Next, the size of the sample is determined (e.g., how many patients, cases). Then the frequency of collection is determined (e.g., concurrently, daily, weekly, monthly). **Concurrent data** are any data collected during the time of care. Data that should be collected and processed on a continuous basis include patient deaths (dependent on the patient mix and regional factors) and serious complications to treatment. The frequency at which data are collected for a specific indicator is reviewed annually to indicate whether the data are adequately capturing the desired information. The final task is to analyze the data and determine how they are manipulated for comparison with the level of expectation or with preestablished criteria. Under CQI, an interdisciplinary team determines the protocol for data collection from various areas of the hospital.

Step 7: Initiate Evaluation. With QA, the staff evaluates the level of performance for an indicator by comparing it with the expectation level. With CQI, the leaders identify areas for evaluation according to the data collected.

Step 8: Take Actions to Improve Care and Service. With QA, individuals are evaluated as to whether expectation levels were achieved and corrective action taken accordingly. The CQI method looks at the process used in providing the care or service rather than at the individual.

Step 9: Assess Effectiveness of Actions and Maintain Improvements. The QA method examines whether the actions taken in Step 8 are effective in ensuring quality, whereas the CQI method shows that improvement is continually being sustained. Documentation of these methods is important.

Step 10: Communicate Results to Affected Individuals and Groups. With the QA method, all results are given to a QA committee and then shared with the department staff and hospital QA committee, whereas with CQI, all results are reported to the leaders and other affected individuals. All data collected must be consolidated for distribution in a final report. A common method of presenting such results is with a storyboard (Fig. 1-1). A storyboard can summarize a whole report or process with photographs and graphs and a minimum of text. The final report should include a description of a process identified for improvement, the method used to identify that process; the department involved; the source of all data collected; any cause of variation that is identified; any corrective action that was taken; the person or persons who implemented this action; the timetable for implementation; whether or not the process was actually improved; future plans to monitor the process; and any plans to restudy, if applicable.

TJC Cycle for Improving Performance. The Joint Commission 10-step monitoring and evaluation process is still valid and is the basis of their "Cycle for Improving Performance," which identifies the steps **design, measure, assess,** and **improve.**

Design. Systematic planning and implementation are key to the design of any function or process. When new functions and processes are being designed and planned, the following factors should be considered:

- The organization's overriding purpose (mission), view of its future (vision), and strategies for carrying out its mission and fulfilling its vision (strategic plan)
- Needs and expectations of patients, staff, accrediting agencies, and payers (customers and suppliers)
- Current knowledge about organizational and clinical activities from both inside and outside the organization
- Current and relevant data, such as the number of patients receiving diagnostic imaging examinations

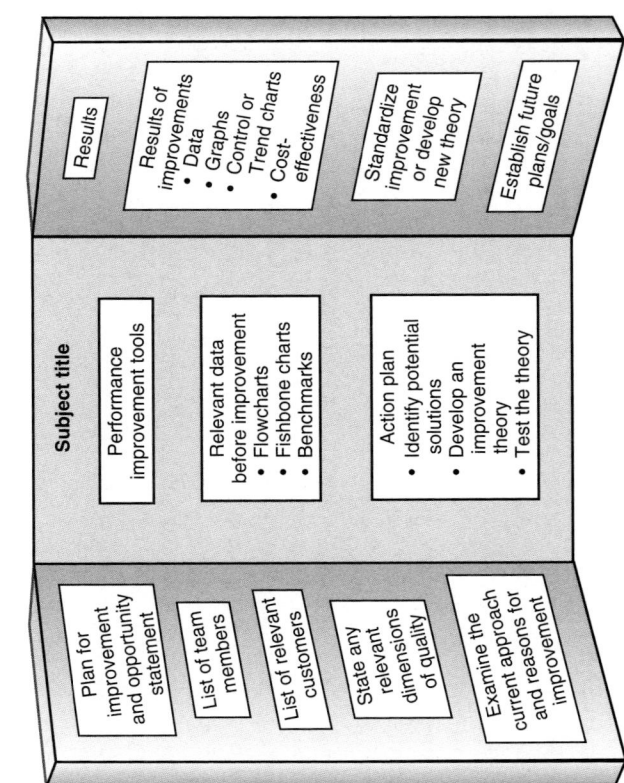

FIGURE 1-1 Model for a storyboard.

per month, the department repeat rate, and the number of practicing physicians
- Availability of resources such as funds, staff time, and equipment

Measure. A *measure* is defined by TJC as a collection of valid and reliable data to demonstrate the effectiveness and efficiency of care and performance improvement. These data can be collected by various means, including focus groups and quality improvement teams.

Assess. *Assessment* is defined by TJC as translating data collected during measurement into information that can be used to change processes and improve performance. Proper assessment usually requires comparing data with a reference point or standard. This includes the following:

Internal:

- *Historical patterns of performance in the organization* (also called *baseline performance*). This is a comparison of current performance levels with those occurring previously, such as comparing current department repeat rates with those of the previous year.
- *Desired performance limits.* The patient population and referring physicians expect a certain level of performance. This should be compared with the level achieved, as indicated by the current data. The healthcare organization also may establish its own control limits, targets, and specifications that can be compared with the data obtained.

External:

- *Practice guidelines and parameters.* These procedures, developed by professional societies, expert panels, or in-house practitioners, represent a consensus of the best practices for a given diagnosis, treatment, or procedure. These are usually described in the form of a *critical path* that documents the basic treatment or action sequence in an effort to eliminate unnecessary variation. A critical path defines the optimal sequence and timing of intervention by healthcare practitioners for a particular diagnosis or process.
- **Performance measurement system.** A performance measurement system is an entity consisting of one or more automated databases that facilitates performance improvement in healthcare organizations through collection and dissemination of process or outcome measures of performance, or both. These systems allow an organization to compare its performance with that of other organizations using information such as patient outcomes, costs, lengths of stay for certain treatments, and mortality and morbidity rates. Examples are the TJC Indicator Measurement System and databases maintained by federal and state governments and third-party payers.
- **Benchmarking.** Benchmarking involves comparing one organization's performance standards with that of another; however, it focuses on the other organization's key processes that achieve performance rather than the numbers and statistical data obtained in an aggregate external reference database. Two main types of benchmarking exist: internal and external. Internal benchmarking compares performance with the best practices within one's own organization. External benchmarking compares an organization's performance with that of other organizations. External benchmarking can be further broken down into two types, competitive and world-class. Competitive external benchmarking involves comparing an organization to competitors marketing the same product or service. The American College of Radiology publishes a National Radiology Data Registry (NRDR) that contains regional and national benchmarks for various diagnostic imaging modalities. This can be accessed online at http://nrdr.acr.org/. World-class external benchmarking involves benchmarking against organizations outside of one's specific industry. A good example might be comparing the billing and collection practices of a healthcare organization with those of a bank or department store. Another commonly used benchmarking site is available from the LeapFrog Group (www.leapfroggroup.org), which will allow you to compare your hospital to other hospitals in terms of assessing quality, resource use, and efficiency.

Improve. Once knowledge is gained through measurement and analysis, action can be taken to improve processes by refining or redesigning a process to improve its level of performance. This cycle of design, measure, assess, and improve should be continuously repeating in a CQI program (Fig. 1-2).

Other Quality Management/Quality Improvement Models

The following are some of the other specific quality management/quality improvement models that are currently in use:

- Evangelical Health Systems CQI Monitoring System
- FADE was created by Organizational Dynamics, a private consulting firm (Fig. 1-3).
- The Five-Stage Plan was developed by Joiner and Associates, a quality consulting group.
- The **SWOT** analysis, developed at Stanford Research Institute in California from 1960 to 1970, analyzes the internal and external environment of a healthcare organization. The environmental factors internal to the organization can be classified as strengths (S) or weaknesses (W), and those external to the organization can be classified as opportunities (O) or threats (T). The SWOT analysis provides information that can be helpful in matching a healthcare organization's resources and capabilities to the competitive environment in which it operates. The four components are placed into a matrix (see Fig. 1-4), and the factors are then placed into each category. The organization's

CHAPTER 1 Introduction to Quality Management

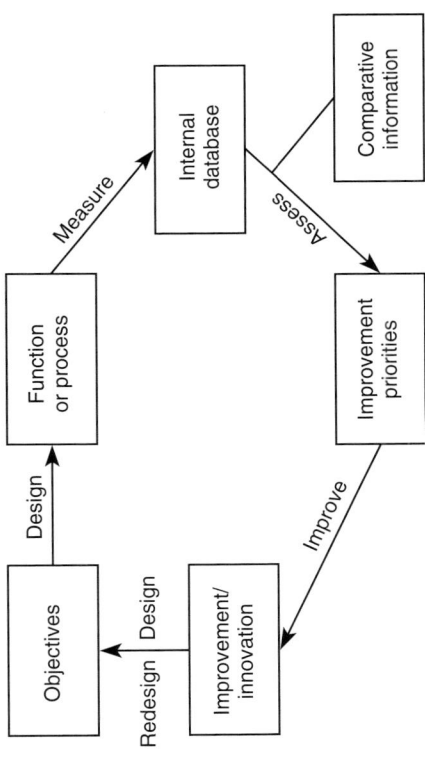

FIGURE 1-2 Cycle for improving performance, showing the important steps, including inputs and outputs, of a systematic approach to improvement. *(From Joint Commission Resources: Forms, charts, & other tools for performance improvement, Oakbrook Terrace, Ill, 1994, JCAHO. Reprinted with permission.)*

FADE

Phases of FADE problem solving

Focus—
Choose a problem and describe it

Analyze—
Learn about a problem by collecting and analyzing pertinent data

Develop—
Develop a solution and a plan

Execute—
Implement the plan, monitor the results, adjust as needed

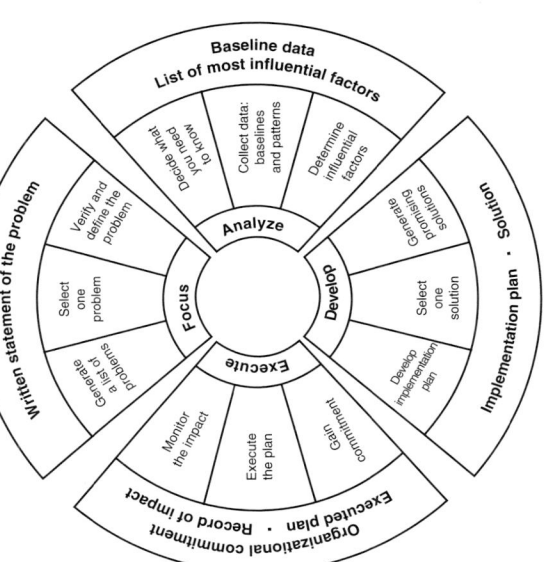

FIGURE 1-3 Phases of FADE problem solving. *(Printed with permission from Quality action teams: team members workbook, Organizational Dynamics, Inc. 1987, www.odionline.com.)*

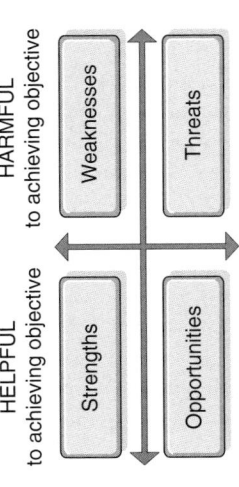

FIGURE 1-4 SWOT analysis matrix.

Strengths and Weaknesses boxes of the matrix contain attributes of the organization (internal in origin). Opportunities for growth might include obtaining the latest equipment or hiring physicians with advanced skills. Threats to the healthcare organization may include competition from a nearby facility or new regulations or reimbursement procedures. The Opportunities and Threats boxes contain attributes from the environment (external in origin).

- The **FOCUS-PDCA** (Fig. 1-5) approach was developed by the Hospital Corporation of America (HCA) in the 1980s, which adapted the "plan, do, check, and act" (PDCA) cycle used by Deming in Japanese industry. The PDCA cycle was initially developed by Walter A. Shewhart at Bell Laboratories, and may be referred to as either the Shewhart cycle Deming cycle, or PDCA cycle. Shewhart originally used the term *PDSA*

strengths are its resources and capabilities such as a good reputation among customers, expertise of physicians and staff, or advanced equipment that may not be available at competing imaging departments. Weaknesses are usually the absence of certain strengths such as a poor reputation among customers or lack of availability of latest equipment and procedures. The

CHAPTER 1 Introduction to Quality Management

FOCUS-PDCA

Hospital Corporation of America

Expands on the PDCA cycle by including "preliminary steps," i.e., FOCUS.

- **F**ind process improvement opportunity
- **O**rganize a team that knows the process
- **C**larify current knowledge of the process
- **U**ncover root causes for process variation
- **S**tart improvement cycle

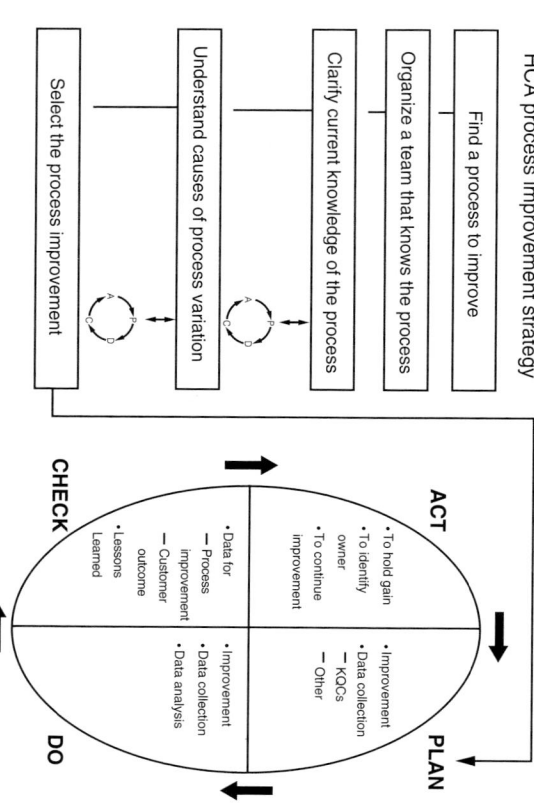

FIGURE 1-5 The FOCUS-PDCA model. (Reprinted with permission from Hospital Corporation of America, Nashville, Tennessee, 1989.)

or *Plan, Do, Study, Act*. The Hospital Corporation of America included the preliminary steps of FOCUS. This model consists of the following tenets:

F Find a process to improve or a problem to solve.
O Organize a team that knows the process and work on improvement.
C Clarify the problem and current knowledge of the process.
U Understand the problem and the causes of process variation.
S Select the method to improve the process.
P Plan to implement a new method to improve the process.
D Do the implementation and measure the change.
C Check the results of the change.
A Act to hold the improvements and continue further improvements.

The whole FOCUS-PDCA approach focuses on the answers to the following questions:

1. What are we trying to accomplish?
2. How will we know when this change is an improvement?
3. What changes can we predict will make an improvement?

4. How shall we pilot test the predicted improvement?
5. What do we expect to learn from the test run?
6. As the data come in, what have we learned?
7. If we get positive results, how do we hold on to the gains?
8. If we get negative results, what needs to be done next?
9. When we review the experience, what can we learn about doing a better job in the future?

- A **Failure Mode and Effects Analysis (FMEA)** is a procedure for analysis of potential failure within a system, classifying the severity or determining the failure's effect upon the system and helping determine remedial actions to overcome these failures. It was first used by the U.S. armed forces in the late 1940s and expanded by NASA in the 1960s to help put a man on the moon. In the late 1970s, the Ford Motor Company implemented FMEA into the automotive industry. Before conducting FMEA, it is necessary to describe the process or system being evaluated. This is best done by using a flowchart (described in the next chapter). The analysis itself occurs in three steps:

  Step 1: Severity. Determine all failure modes and their effects. Each effect is given a severity number (S) ranging from 1 (no danger) to 10 (important). If the severity of an effect has a number of 9 or 10, actions are considered to eliminate the failure mode (such as using only non-ionic contrast media). A severity rating of 9 or 10 is usually reserved for effects that would cause injury or result in litigation.

Step 2: Occurrence. In this step, it is necessary to look at the cause of a failure and how often it occurs. All potential causes for failure should be identified and documented. A failure mode is given a probability number (O), which also ranges from 1 to 10. Actions need to be determined if an occurrence is high (meaning greater than 4 for nonsafety failure and greater than 1 when the severity number from step 1 is 9 or 10).

Step 3: Detection. Whenever actions are taken to minimize failure, it is important to see how efficiently failures can be detected in the system to prevent further failure. Each combination from the first two steps receives a detection number (D), which represents the ability of tests and inspections to detect failure modes. Once these three steps are completed, risk priority numbers (RPN) are calculated by multiplying the numbers from each step: RPN = S × O × D. This number is generally used as a threshold value in the evaluation of any action to reduce failure.

- **Six Sigma** is a management strategy that seeks to identify and remove the causes of errors in business processes. It was originally developed by Motorola in 1986 and is now used in a variety of applications including healthcare management. The term is derived from statistics (discussed in the next chapter) where the word *Sigma* (the lower case Greek letter σ) is used to represent the standard deviation (a measure of variation) of a statistical population. Six Sigma comes from the concept that if there are three standard deviations on either side of the mean of a process and the nearest limit (covering 99% of all variables), then there will be virtually no items that fail to meet the specifications. It allows you to measure how many errors you may have in a process so you can systematically figure out how to eliminate them. Six Sigma starts with process mapping to identify elements that are critical to quality and then focuses on changing these elements. This procedure was inspired by Deming's PDCA cycle and consists of these five steps:

  Define process improvement goals that are consistent with customer demands and the institution's strategy.
  Measure key aspects of the current process and collect relevant data.
  Analyze the data to verify cause-and-effect relationships. Determine what the relationships are, and attempt to ensure that all factors have been considered.
  Improve or optimize the process based on data analysis.
  Control the process to ensure that any deviations from the target are corrected before they result in errors or failure.

- **Lean process improvement** or lean methodology is defined as a systematic approach to identifying and eliminating waste, where waste is defined as any non-valued tasks. Lean process improvement is often used in conjunction with Six Sigma for analyzing, reducing, and eliminating waste in healthcare processes.

SUMMARY

In modern diagnostic imaging departments, the radiologists, department administrators and supervisors, technologists, and support staff should work together to ensure that adequate processes are in place to properly care for the patient, achieve the highest quality image possible, and obtain the correct diagnosis from that image. These processes also are necessary to meet accreditation standards or government requirements, or both. The processes also should be reviewed continuously by all parties and modified as the need arises. Any quality management plan should have specific objectives (what the program is intending to achieve), an outline of the chain of command and responsibilities within the organization, the scope of the program, a mechanism for monitoring various aspects of patient management, evaluation of the program's effectiveness in meeting the objectives, and the efficacy of the program. Having an effective quality management program also has become necessary as a condition of receiving reimbursement for services by the federal government and many private insurance companies.

REVIEW QUESTIONS

1. Which levels of quality control testing can usually be performed by a quality assurance/quality management technologist: level I, level II, or level III?
   a. I and II
   b. I and III
   c. II and III
   d. I, II, and III

2. Which government agency mandates a policy on exposure to blood-borne pathogens?
   a. FDA
   b. EPA
   c. OSHA
   d. CDRH

3. Which of the following terms best describes information or knowledge necessary to achieve a desired outcome?
   a. Supplier
   b. Input
   c. Action
   d. Output

4. How many basic steps are involved in the creation of a TPM?
   a. 3
   b. 5
   c. 7
   d. 10

5. A procedure to identify potential failure within a system is
   a. SWOT
   b. FMEA
   c. Six Sigma
   d. FOCUS-PDCA
6. Which of the following terms best describes a person, department, or organization that needs or wants a desired outcome?
   a. Supplier
   b. Input
   c. Action
   d. Customer
7. Who is considered to be the "Father of Scientific Management"?
   a. W. Edwards Deming
   b. Joseph Juran
   c. Raymond Smith
   d. Frederick Winslow Taylor
8. Which of the following groups is usually responsible for implementing the solutions that the focus groups have determined will improve a particular process?
   a. Quality circle
   b. Work team
   c. Quality improvement team
   d. Problem-solving team
9. Which of the following terms best describes a valid and reliable quantitative process or outcome measure related to one or more dimensions of performance?
   a. External customer
   b. Indicator
   c. Level of expectation
   d. Sentinel event
10. The highest quality of care delivered in the shortest amount of time with the least amount of expense and a positive outcome is termed _____ of care.
    a. appropriateness
    b. continuity
    c. effectiveness
    d. efficiency

CHAPTER 2

Quality Management Tools and Procedures

KEY TERMS

Accuracy
As low as reasonably achievable
Cause-and-effect diagram
Central tendency
Continuous variables
Control chart
Data set
Dependent variable
Dichotomous variables
Dose area product
Dose creep
Flowchart
Frequency
Gaussian distribution
Histogram
Incident
Independent variable
Loss potential
Mean
Median
Mode
Pareto chart
Poisson distribution
Population
Precision
Prejudice
Range
Reliability
Risk
Risk management
Sample
Scatter plot
Standard deviation
Trend chart
Trending
Validity
Variance
Variation

OBJECTIVES

At the completion of this chapter the reader should be able to do the following:

- Describe the four main components of a quality management program
- List and define the basic terms used in statistical analysis
- Discuss the seven types of graphs and charts used to organize and present data in total quality management
- List the basic administrative responsibilities of a quality management program
- Describe the various components of a risk management program
- Describe the radiation safety protocols for patients and radiation personnel

OUTLINE

Information Analysis
Terminology Used in Statistical Analysis
Population
Sample
Data Set
Frequency
Dependent Variables
Independent Variables
Continuous Variables
Dichotomous Variables
Central Tendency
Reliability
Accuracy
Bias
Error
Range
Standard Deviation
Variance
Gaussian Distribution
Poisson Distribution
Variation
Validity
Information Analysis Tools
Flowchart
Cause-and-Effect Diagram
Histogram
Pareto Chart
Scatter Plot
Trend Chart
Control Chart
Miscellaneous Administrative Responsibilities
Threshold of Acceptability
Communication Network
Patient Comfort
Personnel Performance
Record-Keeping System
Corrective Action
Risk Management
Risk Analysis
Policies and Procedures

CHAPTER 2 Quality Management Tools and Procedures

OUTLINE—cont'd

Radiation Safety Program
 Patient Radiation Protection
 Radiographic Examinations
 Fluoroscopic Examinations
 Visitor Protection
 Personnel Protection
 Time
 Distance
 Shielding
 Summary

A comprehensive quality management program consists of many different components, depending on the size and complexity of the healthcare organization. Programs for diagnostic imaging departments, regardless of the size, should contain at least the following components:

- *Equipment quality control.* This aspect of a quality management program involves evaluation of equipment performance to ensure proper image quality, as well as patient and operator safety. These procedures are covered extensively in Chapters 3–15.
- *Administrative responsibilities.* This aspect of the quality management program involves the establishment of various processes to accomplish the specific departmental tasks that are required, such as departmental procedure manuals for performing diagnostic examinations or procedures for scheduling and routing of patients. It also involves data collection and analysis to continuously improve these processes. Other responsibilities include cost control, management of personnel, education of personnel (education for newly hired personnel and continuing education for existing workers), equipment acquisition, communication with various vendors, communication with other departments within the healthcare organization, and various other activities.
- *Risk management.* The ability to identify potential risks to patients, employees, and visitors at the healthcare institution and establish processes that would minimize these risks is extremely important to healthcare organizations. Civil litigation and workers' compensation judgments can severely deplete the financial resources of even the largest healthcare organization.
- *Radiation safety program.* This is to ensure that patient exposure is kept **as low as reasonably achievable (ALARA)** and that department personnel, medical staff, and members of the general public are protected from overexposure to ionizing radiation.

INFORMATION ANALYSIS

To implement the various components of a quality management program, a considerable amount of data must be collected and analyzed, which requires the use of statistics. Statistics is the mathematical science pertaining to the collection, analysis, interpretation, and presentation of data. This data then can be used to verify the success of organizational processes or provide justification for changing and improving these processes. To assist in the implementation of a quality management program, diagnostic imaging personnel need a basic knowledge of the terminology and data presentation tools used in statistical analysis.

Terminology Used in Statistical Analysis

Population. A *population* comprises the entire set or group of items being measured. Identifying the population to be measured is one of the first steps in performing a statistical analysis. For example, if you perform a statistical analysis of the number of repeat chest radiographs during a particular month, you focus on just the patients receiving chest examinations (that particular population) rather than each patient receiving each type of radiographic procedure.

Sample. A *sample* is the number of items actually measured from a population. Some populations may be extremely large and therefore difficult to study. Sampling involves choosing a portion or evaluating a subset of the population that makes data collection more practical, timely, and efficient. An example of sampling is the nationwide measurement of persons watching particular television programs. Only certain persons have their television viewing patterns actually monitored by the ratings services, and the results are extrapolated to be indicative of the entire population. This is known as *statistical inference.* Sampling must be performed carefully to ensure that the sample chosen is representative of the entire population.

Data Set. A *data set* is the information or measurements acquired by evaluating the particular sample.

Frequency. The *frequency* is the number of times a particular value of a variable occurs or the number of observations of an event. For example, during a repeat study of chest examinations, 37 chest views had to be repeated during a particular month. Therefore, the frequency of repeated chest views for that month was 37.

Dependent Variables. *Dependent variables* are those variables that are observed in statistical studies to change in response to independent variables and are not controlled during the study. The dependent variable also can be referred to as response variables, measured variables, or output variables. For example, if one were to study how different brands of contrast media cause allergic reactions in diagnostic imaging patients, a researcher could compare the frequency and intensity of a reaction to the different brands of contrast media. In this study, the frequency and cause of allergic reactions would be the dependent variables.

Independent Variables. Independent variables are those that are deliberately manipulated to invoke a change on the dependent variables. Independent variables also may be referred to as predictor variables or input variables. In the example presented under dependent variables comparing how different brands of contrast media cause allergic reactions in diagnostic imaging patients, the different brands of contrast media given to diagnostic imaging patients would be the independent variable.

Continuous Variables. Continuous variables are those variables being studied that have an infinite range of possible mathematical values. Examples might include the age of patients, weight of patients, height of patients, and time of a particular event.

Dichotomous Variables. Dichotomous variables are those variables being studied that have only two opposing choices, such as male or female and on or off.

Central Tendency. The central tendency is the central position of a sample frequency. In statistical analysis, there are several possible measures of central tendency, three of which are the mean, the median, and the mode.

- *Mean.* The **mean** is the calculated average set of observations and can be denoted by either μ, $\overline{X}$, or M. The mean provides the greatest reliability of the three measures of central tendency.

$$\text{Mean} = \frac{\text{Sum of observed values } (\sum)}{\text{Total number of values } (N)}$$

For example, if the values 7, 3, 6, and 4 are observed, the mean is determined by taking 20 (the sum of the observed values) divided by 4 (the total number of values observed), which yields a mean of 5.

- The **median** is a point on a scale of measurement above which are exactly one half of the values and below which are the other half. In other words, it is the numeric middle. For example, if the values 4, 6, 8, 10, and 12 are observed, the median is 8.
- The **mode** is the one value that occurs with the greatest frequency in the data set. For example, if the values 2, 3, 4, 4, 4, 5, and 5 are observed, the mode is 4. The mode provides information about the most typical occurrence, but this is usually just a rough estimate of central value.

Reliability. Reliability refers to the consistency of repeated measurements of the same thing or the reproducibility of a result and is sometimes known as **precision**. Many factors, such as the sample size (larger samples are usually more reliable), the design of the data collection process (e.g., Are the questions on a survey worded in a "biased" way?), and the collection and interpretation of the data (e.g., Is the person collecting the data including all of the information given?), can affect the reliability of statistical information. A new quality management program may have unreliable data at first because of the "start-up effect." This effect can cause an unusually high or low data result because the human tendency is to be hyperaware when new studies are begun. To counteract the start-up effect, a sufficient period of time needs to elapse to allow the data to change and stabilize before reliable data analysis is obtained. Reliability or precision does not imply accuracy.

Accuracy. Accuracy refers to the ability to measure what is purported to be measured and is sometimes referred to as **validity**. In other words, do the data collected reflect the reality of the situation being studied? One also can think of accuracy as how well a value that has been studied and measured agrees with the true value.

Bias. Bias is a systematic or nonrandom difference between the true value of a property and individual measurements of that property or the presence of a systematic error. Sometimes bias in a statistical context is thought of as being synonymous with the term **prejudice**. This is an incorrect assumption because prejudice refers to an individual's state of mind that would create a desire for a particular outcome.

Error. Measurement error refers to the difference between the measured value and the true value of the variable being measured. Errors of measurement can be divided into two categories, systematic errors and random errors. Systematic errors, also known as determinate errors, result from factors such as malfunctioning equipment, not correcting all outside influences, and poor design of the data collection process. Examples in imaging would include equipment not calibrated properly or incorrect exposure factors selected by a technologist. Random errors, also known as indeterminate errors, are caused by statistical fluctuations or uncertainties such as quantum mottle.

Range. Range refers to the difference between the highest and lowest values and is a measure of the dispersion of the data distribution.

Standard Deviation. The **standard deviation** is the range of variation or dispersion of a set of values surrounding the mean, or the spread or distribution of a data set. It can apply to a random variable, a population, a probability distribution, or a multiset. This can be symbolized by the capital letters SD or the small Greek letter *sigma* (σ). It is defined as the root-mean-square deviation of the values from their mean. Since standard deviation is a measure of statistical dispersion, it measures how widely spread the values in a data set are from the mean. If many data points are close to the mean, then the standard deviation is small; if many data points are far from the mean, then the standard deviation is large. If all data values are equal, then the standard deviation is zero.

$$SD = \sqrt{\frac{\sum x^2}{M}}$$

The small letter x is the amount of deviation of a value X from the mean (M). $x = X - M$. For example, with the values 7, 3, 6, and 4, the mean is 5. The standard deviation is determined with the following equation:

$$SD = \sqrt{\frac{(7-5)^2 + (3-5)^2 + (6-5)^2 + (4-5)^2}{5}}$$

The standard deviation is 1.41.

When a large standard deviation is obtained (i.e., a large variation has occurred from the mean), it is important to analyze why this may have occurred. Possibilities to consider include that this may be a normal occurrence and that the data are valid. It is also possible that the ways in which the measurements were obtained, calculated, or determined were not correctly performed. The validity of the standard deviation value must be determined before the results of the study being performed can be considered valid.

Variance. Variance is the square of the standard deviation in Poisson statistics (discussed below) and is used to determine if the separate means of several different groups differ significantly from each other (e.g., between male and female patients, different age groups). Like standard deviation, it is used as a measure of the dispersion or spread of a set of values. As the mean increases, the variance will increase as well.

Gaussian Distribution. A Gaussian distribution, named after German mathematician Carl Friedrich Gauss, is also known as a *normal distribution* and creates a bell-shaped curve that is continuous with both tails extending to infinity (Fig. 2-1). The distribution is symmetric about the mean value of the measurement set with the spread of the measurements characterized by the standard deviation of the measurements. With this distribution, 68% of all values will fall within one standard deviation on either side of the mean, 95% will fall within two standard deviations, and 99% will fall within three standard deviations. (This is the basis of **Six Sigma**, discussed in the last chapter, whereby 99% of all variables are covered.)

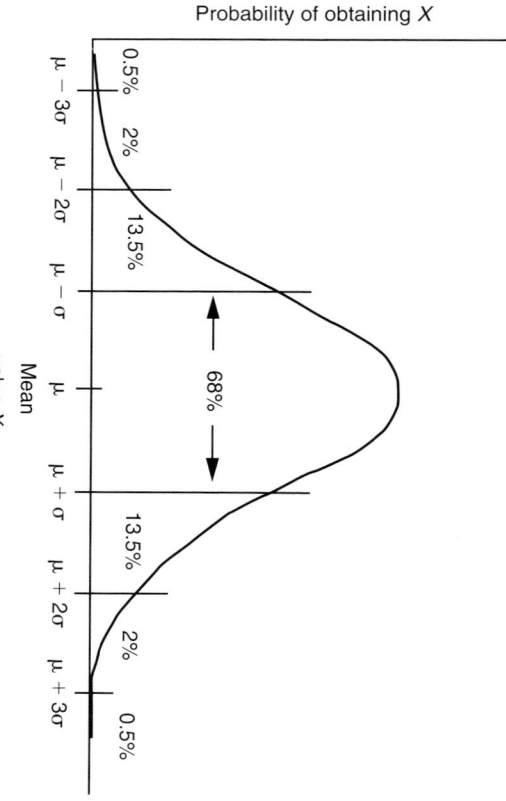

FIGURE 2-1 Gaussian probability (normal) distribution.

Poisson Distribution. A Poisson distribution, named after French mathematician Simeon Poisson, is a discrete probability distribution that is used to determine whether events occur randomly or not (such as the number of particles emitted by a radioactive source in a given period of time). In this type of distribution, the variance is equal to the mean. This distribution is generally asymmetrical (the opposite of Gaussian distribution) for low mean values (<10). In Poisson statistics, the standard deviation can be estimated by taking the square root of the mean. For example, if a sample has a mean of 144, the standard deviation is 12. This method is used in nuclear medicine.

Variation. Variation refers to anything that would cause a process to deviate from acceptable standards (or the norm). It is related to the statistical concepts of variance and standard deviation, since it describes the range of output around the central measure of a process. For example, a chest X-ray examination on a patient in a hospital radiology department may average 16 min to complete. However, the exam may take as few as 11 min or as long as 25 min. This range would indicate the extent of variation of the process. Sources of variation in diagnostic imaging might include materials and supplies, equipment, procedures and methods, personnel, and management. Two basic types of variation are encountered in diagnostic imaging, special cause variation and common cause variation. Common cause variation is generally due to the process or system in place, as well as the people within the system (i.e., personnel or patient population). Special cause variation is assignable to a specific cause or causes and arises because of special circumstances.

Validity. As mentioned previously, **validity** is sometimes referred to as *accuracy*. In survey measurement, there are three main types of validity of concern: construct validity, content validity, and criterion validity. Construct validity is the extent to which a measure would agree with other survey instruments that have been used to measure the same parameters and have a proven accuracy. Content validity is the extent to which a survey will cover all of the content area. Criterion validity compares the results obtained in a survey to an established criterion measure.

Information Analysis Tools

As mentioned previously, total quality management (TQM) is devoted to process improvement so that goods and services can be delivered more efficiently to increase customer satisfaction. This means that data must be collected about how well the various processes are being implemented, identify sources of variation, conduct in-depth analysis to clarify knowledge and present results, measure improvements, and monitor progress. Customer satisfaction surveys and repeat analysis of radiographic images are examples of data collection. Once these data are collected, they then must be organized and presented in a format that is easy to analyze. Seven basic statistical tools can be used to display data for interpretation and analysis: flowcharts, cause-and-effect diagrams, histograms, Pareto charts, scatter plots, trend charts, and control charts.

Flowchart. A flowchart is a pictorial representation of the individual steps that can be contained in a process. It is designed to present the sequence of events in the process from its beginning point to its end point. When correctly constructed, it can demonstrate potential problem areas, inconsistencies, or redundancies that can produce variations in the output of the process, which may result in system failure. It also can help document current processes, redesign current processes, and design new processes. Flowcharts are relatively easy to construct but are best developed by persons who are directly involved in or have knowledge of the particular process to be presented.

Before constructing a flowchart, one must identify all of the inputs, outputs, and actions within the process, as well as the sequence in which they occur. Then the appropriate symbol must be chosen to characterize each step within the process. For an explanation of the symbols used in a flowchart, see Box 2-1. Computer software programs are available for help in constructing a satisfactory flowchart. With all of the steps in a process accurately diagrammed, it should be easier to communicate the process and its outcomes to all staff (especially new hires). It should also allow a project improvement team to examine the process in order to be able to improve it. An example of a flowchart is shown in Fig. 2-2.

Cause-and-Effect Diagram. A cause-and-effect diagram is a causal analysis tool (also called a *fishbone chart* or *Ishikawa diagram*). This tool was developed by Kaoru Ishikawa of the University of Tokyo in 1943. It is used to demonstrate graphically the causes and effects of different variables or conditions on a key quality characteristic and, thereby, potential areas for improvement. It is most useful in identifying sources of variation within a process. It is especially useful in identifying multiple causes of problems during root cause analysis studies.

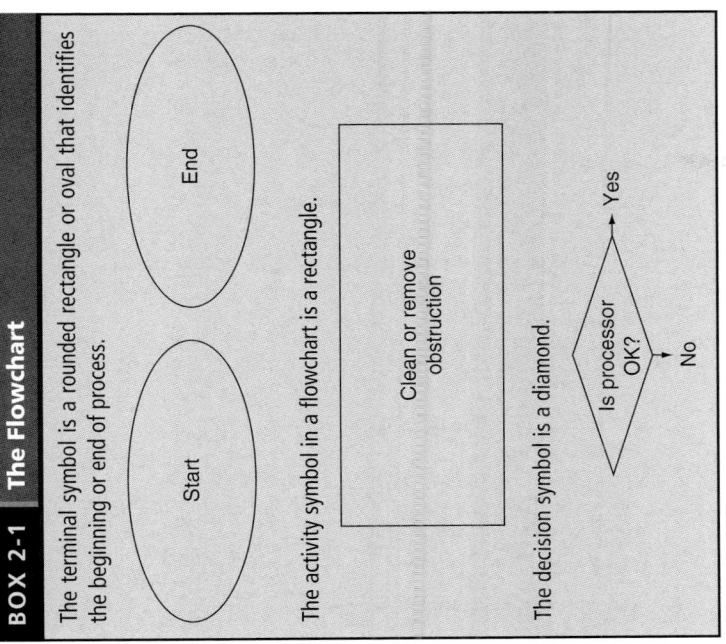

BOX 2-1 | The Flowchart

The terminal symbol is a rounded rectangle or oval that identifies the beginning or end of process.

The activity symbol in a flowchart is a rectangle.

The decision symbol is a diamond.

To construct a cause-and-effect diagram, you must first determine the key quality characteristic to be improved. Then potential causes of the effect must be identified so they are included in the chart. Brainstorming by a quality improvement team or similar group may be helpful in this identification. The main ideas are listed on branches flowing toward the main branch of the diagram and grouped according to categories. All possible problems or causes for each of these main ideas must then be listed as subcauses within each branch. An example of a cause-and-effect diagram is shown in Fig. 2-3.

Histogram. A histogram is a data display tool in the form of a bar graph that often plots the most frequent occurrence of a quantity in the center. After a cause-and-effect diagram has been created, data is usually collected to see how often different causes of process variation are occurring. A histogram differs from a bar graph in that it is the area of the bar/s that denotes the value and not the height of the bars. The distribution of continuous data is often best accomplished with a histogram. It also can help demonstrate the amount of variation within an individual process. Histograms often are used in diagnostic imaging to depict such continuous variables as the monthly repeat rate of a department or the number of examinations performed monthly. They also are programmed into computerized radiography systems to create satisfactory images (see Chapter 9). Software programs such as *Microsoft Excel* can generate histograms from information contained in a spreadsheet. Figure 2-4 shows an example of a histogram. Histograms can also be adapted in a "scorecard display," in which the bars are color coded to indicate whether certain goals

CHAPTER 2 Quality Management Tools and Procedures

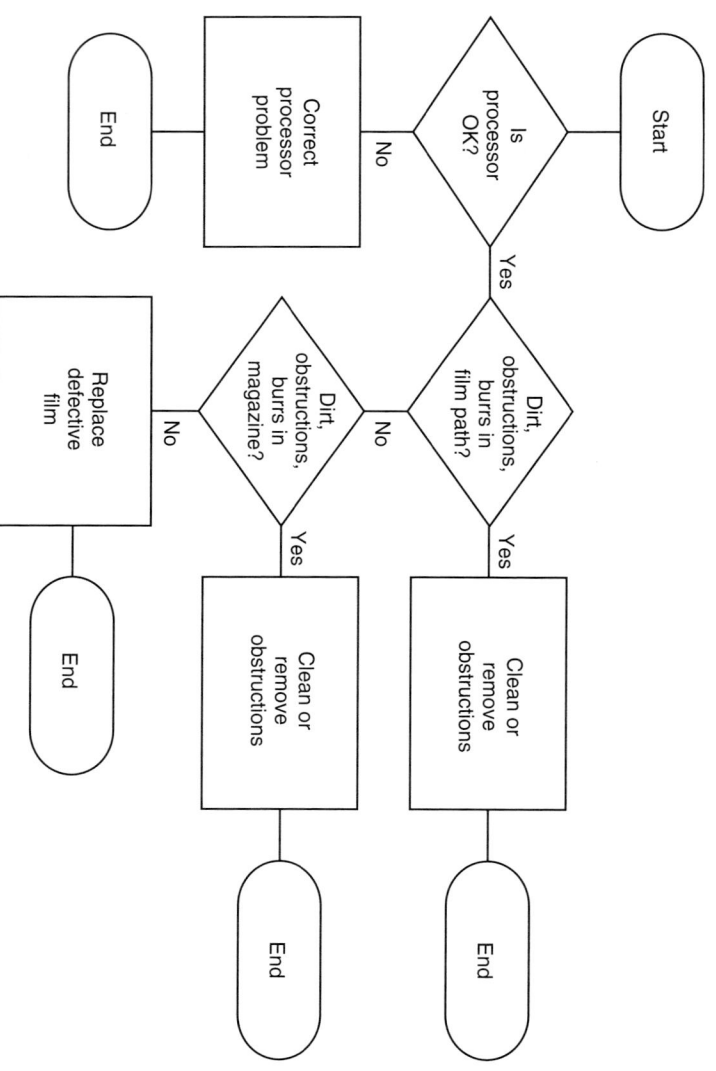

FIGURE 2-2 Flowchart diagrams the process of eliminating scratches on images caused by film processors.

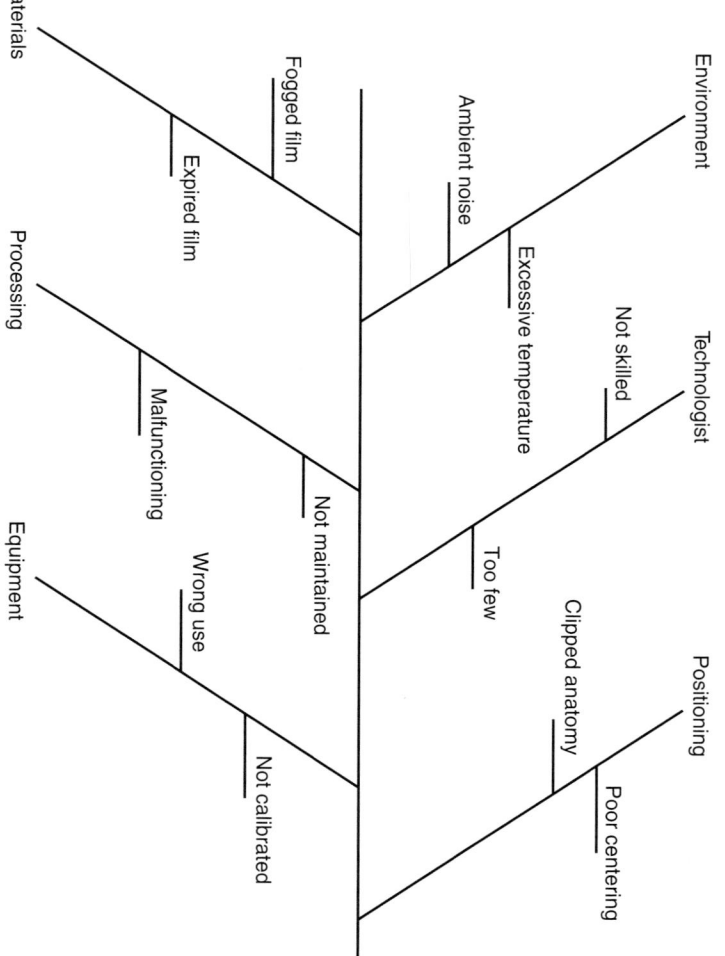

FIGURE 2-3 A fishbone chart shows the effect of various parameters on key quality characteristics or outcomes of proper image quality.

or benchmarks have been achieved. Green is used if the goal or benchmark has been met or exceeded, yellow is used if it is within a certain percentage of the goal, and red would indicate that the goal or benchmark has not been met.

Pareto Chart. A Pareto chart is a causal analysis tool that is named after Wilfredo Pareto, a seventeenth-century Italian political economist. The Pareto chart is a variation of the histogram or bar graph, which prioritizes the most frequent problems at the y-axis (far left)

CHAPTER 2 Quality Management Tools and Procedures

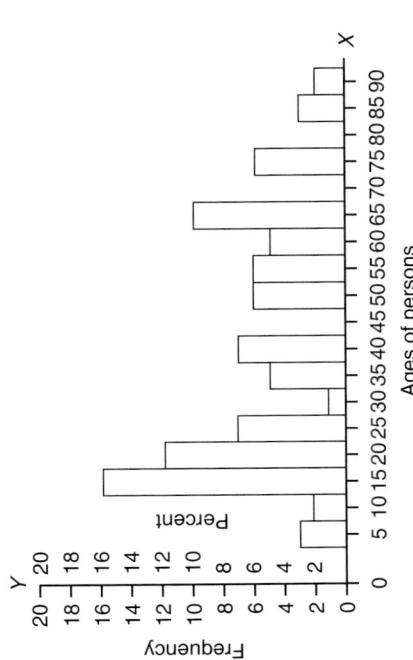

FIGURE 2-4 Histogram. Frequency of occurrence is demonstrated on the y-axis, and category or class interval is demonstrated on the x-axis. This example plots percentage of patients undergoing diagnostic procedures versus ages of patients.

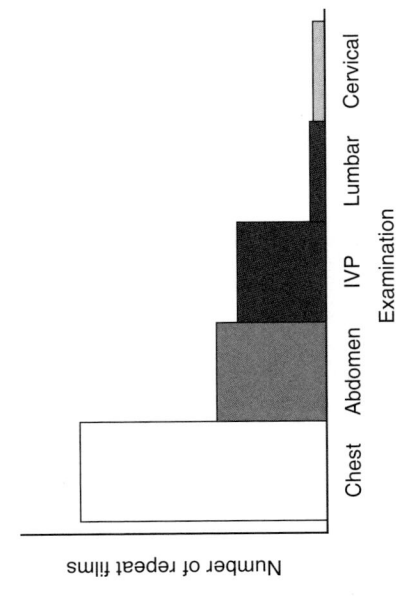

FIGURE 2-5 A Pareto chart indicates specific areas that cause unsatisfactory outcomes so improvement actions can be appropriately directed. IVP, Intravenous pyelography.

of the graph and the other problems in decreasing order to the right. The Pareto chart was developed to illustrate the 80/20 Rule (that 80% of the problems stem from 20% of the causes). The horizontal axis, or x-axis, indicates the factors or problems to be evaluated, whereas the vertical axis, or y-axis, demonstrates the frequency of occurrence. Pareto charts also may include a horizontal reference, or norm (normal occurrence). The Pareto chart is useful in identifying the main causes (i.e., those that occur with the greatest frequency) of problems and in demonstrating the results of improvement strategies that have been implemented. It is important to note that Pareto charts document the frequency of causes and not necessarily the severity of a cause. An example of a Pareto chart is shown in Fig. 2-5.

Scatter Plot. A **scatter plot** (also called a *scatter diagram*) is a traditional two-axis graph (x-axis and y-axis), with several data points that have been plotted throughout. It is designed to determine whether a relationship exists between two different variables in a process. When looking for ideas for improvement or the causes of problems, it can be important to determine whether or not

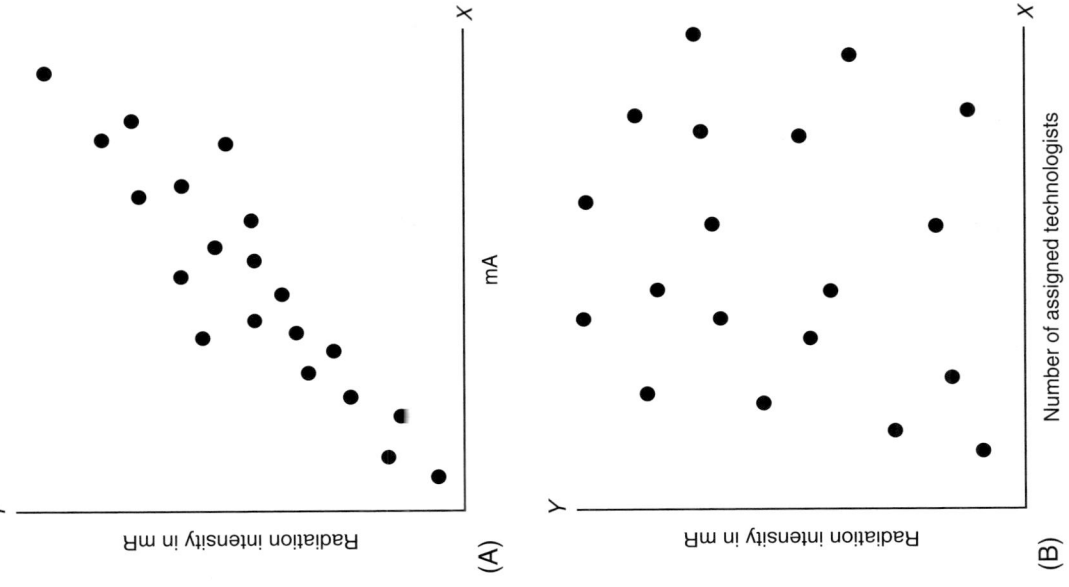

FIGURE 2-6 A scatter plot graph shows relationship between a key outcome or characteristic (y-axis) and a key process variable (x-axis). Graph (A) indicates a positive correlation between two values, and graph (B) indicates that no correlation exists. mA, Milliampere; mR, milliroentgen.

one event or variable is related to another. Once the data points are plotted, the scatter plot then is examined to see if these points are scattered in any particular pattern. If so, a correlation may exist between the two variables. A positive correlation is indicated when both the x and y values increase in relation to each other. A negative correlation is demonstrated when there is an increase in the x variable in relation to a decrease in the y variable. Scatter plots are often used in regression analysis studies, which are statistical forecasting models based on data demonstrated in scatter plots. An example of a scatter plot is shown in Fig. 2-6.

Trend Chart. A **trend chart** (also called a *run chart* or *run-sequence plot*) pictorially demonstrates whether key indicators are moving up or down over a given period of time, on an ongoing basis. *Trending* refers to the evaluation of data collected over a period of time for the

is considered unstable. The control chart was invented by Walter A. Shewhart while working at Bell Labs in the 1920s, so it is sometimes referred to as the Shewhart chart or process/behavior chart. Like the trend chart, the control chart cannot identify a specific cause of a problem, but rather if and when they have occurred. The control chart is often used for demonstrating phantom image analysis in mammographic units over time (see Chapter 11). An example of a control chart is shown in Fig. 2-8.

MISCELLANEOUS ADMINISTRATIVE RESPONSIBILITIES

In Chapter 1, a distinction between quality assurance (which deals with human factors) and quality control (which deals with equipment factors) is made. Merging these entities in a TQM program requires certain administrative procedures (Box 2-2) to be implemented by radiologists, department administrators, quality control technologists (Box 2-3), quality improvement committees, and imaging professionals (since they have direct patient contact and are therefore on the front line in demonstrating quality of care). Some of the more important administrative procedures follow.

Threshold of Acceptability

The threshold of acceptability includes levels of accuracy, sensitivity, and specificity of diagnosis (see Chapter 10). It also should include such items as the number of radiographs per examination, the amount of radiation per examination, and the performance thresholds of the equipment. These should be established according to both external factors (such as federal and state guidelines or professional and accrediting agencies) and internal factors, which are based on the needs and resources of the individual department.

Communication Network

Proper communication among all members of a diagnostic imaging department is essential for a successful

purpose of identifying patterns or changes. The variable being measured is placed on the vertical axis, or y-axis, and the time factor is placed on the horizontal axis, or x-axis. Often, some measure of central tendency (mean or median) of the data is indicated by a horizontal reference line. The trend chart can display the performance of, and any variation in, a process over a given period of time. For a trend chart to be constructed, the measurement or indicator to be measured must first be identified. Then all relevant data must be collected and analyzed. Next, all data points are plotted and connected with a linear line. Once the chart has been constructed, the plotted points and lines must be analyzed to determine the degree of variation within the indicator. If there are no large spikes (upward or downward) and the line is relatively flat, then the process is considered to be under control. If unusual trends are observed, then the potential causes must be investigated and corrected. Trend charts cannot determine the source of any problem within a process, only if and when they have occurred. An example of a trend chart is shown in Fig. 2-7.

Control Chart. A control chart is a modification of the trend chart, in which statistically determined upper and lower control limits are placed with a central line that indicates an accepted norm. If the plotted data points fall above or below these control limits, then the process

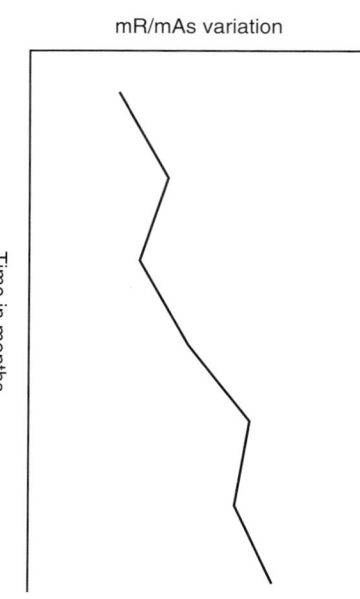

FIGURE 2-7 A trend graph displays amount of variation of indicator (radiation emitted from an X-ray generator) as a function of time. mAs, Milliampere-second; mR, milliroentgen.

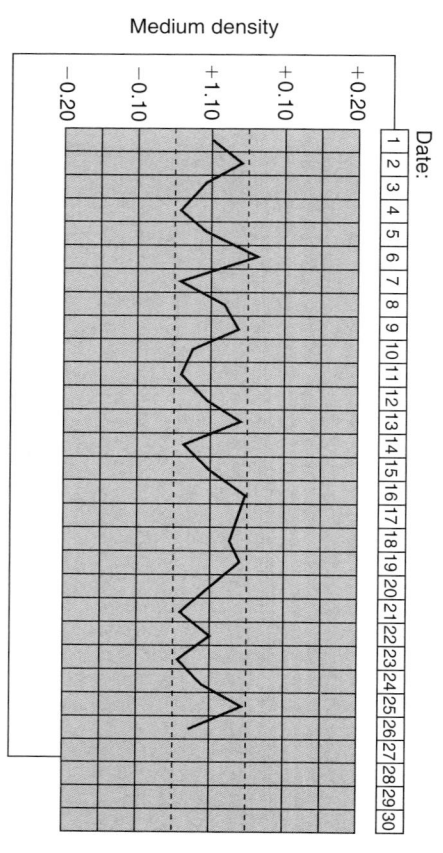

FIGURE 2-8 A control graph displays amount of variation of indicator (speed or medium density of a sensitometry film) as a function of time, with upper and lower control limits indicated.

CHAPTER 2 Quality Management Tools and Procedures

quality management program. Items such as the proper examination ordered for a particular patient must be supplied to the technologist from the ordering physician and office support staff. The technologist also must communicate the appropriate patient history to the radiologist and ensure proper film identification and marking. Administrative personnel and radiologists must then communicate with technologists about proper procedures and guidelines for patient care and image parameters. Diagnostic imaging departments also should have proper communication with other departments within the healthcare setting such as the emergency department staff or floor nurses so the patient can be cared for properly. Proper communication also includes report dictation, transcription, and distribution to the ordering physician and other interested parties. Modern imaging departments rely on electronic reporting and electronic record keeping (i.e., Hospital Information Systems and Radiology Information Systems), so a major administrative responsibility is making sure that all personnel have competency in computer usage and knowledge of HIPAA requirements.

Patient Comfort

Patient comfort, convenience, and privacy should be provided within reasonable limits in diagnostic imaging departments. Factors such as patient scheduling, preparation, waiting time, ambient room temperature, and politeness and consideration of personnel should be monitored regularly. This is best accomplished by a patient survey or questionnaire, which should be sent to patients 3–7 days after the procedure for maximum reliability. These can be administered in various formats including comment cards, mail surveys, web-based or social network surveys (using tools such as SurveyMonkey, etc.), or telephone interviews (personal interviews with patients via telephone by trained interviewers). Some healthcare organizations may also utilize point-of-service interviews, which are either self-administered or interviewer-administered questionnaires that are usually completed following service delivery at the clinical site. The method of delivery of patient satisfaction surveys is usually determined by which method will yield the greatest response rate. As mentioned in Chapter 1, respect and caring and timeliness of care are key clinical performance indicators that require measurement by accrediting agencies. Acute care hospitals subject to the Inpatient Prospective Payment System must survey recently discharged patients on their hospital experience using the Hospital Care Quality Information from the Consumer Perspective (HCAHPS) survey. This survey was developed by the Centers for Medicare and Medicaid Services and the Agency for Healthcare Research and Quality in 2002. The core of the survey consists of 21 items that ask whether patients experienced a critical aspect of hospital care, rather than whether they were "satisfied" with their care. Also included in the survey are four screener items that direct patients to relevant questions, five items to adjust for the mix of patients across hospitals, and two items that support Congressionally mandated reports. Hospitals may include additional questions after the core HCAHPS items. Further information can be found at www.hcahpsonline.org.

Personnel Performance

Policies should be developed to ensure that diagnostic personnel are performing their duties within accepted professional standards for areas such as proper equipment operation, critical thinking, and interaction with patients and other personnel. Information obtained from repeat analysis studies and patient surveys can be useful in assessing performance. Documentation of

---

BOX 2-2 Administrative Procedures

Establish thresholds of acceptability.
Establish an effective communication network.
Provide for patient comfort.
Ensure accepted performance of diagnostic imaging personnel.
Develop a record-keeping system.
Establish corrective action procedures.

BOX 2-3 Quality Management Technologist Duties

1. Coordinating, performing and monitoring quality control procedures for all types of equipment.
2. Determining and monitoring exposure factors and/or procedural protocols in accordance with ALARA principles.
3. Ensuring adherence to federal, state and local regulatory requirements.
4. Ensuring adherence to accreditation requirements.
5. Providing input for equipment and software purchase and supply decisions when appropriate or requested.
6. Facilitating performance improvement processes.
7. Providing practical information regarding quality management topics.
8. Facilitating the department's quality assessment and improvement plan.
9. Performing physics surveys independently on general radiographic and fluoroscopic equipment. Medical physicist oversight is required.
10. Supporting and assisting a medical physicist for special modality physics surveys such as CT, mammography, MRI, nuclear medicine, radiation therapy, and positron emission tomography.
11. Providing assistance to staff for image optimization, including patient positioning, proper equipment use, and image critique.
12. Creating policies and procedures to meet regulatory and accreditation requirements.
13. Serving as a resource regarding regulatory and accreditation requirements.

Data from American Society of Radiologic Technologists: *Practice standards for medical imaging and radiation therapy*, Albuquerque, 2012, ASRT.

Record-Keeping System

A record-keeping system is necessary to document that quality management and quality control procedures are being implemented and that they are in compliance with accepted norms. Items that should be included are processor control charts (film/screen departments only), phantom image results, equipment checklists, examination requisitions, equipment service records, incident reports, personnel dosimetry reports of radiation exposure, and image interpretation reports.

A record-keeping system is necessary to document data, periodic review of these data, and any corrective actions that have been taken also should be included. Personnel education programs also should be offered and documented to improve performance and maintain staff competency. In addition to continuing education in topics that are specific to each modality (i.e., new equipment operation, radiation safety, etc.), departments should also try to educate their personnel in quality management topics such as working in interdisciplinary teams, applying quality improvement activities, and using informatics.

Corrective Action

If equipment or personnel are not performing to accepted standards, corrective action must be taken and documented. Equipment downtime and failure should be documented using established forms and procedures. In-service education or other corrective action procedures may be necessary for department personnel. A flowchart is a useful tool in demonstrating corrective actions for possible problems.

RISK MANAGEMENT

An important aspect of a quality management program for diagnostic imaging departments is **risk management**. This is the system or process for the identification, analysis, and evaluation of risks and the selection of the most advantageous method for minimizing them. Other names for risk management include *safety* and *loss prevention*, *total loss control*, or *loss control management*. **Risk** can be defined as the chance of an event or incident happening that may threaten or damage an organization. Measuring risk can take place in the form of either the likelihood of something happening or the consequences should something actually happen. The purpose of a risk management program is to maintain quality patient care and a safe environment for employees and visitors, while conserving the healthcare institution's financial resources. Therefore, processes need to be in place to reduce the likelihood of an event occurring (risk reduction) as well as to minimize the consequences of an event, should one occur. The overall responsibility for risk management may lie with a risk management coordinator, a risk management team, the individual department manager, or the department quality management person, depending on the size and structure of the institution. However, all employees must be made aware of their role in the risk management process. This includes proper education in both departmental and institutional policies and procedures, awareness of safety issues, and the immediate reporting of incidents and hazardous conditions to the appropriate person.

Risk Analysis

The first step in developing risk management policies and procedures for diagnostic imaging departments is to perform a risk analysis. This means identifying the potential risks to patients, employees, students, and visitors to the diagnostic imaging department.

- *Risks to patients*. The potential risks to patients in diagnostic imaging departments are considerable. For example, patients may slip and fall, be hit by equipment, have a reaction to contrast media, have entered the department with a traumatic injury and be improperly manipulated, or receive the wrong diagnostic procedure (all are considered to be sentinel events). Other more subtle risks can include excess radiation exposure (due to failure to adequately shield the patient from repeat images), exposure to infectious disease (due to failure of the technologist to maintain room cleanliness), and breach of confidentiality (due to technologists discussing patient information near waiting areas or other unauthorized persons). These potential risks can be reduced by having the appropriate policies and procedures in place and making sure that employees have knowledge of and follow these procedures. Accrediting agencies such as The Joint Commission and DNV Healthcare publish extensive safety guidelines for patients for various types of healthcare institutions on their websites. Documentation of adherence to these guidelines is essential in obtaining and maintaining accreditation.

- *Risks to employees and medical staff*. Risks to employees and professional staff include injuries from falls, back injury from lifting patients or heavy equipment, repetitive stress injuries, needle sticks, exposure to infectious diseases, exposure to ionizing radiation, and exposure to toxic chemicals such as processing solutions. Most of the risks to employees and medical staff (like those to the patient) also can be reduced by implementing appropriate policies and procedures. Information concerning work-related employee injuries and illness is available in the Occupational and Safety Health Administration (OSHA) 2000 Log. This report must be posted at the work site each year during the month of February. These reports may be maintained by the human resources department, risk manager, or employee health department, depending on the institution.

CHAPTER 2 Quality Management Tools and Procedures

- *Risk to others.* This category includes such persons as students, visitors, and volunteers and is probably the most difficult category to assess. This is due to the potential size of this group and the variety of persons that can be included. Another potential difficulty is that the individuals within this group probably have little or no knowledge of the policies and procedures of the healthcare institution. The greatest potential risks to members of this group are injuries from falling, exposure to infectious disease, and HIPAA violations (such as they may not have knowledge of privacy concerns). It is imperative to have appropriate policies and procedures in place to address these risks and to encourage employees (because they should have been educated in risk management) to report any hazardous conditions (e.g., liquid spills) immediately.

- Once a risk analysis is performed and policies and procedures have been created to reduce any potential risks, the next step in a risk management program is to create an investigation procedure for any incidents that may occur. An **incident** is any occurrence that is not consistent with the routine care of a patient or the normal course of events at a particular facility. Facilities should have some type of "incident report" form that is to be completed as soon as possible after an incident. The completed reports should be reviewed immediately by the department manager and then forwarded to the risk manager for additional review. The risk manager should then determine whether any follow-up action is necessary. This can include additional investigation, notification of government agencies (e.g., the Food and Drug Administration [FDA], OSHA, the Nuclear Regulatory Commission [NRC], or the Environmental Protection Agency), or the obtainment of legal counsel. A risk management program also should include policies and procedures addressing claims prevention and loss potential. **Loss potential** refers to any activity that costs a facility either money or its reputation. Educating employees on safety policies and procedures, emphasizing quality patient care, and communicating effectively within the healthcare facility can greatly reduce the occurrence of incidents and therefore the cost of defending any claims that may result from these incidents. With these policies in place and documentation that they are being implemented, loss potential can be reduced, first by minimizing the chance of an incident and second by showing that the healthcare facility did all that it could to minimize risk, which should cast a more favorable opinion if litigation becomes necessary.

bills for a patient or employee who is injured in a diagnostic imaging department. Having effective policies and procedures addressing this type of responsibility and loss can often prevent the filing of a claim or reduce the amount of a claim after litigation. As with all quality management components, keeping proper records of all incidents, documents, reports, and policies is imperative for the process to be successful. The following list summarizes the key concepts of an effective risk management program:

1. *Risk analysis*—to identify all potential hazards and risks that can occur
2. *Written policies and procedures*—to reduce all risks and deal with incidents as they occur
3. *Employee education*—to inform employees of all policies and procedures, as well as seek input from employees (such as a brainstorming session) to identify and reduce further risks
4. *Periodic inspection*—to make sure that all policies and procedures are being implemented
5. *Record keeping*—to document that all policies and procedures have been implemented

Policies and Procedures

Finally, if an incident does occur, a risk management program should have policies and procedures in place that address responsibility of the healthcare institution for the outcome of the incident, for example, paying the medical

RADIATION SAFETY PROGRAM

Diagnostic imaging procedures (with the exception of magnetic resonance imaging and sonography) contribute the largest single exposure to artificial radiation (more than 90%) in the United States. The average effective dose equivalent for diagnostic radiographs is 39 millirem (mrem) (0.39 millisievert (mSv)) and 14 mrem (0.14 mSv) for nuclear medicine procedures. This is in addition to the 360 mrem (3.6 mSv) per year that is received from natural sources such as cosmic radiation (from outer space), terrestrial radiation (from the earth, air, and drinking water), and internal radiation (from our own body tissues). The 360 mrem (3.6 mSv) per year is an average for the United States and can vary considerably from one location to the next. Persons who live in areas where the altitude is high or where exposure to radon-222 is common may experience considerably more than 360 mrem per year. It is therefore imperative that patients, visitors, hospital staff, and radiographers themselves receive as little radiation exposure as possible. It is the primary responsibility of each radiographer to ensure that this indeed occurs. A quality management program should have radiation safety policies and procedures in place to make sure that all employees who administer ionizing radiation to patients are aware of this responsibility. The NRC (or state radiation governing body) and The Joint Commission require a radiation safety committee, administered by a radiation safety officer, to implement these policies. Additional responsibilities of this committee would include creating policies and procedures for the safe handling and disposal of radioactive materials, radiation accidents, and care of patients exposed to radiation.

Implementation of proper radiation safety protocols is mandated by the federal government and most state governments. The more important federal laws are described in Chapter 1. The enactment of the laws mentioned in Chapter 1 means that radiographers may have to interact with one or more regulatory agencies that oversee compliance. These federal agencies include the following:

- *The FDA.* As mentioned previously, the FDA, through the Center for Devices and Radiological Health, regulates the design and manufacture of X-ray equipment. These regulations are contained in the document Title 21 of the Code of Federal Regulations Part 1020 (21 CFR 1020). Title 21 refers to the FDA. The FDA also must certify the administrative, professional, and technical aspects of mammographic services in order to obtain Medicare and most private insurance reimbursement. The FDA uses three classifications of all medical devices:

  Class I—general controls: class I devices are subject to the least regulatory control and present minimal potential for harm to the user. Examples would include image receptors, grids, and lead aprons.

  Class II—special controls: class II devices are those for which general controls alone are insufficient to assure safety and effectiveness. In addition to complying with general controls, class II devices also are subject to special controls. Examples would include collimators, pressure injectors for contrast media, and barium enema tips.

  Class III—premarket approval: class III is the most stringent regulatory category for devices. Class III devices are those for which insufficient information exists to ensure safety and effectiveness solely through general or special controls. Class III devices are usually those that support or sustain human life; are of substantial importance in preventing impairment of human health; or present a potential, unreasonable risk of illness or injury. Examples include angioplasty catheters and cardiovascular stents.

- *The NRC.* This agency is responsible for enforcing both equipment standards and radiation safety practices. This information is published in Title 10 of the Code of Federal Regulations Part 20 (10 CFR 20). Title 10 refers to the Department of Energy, which contains the NRC. In some states called *agreement states,* the NRC allows the state to have the responsibility to enforce equipment standards and radiation safety practices. As of the writing of this edition, there are currently 37 agreement states. The nonagreement states are Montana, Idaho, Wyoming, South Dakota, Missouri, Indiana, Michigan, West Virginia, Connecticut, Delaware, Vermont, Alaska, Hawaii, as well as Washington, DC.

- *OSHA.* This agency is responsible for establishing standards for safety and monitoring the workplace environment, including the requirements for occupational exposure to radiation, handling and disposal of hazardous materials, universal precautions (Tier 1) for protection of employees from infectious diseases, and personal protective equipment. This information is contained in Title 29 of the Code of Federal Regulations Part 1910 (29 CFR 1910). Title 29 refers to OSHA.

Patient Radiation Protection

Radiographic Examinations. The federal government recommends that the "As Low As Reasonably Achievable" (ALARA) concept be used during all diagnostic X-ray procedures. ALARA is covered in detail in the National Council on Radiation Protection (NCRP) Report #107. Some of the main recommendations of the ALARA program for radiographic examinations include the following:

1. *Use of high kilovolt (peak) (kVp) and low milliampere-second (mAs) exposure factors.* This is the most effective method of reducing patient exposure because milliampere-second selection is the primary control of the quantity of radiation emitted by the X-ray source. This is even more critical with computerized radiographic (CR) systems and direct-to-digital radiographic (DR) systems. With these systems, the computer can compensate for overexposure to radiation when it creates the final image on the monitor. This can lead technologists to become careless in their milliampere-second selection; they can overexpose the patient, resulting in **dose creep.** This is an increase in patient radiation exposure that occurs in CR and DR imaging, since these systems can compensate for overexposure up to 500% above the ideal amount but only compensate for underexposure of about 60% below the ideal value. It is extremely important to adhere to your system's recommended exposure indicator values (e.g., the S-numbers in the Fuji CR system, logM in Agfa CR system, etc.) to avoid overexposure to your patient. The radiographer must keep in mind that the kilovolt (peak) that is used must be kept in an optimum range for the particular part of the body that is being radiographed, because excessive kilovolt (peak) can produce images that may be of poor diagnostic quality (especially with film/screen image receptors).

2. *Use of high-speed image receptor systems.* This is the second most effective method of reducing patient exposure, because a faster speed system requires a lower mAs value to obtain a diagnostic image. With conventional film/screen imaging systems, most departments use rare-earth phosphors that are high speed and demonstrate acceptable recorded detail. When deciding which image receptor to use, one must consider that faster speed film/screen systems

CHAPTER 2 Quality Management Tools and Procedures

REVIEW QUESTIONS

1. Which of the following terms best describes the entire set or group of items being measured?
   a. Population
   b. Sample
   c. Frequency
   d. Central tendency

2. Which of the following terms best describes the average set of observations?
   a. Mean
   b. Median
   c. Mode
   d. Variance

3. Which of the following terms best describes variables that have only two values or choices?
   a. Continuous variables
   b. Dichotomous variables
   c. Stochastic variables
   d. Statistical variables

4. A cause-and-effect diagram is also known as which of the following?
   a. Fishbone chart
   b. Pareto chart
   c. Trend chart
   d. Scatter plot

5. Which of the following terms best describes a chart that pictorially demonstrates whether key indicators are moving up or down over a given period of time?
   a. Histogram
   b. Pareto chart
   c. Trend chart
   d. Scatter plot

6. The distribution of continuous data can best be demonstrated by the use which of the following?
   a. Histograms
   b. Control charts
   c. Scatter diagrams
   d. Pareto charts

7. Which of the following is not a tool for data presentation?
   a. Control charts
   b. Brainstorming
   c. Pareto charts
   d. Cause-and-effect diagrams

8. The unit of measure used to express the dose equivalent to occupational workers is which of the following?
   a. Roentgen
   b. Rad
   c. Rad equivalent, man
   d. Relative biological effectiveness (RBE)

9. Which of the following terms best describes the square of the standard deviation?
   a. Range
   b. Mode
   c. Variance
   d. Frequency

10. Which of the following does not affect patient dose during diagnostic radiography?
    a. Inherent filtration
    b. Added filtration
    c. Focal spot size
    d. Source-to-image distance (SID)

will also issue a second dosimeter to act as a fetal dose monitor. This should be worn at the waist level under a lead apron. The institution should also provide the pregnant employee a full explanation of the potential risks of radiation exposure, dose limits, as well as any state, local, or institutional policies. Technologists who become pregnant should not work with patients who have been treated with radionuclides since these materials could deliver a dose that would exceed acceptable limits.

Medical facilities must have an orientation program on radiation safety for newly employed technologists and a continuing education program to update the skills of all department personnel. Personnel who work in proximity to radiographic and fluoroscopic procedures (e.g., emergency department, operating room, intensive care unit) also should have the same in-service training.

Periodic surveys with properly calibrated instruments such as Geiger Müller counters and ionization chambers should be performed to assess that radiation in the workplace does not exceed accepted standards. Warning signs marked "Caution: Radiation Area" should be posted for any areas where dosage can exceed 5 milliroentgen (mR)/h. The cardinal principles of radiation protection (time, distance, and shielding) should be followed by all radiologic technologists to minimize their occupational exposure.

Time. Radiographers should keep the time of exposure to radiation as short as possible because the amount of exposure is directly proportional to the time of exposure, as indicated by the following equation:

$$\text{Total exposure} = \text{exposure rate} \times \text{time}$$

The exposure rate is the output of radiation from the source per unit time. For example, if a radiation source creates an exposure rate of 225 mR/h at a position occupied by an occupational worker, and the worker remains at that position for 36 min, what is the total exposure?

$$\text{Total exposure} = \frac{(225 \text{ mR/h})}{(36/60 \text{ h})} = 135 \text{ mR}$$

The factor of time is especially important during fluoroscopic, angiographic, and interventional procedures.

Distance. Radiographers should always maintain as large a distance as possible between the source of radiation and themselves. The reason is that radiation continually diverges from its source, so as distance is increased, less radiation exists per unit area. Reduction in radiation intensity follows an inverse square relationship and can be determined from the following equation:

$$\frac{\text{New intensity}}{\text{Old intensity}} = \frac{\text{Old distance}^2}{\text{New distance}^2}$$

For example, if the radiation intensity at 90 cm from a radiation source is 1.3 R/min, at 270 cm (3 times the distance as 90 cm), the radiation intensity is reduced to only 0.14 R/min (nine times less than the amount received at 90 cm). Therefore, a small increase in the distance from the source causes a large decrease in the amount of radiation exposure that is received. This factor is especially important in fluoroscopy because it may require the operator of the X-ray equipment to remain in the examination room. As a rule of thumb, the occupational radiation exposure during tableside fluoroscopy is about 1 mrem/min. Moving back away from the side of the examination table (if possible) can significantly reduce this amount according to the inverse square law. Standing on the image receptor side of a C-arm fluoroscopic unit rather than the X-ray tube side will also minimize radiation dose.

Shielding. Any material that can be placed between you and a source of radiation is considered shielding. Materials with a high atomic number (such as lead) that are not naturally radioactive are best for shielding because the greatest amount of photoelectric absorption occurs in these materials. Shielded booths are required for protecting the area around the control panel of radiographic units. The walls of the examination room are designed to protect personnel, other hospital employees, and the general public from unnecessary exposure. Lead aprons and gloves must be provided to employees when the possibility of exposure rate could exceed 5 mR/h (i.e., technologists who must be outside of the control booth during fluoroscopic or mobile procedures). Lead aprons must have a minimum lead equivalent thickness of at least 0.25 mm and cover 75–80% of the active bone marrow of the person wearing it. Protective gloves require a minimum lead equivalent thickness of 0.25 mm, with 0.5 mm preferred. Thyroid shields are available for general fluoroscopic, angiographic, and interventional procedures and must have a minimum lead equivalent thickness of 0.5 mm. Protective eyeglasses with a minimum lead equivalence of 0.35 mm or 0.5 mm are also available. Fluoroscopic and cardiovascular/interventional suites can also be equipped with leaded shields made of either radiation-absorbing acrylic or glass panels that are mounted on wheels for portability or are suspended from the ceiling.

SUMMARY

Implementing a quality management program requires considerably more than just equipment monitoring and maintenance. A basic knowledge of statistics and data collection, data presentation tools, administrative responsibilities, risk management, and radiation safety practices is essential in order for a quality management technologist to implement a successful quality management program.

Refer to the Evolve website at https://evolve.elsevier.com for Student Experiment 2.1: Attenuation or Transmission of Radiation.

4. *Use intermittent fluoroscopy (periodic activation of the fluoroscopic X-ray tube rather than continuous activation).* This can reduce patient dose by as much as 90%. Many departments have incorporated a procedure of recording the total fluoroscopic exposure time of a patient in their medical records or in a department log sheet. This information also should include the name of the radiologist/physician who performed the fluoroscopy, along with the patient case number.
5. *Use the last-image-hold feature.* This feature holds the last image obtained in digital storage and displays it on the monitor. This can reduce total fluoroscopic time by 50–80%.
6. *Avoid the magnification mode.* The magnification mode found with multifield tube type image intensifiers can increase patient dose 2–10 times that of the standard mode. This is because the magnification mode reduces the brightness gain of the image intensifier tube, requiring an increase in fluoroscopic milliampere to compensate.
7. *Keep the patient-to-image intensifier distance as short as possible during mobile fluoroscopic studies with a C-arm.* This reduces the source-to-skin distance to the patient.
8. *Reduce the number of spot images, and reduce the spot image size.* Patient dose increases as the number of spot images increases. In addition, larger spot size formats require more radiation; therefore, patient dose is increased.

During mobile radiographic procedures, visitors should leave the area if possible or move at least 8 ft away from the source of radiation. Visitors who want to accompany patients or observe a radiographic examination (such as a prospective radiography student or a radiology resident) should remain behind a protective barrier or wear protective apparel, or both. In some cases (e.g., pediatric patients), a visitor (nurse, patient care technician, parent or other relative) may be asked to help hold a patient during a radiographic procedure. These persons should be provided with protective apparel (such as lead aprons and gloves) to prevent overexposure to radiation that can occur during the procedure. Avoiding repeat exposure is also important in these instances because repeat exposure increases the patient's and visitor's dose.

Personnel Protection

Personnel who perform diagnostic procedures using ionizing radiation can potentially receive significant amounts of radiation and must therefore follow proper radiation practices. According to NCRP report number 116, maximum total effective dose equivalent for occupational personnel are as follows:

Whole body exposure	5 rem (50 mSv) per year
Eye lens	15 rem (150 mSv) per year
All other body parts (such as hands)	50 rem (500 mSv) per year

Examinations in which mobile equipment, fluoroscopy, cardiac catheterization, and interventional procedures are used pose a greater risk of higher dosages to radiographers and radiologists assistants than traditional radiographic procedures. Occupational radiation dosage should be monitored with a dosimeter obtained from a licensed provider. The most common of these are film badges, optically stimulated luminescent dosimeters, and thermoluminescent dosimeters. These are checked at either 1- or 3-month intervals with a report sent back to the institution indicating the dosage measured. For whole body measurement, these dosimeters are worn at either the waist or collar area. Finger dosimeters can also be issued in cases where the hands may receive relatively high dosages (i.e., nuclear medicine technologists and interventional technologists).

The embryonic/fetal dose of occupational workers should not exceed 0.0025 mrem (0.025 mSv) per day, 0.05 rem (0.5 mSv) in any 1 month of the 9-month gestation period and 0.5 rem (5 mSv) for the entire gestation period. When a radiographer, radiologist, or radiologist assistant has confirmation that they are pregnant, they must first declare their pregnancy to their employer or many institutions will not accept liability for proper precautions to protect a pregnant worker from radiation. Once the declaration is on file, the fetus is treated like a member of the general population. Most institutions

Visitor Protection

"Visitors" to diagnostic imaging departments are persons other than patients or radiology department staff. They may include relatives or friends of patients, hospital volunteers, security personnel, or other hospital employees who do not normally work in radiation areas (e.g., nurses, patient care technicians, respiratory therapists). While these persons are in the diagnostic imaging department or near mobile X-ray equipment in use (e.g., the emergency department or surgical suite), they are entitled to a safe environment with no unnecessary exposure to ionizing radiation. The NCRP lists maximum effective dose equivalent limits for members of the general population in its report, number 116. For members of the general population who may be exposed to frequent or continuous exposure from artificial sources other than medical irradiation (this includes radiography students younger than the age of 18), the NCRP recommends a maximum effective dose equivalent limit of 0.1 rad equivalent, man (rem) (1 mSv) per year. For those who may receive infrequent exposure (e.g., a parent who may be asked to hold a child for an X-ray procedure), a maximum of 0.5 rem (5 mSv) per year is recommended. To help minimize exposure to department visitors, radiographers can make sure that all examination room doors remain closed during radiographic procedures.

can demonstrate poorer resolution than slower speed systems. Most current CR and DR systems possess a system speed that is comparable to a 200- to 300-speed film/screen system.

3. *Use of proper filtration.* Filtration removes lower energy X-rays from the primary beam before contact with the patient. This can reduce the patient's entrance skin dose by as much as 90%. There is usually a certain amount of inherent filtration (filtering performed by the window of the X-ray tube, as well as any cooling oil) present and added aluminum between the X-ray tube window and the top of the collimating device.

4. *Use of the smallest field size possible, along with proper collimation.* This reduces the amount of the patient's body that is exposed to radiation, thereby reducing the total dose. The effect of field size can be seen by calculating a value known as the **dose area product (DAP)**; this calculation incorporates the total dose of radiation along with the area of field that is being used. The units used to measure this value can be roentgen (R) × square centimeter (R × cm^2), coulomb per kilogram (C/kg) × square centimeter (C/kg × cm^2), Rad × square centimeter (R × cm^2) or milliGray × square centimeter (mGy × cm^2). For example, a field size of 5 × 5 cm (25 cm^2) can receive a dosage of 4 R, yielding a DAP of 100 R × square centimeter. A field size of 20 × 20 cm (400 cm^2) can receive a much lower dose of only 0.25 R but still yield the same DAP of 100 R × square centimeter because of the increase in the size of the X-ray field.

5. *Use of optimum processing conditions.* Regardless of whether one is using film/screen radiography or a digital radiographic imaging system, proper image processing must exist in order to obtain consistent image quality. Automatic film processor quality control is extremely important in lowering the patient dose in conventional film/screen radiography. For example, if the developer temperature were too low, the resulting radiographs would appear to lack optical density. This can lead to a repeat image (increasing the dose for that particular patient) or to an increase in technical factors for subsequent images (increasing patient dose for all subsequent patients). For CR and DR systems, proper manipulation of both preprocessing and postprocessing software factors by the radiographer is necessary to obtain proper image quality.

6. *Avoidance of repeat examinations.* The ideal overall repeat rate for diagnostic imaging departments is no greater than 4–6% (2% for mammographic procedures). This figure can vary depending on the patient population and acceptance standards of a particular imaging department but should never exceed 10–12%. Proper patient instructions, along with correct positioning and technique selection by the radiographer, should help reduce the need for repeat examinations. Digital radiographic systems can reduce the repeat rate due to technique error because postprocessing software can yield some correction of image brightness (optical density in film/screen imaging) and image gray scale (contrast in film/screen imaging). Proper positioning is extremely important when automatic exposure control devices are used with both film/screen imaging (to be sure the correct portion of the anatomy is over the cell that has been selected) and with CR and DR systems (because the computer must compare the image obtained with its preprogrammed ideal image to obtain the correct image).

7. *Use of a posteroanterior (PA) projection instead of an anteroposterior (AP) projection for scoliosis series on young female patients.* Normally, radiographic views of the spine are performed with an AP projection to place the spine as close to the image receptor as possible. However, the breast tissue in female adolescents is extremely sensitive to the development of radiation-induced breast cancer (with a latent period of 5–15 years). When the examination is performed with the PA projection instead of the AP projection, the breast tissue receives the exit dose instead of the entrance dose of radiation. This can reduce the mean glandular dose to the breast tissue by as much as 98%. Shielding of the breast areas with specialized devices also should be used to reduce the dose even further.

8. *Use of gonadal shielding.* Gonadal shielding with at least 0.5-mm lead equivalence should be used whenever the gonads lie within 5 cm of the collimation line and do not interfere with the anatomy of interest. This can reduce the dose to the reproductive organs by as much as 90%. Gonadal shielding may be a flat contact, a shaped contact, or a shadow type of shield.

Fluoroscopic Examinations. Fluoroscopic examinations have the potential to deliver a considerable dose of radiation to the patient. Therefore, ALARA protocols including the following should be in place for these examinations:

1. *Keep fluoroscopic milliampere (mA) and time as low as possible when performing fluoroscopy.* The mA is usually kept in a relatively narrow range (0.5–3 mA), so reducing the fluoroscopic time is one of the most effective means of reducing patient dose during fluoroscopic procedures.

2. *Use high kilovolt (peak) if possible.* Fluoroscopic examinations should be performed in the 85- to 125-kVp range (depending on the contrast media being used). The use of a higher kilovolt (peak) reduces the fluoroscopic mA required to obtain adequate image brightness, thereby reducing the patient's dose.

3. *Limit field size as much as possible.* This is done with the fluoroscopic collimation shutters and with a smaller size image intensifier. This has the same effect as collimation, which was previously discussed.

CHAPTER 3

Film/Screen Image Receptors, Darkrooms, and Viewing Conditions

KEY TERMS

Contrast-to-noise ratio
Contrast resolution
Darkroom
Densitometer
Edge spread function
Fluorescence
Foot-candle
Full-width half maximum
Humidity
Illuminance
Intensification factor
Latensification
Line spread function
Luminance
Luminescence
Modulation transfer function
Nit
Nyquist frequency
Orthochromatic
Panchromatic
Phosphorescence
Photometry
Point spread function
Psychrometer
Quantum mottle
Relative speed
Safelight
Screen speed
Sensitometer
Signal-to-noise ratio
Solarization
Spatial resolution
Spectral matching
Static electricity
Temperature
Ultraviolet
Ventilation
Viewbox illuminator

OBJECTIVES

At the completion of this chapter, the reader should be able to do the following:

- State the function and characteristics of a darkroom used for diagnostic imaging
- Explain the importance of proper safelight type and function
- Perform a safelight evaluation test
- Perform an evaluation of white light leakage and processing area condition
- Explain the conditions for proper film and chemical storage
- Discuss the importance of proper viewbox illuminator function on image quality
- Perform a viewbox quality control test
- Explain the evaluation process of image duplicators
- Explain the factors affecting screen speed
- Describe the importance of spectral matching of intensifying screens and film
- Describe the different types of image resolution

OUTLINE

Darkroom Function
Darkroom Environment
  Darkroom Characteristics
  Darkroom Lighting
    Overhead Lighting
    Safelight
  Light and Leakage Testing
    Safelight Testing
    Leakage Testing and Processing Area Condition
  Film and Chemical Storage
Viewbox Quality Control
  Viewbox Illuminators
  Viewbox Quality Control Test
Image Duplicating Units
Film/Screen Image Receptors
  Intensifying Screen Speed
    Intensification Factor
    Relative Speed Value
    Name of Screen
    Factors Affecting Screen Speed
  Quality Control Testing of Screen Speed
  Spectral Matching
  Screen Resolution
    Contrast Resolution
    Spatial Resolution
  Screen Condition
Summary

Despite the digital revolution that has recently occurred in diagnostic imaging, many radiographic images may still recorded on film. Even with digital imaging, hard copy imaging may be desired, and this necessitates the use of silver-based film. Because all traditional film is light sensitive, it must be handled in a safe area where no light or ionizing radiation is present. Most diagnostic imaging departments use a **darkroom** area for this purpose, whereas other nondigital departments may use some form of a daylight system (discussed in Chapter 5). Even departments with daylight systems usually have a traditional darkroom that can be used for duplicating existing radiographs or used as a backup in case of a malfunction in the daylight system.

DARKROOM FUNCTION

The function of a radiographic darkroom is to protect the film from white light and ionizing radiation during handling and processing. After a film has been exposed to light or ionizing radiation (such as in a cassette during a radiographic examination), it can be as much as two to eight times more sensitive to subsequent exposure than an unexposed film (depending on the type of emulsion). This increase in sensitivity is formally known as **latensification**. As a result of this phenomenon, any accidental exposure from an unwanted source (such as a darkroom light leak) can destroy a diagnostic image. Film can also be affected by excess heat, humidity, static electricity, pressure, and chemical fumes. All of these variables must be carefully controlled to obtain a diagnostic quality image. If they are not controlled, the most common result is the presence of fog on the manifest image. Fog is defined as noninformational density that occurs because silver grains are formed and do not represent any of the anatomic structures within the patient.

DARKROOM ENVIRONMENT

A darkroom is considered a scientific laboratory by common practice standards and the Occupational Safety and Health Administration (OSHA) and should meet all of the requirements and possess all of the equipment of a laboratory. It also should be clean, well ventilated, well organized, and safe. Eating, drinking, and smoking must be prohibited in the darkroom because bits of food or ashes from cigarettes can get into image receptors as they are being loaded and unloaded. These can cause artifacts on the image that can mimic pathologic conditions (especially in mammography cassettes) or otherwise degrade the diagnostic quality of the image. These artifacts are discussed in detail in Chapter 10.

Darkroom Characteristics

Countertops or other work surfaces and rubber floor mats should be grounded to reduce the risk of **static**

electricity. Static electricity creates sparks that emit white light (all colors of the visible spectrum). Because all imaging films are sensitive to some portion of the visible light spectrum, this light creates artifacts that appear on the processed image. The types of static artifacts are tree, crown, and smudge (see Chapter 10). In addition to the work surfaces being grounded, static can be minimized by the following:

1. Handle film properly. Proper film handling, placing a film into and out of a cassette or onto a film tray rather than sliding it, reduces the risk of static electricity because friction is a primary cause of static electricity.
2. Wear natural-fiber clothing (cotton) versus synthetic-fiber clothing (e.g., nylon, polyester).
3. Maintain a proper **humidity** range (30–60% relative humidity). Moisture in the air absorbs the buildup of static charges. This is why static is less of a problem in the summer, when the relative humidity is greater. In some darkrooms, installation of a humidifier or ion generator may be necessary to maintain the recommended level of humidity. A **psychrometer**, which measures humidity, should be available or installed in the darkroom. A psychrometer is a type of hygrometer (a device that measures atmospheric humidity) for calculating relative humidity (Fig. 3-1). It consists of a thermometer with wet and dry bulbs, the readings of which are compared, giving the rate of evaporation of water from which the water vapor saturation

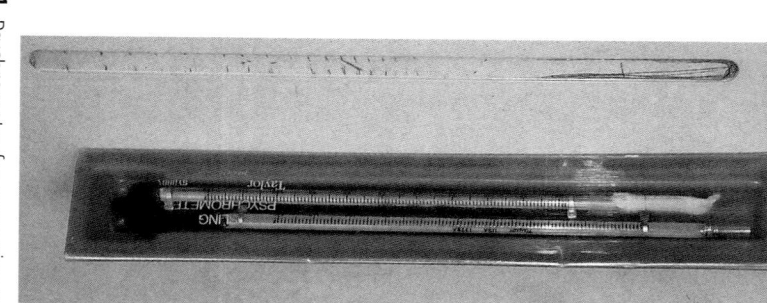

FIGURE 3-1 Psychrometer for measuring relative humidity.

of the atmosphere can be calculated. At low relative humidity, moisture evaporates from the wet bulb more rapidly, causing the wet bulb to have a lower reading than the dry bulb. The temperature difference between the two bulbs is used to calculate the relative humidity. Excessive humidity could cause the films to stick together, and the emulsion from the films could be removed when they are pulled apart. Excessive humidity also could cause a condensation problem, and the result could be artifacts (see Chapter 10).

4. *Clean screens regularly with an antistatic nonabrasive cleaner.* Appropriate screen cleaners are available from the manufacturers from whom the screen is purchased (it is important to match these products to the particular brand of screen). The proper procedure for cleaning intensifying screens is covered in Chapter 7. This is especially critical with film/screen mammography cassettes since any dirt or debris in the cassette can leave artifacts that can mimic microcalcifications (an early sign of breast cancer).

The darkroom must be well ventilated to prevent buildup of heat and humidity, which degrade the film. Proper ventilation also removes excessive fumes from the processing solutions that may sensitize film emulsions. The presence of these fumes also can cause condensation of processing chemicals onto work surfaces in the darkroom (e.g., underneath cabinets or shelves). Over time, the residue created by this condensation may fall into open cassettes, causing artifacts to appear in the final images. Removing these fumes, along with periodically wiping these areas with a damp cloth, should minimize the occurrence of these artifacts. **Temperature** should be maintained in a range of 65–75 °F (18–24 °C). The fumes from the processing solutions are considered toxic, corrosive, and potentially carcinogenic by OSHA, the Environmental Protection Agency, and the Department of Transportation. OSHA maintains a listing of permissible exposure limits (PELs), which are the chemical levels to which employees can be exposed in the workplace without risk or harm. An environmental engineer can be consulted to monitor the level of a darkroom area. The following are PELs for some of the components found in processing solutions:

Acetic acid: 25 mg/m^3 (10 parts per million [ppm])
Ammonium thiosulfate (as ammonia): 35 mg/m^3 (50 ppm)
Hydroquinone: 2 mg/m^3 (0.44 ppm)
Phenol: 19 mg/m^3 (5 ppm)
Sulfur dioxide: 13 mg/m^3 (5 ppm)
Glutaraldehyde: 0.7 mg/m^3 (0.2 ppm)
Silver: 0.01 mg/m^3

The values just listed were established in 1968, and discussion to revise these figures is taking place. In recent years, many technologists and darkroom technicians have complained of hypersensitivity to darkroom chemicals, a condition sometimes called *darkroom disease,* which manifests in a variety of symptoms ranging from hives to severe fatigue and impairment of the immune system. The Society of Toxicology and the American Society of Radiologic Technologists are currently collecting data on this phenomenon. Proper **ventilation** in a darkroom should keep the levels of chemical vapors well below PELs and should include a source of fresh air, slight positive air pressure (so that chemical fumes are not sucked out of the processor), and ventilation to the outside atmosphere. *This should yield about 8 to 10 room changes of air per hour.* A ventilator duct should be placed near the floor, in either the lower portion of the entrance door or the wall.

Many darkrooms have interior walls that are mistakenly painted black, and these walls can make the room too dark. Instead, darkroom walls should be painted in pastels and light colors to increase the reflectance of the light emitted from the safelight. Enamels or epoxy paints are best because they are easy to clean and more durable. However, a matte finish must be used, because a high-gloss finish could reflect and amplify light leaks. Should any darkroom wall lie adjacent to a radiation area (e.g., radiographic room, nuclear medicine area), proper lead shielding that is appropriate to the type and energy of radiation used must be present in the walls to protect darkroom personnel and prevent fogging of the film.

The processing of most diagnostic images requires a large quantity of clean water. Today, in most automatic film processors, only cold water is used, because the processors have built-in heating systems to regulate solution temperatures (see Chapter 4). Older processors and many cine film processors may require a hot water supply in addition to the cold water and have a mixing valve to regulate the temperature. Adequate drainage must be in place to remove the dirty water and used chemicals after processing is completed. *Adequate drainage* is generally defined as the capacity to handle 2.5 times the maximum outflow of the processor when all drains are open. For most automatic film processors this is about 10 gallons per minute (38 l/min). A floor drain is generally desired for maximum efficiency, with a 3-inch-diameter cast iron or plastic (polyvinylchloride [PVC]) pipe. Local building codes should be referenced before choosing PVC pipe because some municipalities have restrictions on its use. Copper or brass pipes and fittings should be avoided because of the corrosive effect of the processing chemicals. These drains should be dedicated only to film processors and should not share a common line with sinks and toilets, to reduce the chance of blockage. They also must be cleaned on a regular basis with a commercial drain cleaner because buildup forms over time. This is especially important when metallic replacement silver recovery units (see Chapter 6) are used. Flooring around the drain must be easy to clean, moisture resistant, and of a light color to allow identification of objects that may have been dropped in the dark.

38 CHAPTER 3 Film/Screen Image Receptors, Darkrooms, and Viewing Conditions

Darkrooms should have adequate storage space for film and chemicals. Film must be stored in an upright position (with no heavy objects or other boxes of film stacked on top) to avoid pressure marks. Open boxes of film should be kept in a metal film bin (usually mounted under the work counter) to minimize the chance of being exposed to white light (Fig. 3-2). Passboxes, also known as *film transfer systems*, also should be present to prohibit white light from entering. These are special boxes whereby one side of them has a door inside of the darkroom while the other side of the passbox has another door on the outside. If one of the doors is open, the other cannot be opened. This allows a person on the outside to place a cassette in the box, close the door, and then the person inside of the darkroom can open their door without allowing light into the darkroom. The darkroom door should be double interlocked or revolving, or a lightproof maze can be installed if floor space permits.

Darkroom Lighting

A darkroom should have two types of lighting, overhead lights and safelights.

Overhead Lighting. Overhead lighting is the standard white light that normally illuminates the interior rooms of hospitals and clinics. This standard lighting is necessary for cleaning, maintenance, and possible emergencies (e.g., darkroom personnel becoming ill). Proper overhead lighting normally requires a standard fluorescent fixture (two to four 48-inch fluorescent tubes) per eight square feet (0.74 m²) of floor space. The overhead light should be interlocked with the film bin(s) so that if a bin is open, the light cannot be energized. If this is not practical, a cover should be placed over the switch to prevent accidental activation. Film bin alerts also are available (at a minimal cost) that sound a continuous alarm while the film bin is open to prevent accidental exposure to white light.

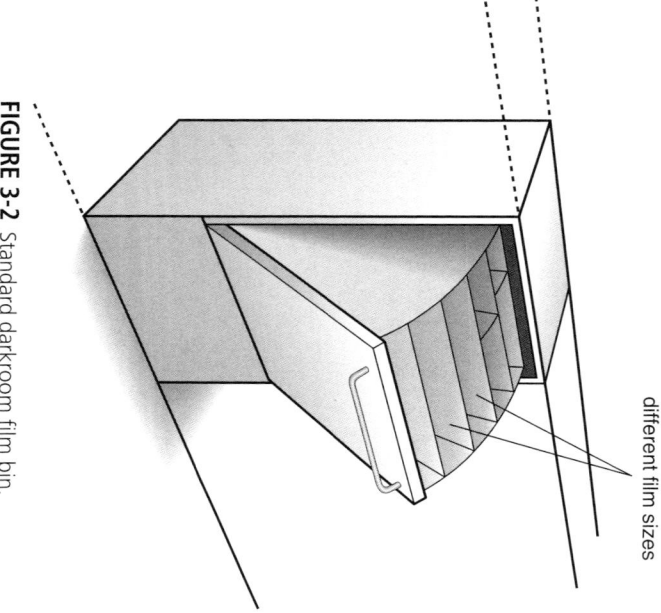

Compartments for the different film sizes

FIGURE 3-2 Standard darkroom film bin.

| Red | Orange | Yellow | Green | Blue | Indigo | Violet |

FIGURE 3-3 Visible light spectrum.

Safelight. A safelight is a light source that emits wavelengths to which particular types of film are not sensitive. Ordinary room light (known as white light) is really a mixture of all of the colors in the visible light spectrum mixed together, as shown in Fig. 3-3. Each individual color is determined by the wavelength of the light photon, which is measured in units called angstroms (Å). One angstrom is equal to 10^{-10} m of 10^{-8} cm. Wavelengths range from about 4000 Å for violet light to 8000 Å for red light. In comparison, the wavelengths of diagnostic radiographs generally range from only 0.1 to about 0.5 Å.

Even the best safelights emit some white light (only lasers emit a pure light of one specific wavelength), so it is important not to leave film in safelight indefinitely. Also, remember the concept of latensification whereby a film that has been previously exposed is more sensitive than film that has not been exposed. A typical radiographic film (exposed) should be able to remain in safelight for at least 40 seconds without becoming fogged. Mounting safelights at least three to four feet from feed trays or loading counters also helps minimize safelight fog.

The type of film to be processed in the darkroom determines the type of safelight to be used.

Blue-Violet-Sensitive Film. Blue-violet-sensitive film is a common type of film used in screen cassettes, and, as its name implies, is primarily sensitive to the colors blue, indigo, and violet. An amber-colored safelight (a mixture of red, orange, and some yellow) is normally used, with two options available. For the average-sized darkroom, a fixture type of safelight containing either a 7.5- or 15-watt (W) light bulb is sufficient (Fig. 3-4). A 7.5-W bulb is recommended for single-emulsion film. The light bulb is covered by a colored piece of plastic or glass called a *filter*. The most common types of filters for blue-violet-sensitive film are the Kodak Wratten 6B or the Kodak Mor-Lite (which is slightly brighter). Both of these filters emit an amber- or brownish-colored light. The other option, called a *sodium vapor lamp* (Fig. 3-5), is used in a large darkroom or when bright safelight conditions are desired. This works on the same principle as mercury streetlights; however, sodium yields a bright amber color when energized, instead of the bright white color of the mercury lamps. These lights are large, expensive, and require a long warm-up time to reach maximum brightness. They must be mounted on the darkroom ceiling (at least six feet above counters and film bins) because of their brightness level and to provide indirect lighting. Shutter or door openings on top are adjusted with a pull chain to regulate the level of brightness.

Orthochromatic Film. Orthochromatic film is mainly sensitive to the green portion of the visible spectrum, in addition to the blue-violet portion. A red or magenta dye is added to the film emulsion to increase the absorption of green light by the silver halide crystals. Amber is a mixture of red, orange, and yellow; therefore, the safelights discussed previously are not compatible with this type of film because orange and yellow are too close to green in the spectrum. It is therefore necessary to use a safelight with the same fixture and light bulb combination mentioned previously, but to use a safelight filter that emits light that is pure red. The most common of this type is the Kodak GBX Series of all-purpose filters (GBX stands for green/blue/X-ray). In addition, all Kodak duplicating film requires a GBX-2 filter. An older type of safelight filter that is still acceptable for **orthochromatic** film is the Kodak 2 filter, which is dark red. Another option is an LED safelight, which uses a light-emitting diode that consumes low power and can last up to 15 years. These safelights are perfectly compatible for use with blue-violet-sensitive film but are not as bright as safelights with amber filters. Facilities should avoid the use of red-colored light bulbs such as those found in Christmas decorations. Although considerably less expensive than actual safelight fixtures, they can emit too much white light, resulting in safelight fog.

New Modality Film. New modality film is designed to obtain images from either a cathode-ray tube (multiformat camera) or a laser camera (often used in computed tomography [CT], sonography, nuclear medicine, magnetic resonance imaging [MRI], and older digital radiographic systems [hence the name]). The light source for many of these devices usually emits light that is red or amber colored, so the film emulsion is designed accordingly (it is also sensitive to infrared). A fixture and light bulb combination safelight with a dark green filter (Kodak Number 7) can be used with these emulsions. This filter is dark, and some time is necessary for the eyes of technologists or darkroom personnel to adapt. Some types of new modality film are **panchromatic** (sensitive to all colors of the visible spectrum) and therefore cannot be exposed to any safelight. It is best to consult the literature accompanying the box of film or the manufacturer's technical representative before dark green safelight is used. The dry laser printer has virtually replaced the need for this type of film.

Other Film Types. Most other types of film (e.g., duplicating, subtraction, spot, industrial) can be processed in darkrooms with the safelights just discussed. It is best to consult the film manufacturer to determine the correct type of safelight for these films. Cine film used in cardiac catheterization studies is black-and-white motion picture film (panchromatic) and cannot be exposed to safelights. It normally requires its own dedicated processor (see Chapter 9).

Dry Laser Printer Film. Film used in dry laser printers (discussed in Chapter 9) may need to be handled in darkroom conditions, depending on whether or not it has a special dye added to the top-coating layer. If present, this dye will block ordinary room light from exposing the emulsion (the laser from the printer can still penetrate the dye) so it can be loaded into the printer in ordinary room light. Film that does not have this coating will have to be loaded under darkroom conditions.

Light and Leakage Testing

Safelight Testing. Safelights may become unsafe over time as a result of cracks or pinholes in the filter (resulting from expansion and contraction with heat), the wrong wattage of the bulb being installed, or the doors on a sodium vapor lamp being open too far; therefore, a safelight test should be performed at least semiannually or more frequently if problems are discovered. Testing also should be performed when the safelight bulb or filter is

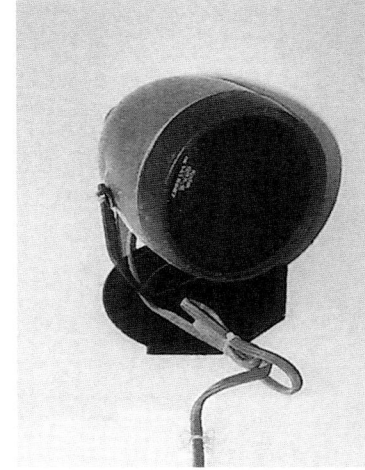

FIGURE 3-4 Fixture type of darkroom safelight.

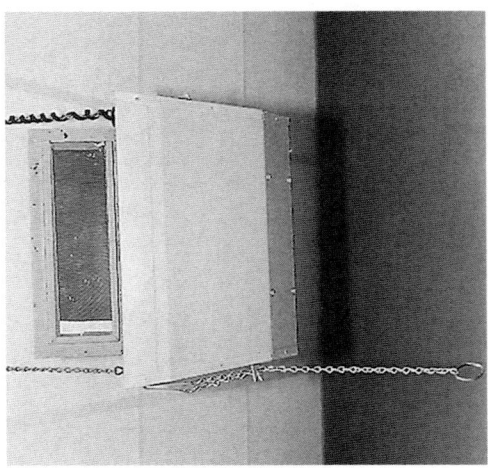

FIGURE 3-5 Sodium vapor lamp darkroom safelight.

changed. Safelights that are turned on for 24 hours a day, 7 days a week, should have their filters changed annually. If safelights are turned on an average of 12 hours a day, 7 days a week, the filter should be changed every 2 years. Testing requires a sensitized film (preexposed) because this makes it more sensitive to safelight fog.

Safelight testing (Fig. 3-6) can be accomplished by either of the procedures discussed in the following paragraph.

PROCEDURE

This procedure is performed with a penetrometer (step wedge) on dual-emulsion films only.

1. Use a tape measure to verify the proper distance from the safelight to the work counters or feed trays. Also check the wattage of light bulbs, and inspect the filter for cracks or pinholes. Make sure that the filter type matches the film type.
2. Load an 8 × 10 inches (20 × 25 cm) cassette with film from a fresh box of film. If more than one type of film is used by the facility, a separate test should be performed for each type of film.
3. Take the loaded cassette to a radiographic room, and center the cassette on a radiographic table at a source-to-image distance (SID) of 40 inches (100 cm). Place a penetrometer (step wedge) in the center of the cassette, aligning the long dimension of the wedge with the long axis of the cassette. Collimate the light field to the edges of the step wedge.
4. Expose the cassette at approximately 70 kilovolts (peak) (kVp) and 5 milliamperes-second (mAs). Ideally, the image of the step wedge on the film should have an optical density of approximately 1 when measured with a densitometer. The kilovolt (peak) and milliampere-second can be adjusted depending on the speed of the image receptors that are used.
5. Bring the cassette back into the darkroom, lay the exposed film on the counter, and cover one-half of the film with an opaque material such as cardboard. Be sure to bisect the latent image of the penetrometer into right and left halves and not top and bottom.
6. Expose the film to normal safelight conditions for 2 min, and then process the film.
7. Place the film on a viewbox illuminator and observe if there is a defined line or break between the halves (see Fig. 3-6). If there is no defined line between the halves, then there is no safelight fog because the human eye can observe differences of as little as 0.01 optical density units. If a discernible line is present, use a **densitometer** to measure the optical density on each side of the line. The difference between the two sides is a measure of darkroom fog. Because the difference in optical density measurements varies for each step, the step with the maximum density difference must be found. Record the density difference value and the step on which it was measured. This same step should be used for all future safelight tests. The maximum density difference (or darkroom fog level) should be less than 0.05 optical density units. Levels in excess of this value indicate serious safelight fog, which can reduce the image contrast of any films that are exposed to these conditions. If the fog levels are greater than 0.05, readjusting the position of the safelight, replacing the safelight filter, checking to see that the proper wattage bulb has been installed into the safelight, or closing the shutters on a sodium vapor lamp can usually correct the situation.

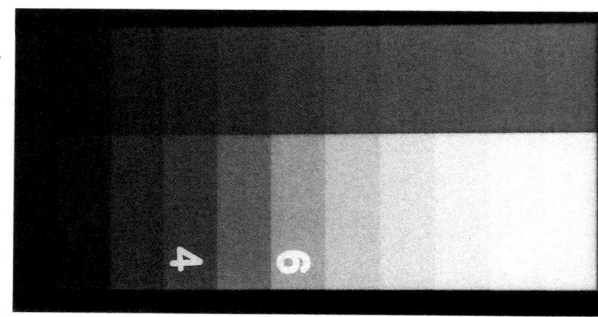

FIGURE 3-6 Image of penetrometer showing safelight fog. (Courtesy Nuclear Associates, Carle Place, N.Y.)

PROCEDURE

This procedure is performed with a sensitometer and is acceptable for both single-emulsion (which is usually slower speed) and dual-emulsion film, if one does not want to use the previous procedure.

1. In the darkroom (in complete darkness with the safelights turned off), remove a sheet of film from a fresh box of film.
2. Expose this sheet of film with a **sensitometer**, and place it on the counter in the darkroom. Place an opaque card over one-half of the exposed wedge pattern on the film, just as in the first procedure.
3. Expose the film to normal safelight conditions for 2 min, and then process the film.
4. Use a densitometer to determine the step that will have an optical density closest to 1.4 optical density units (using the side that was covered with the opaque card).
5. Determine the maximum density difference (the difference in optical density between the covered side and the uncovered side) for this step and record for future use. For dual-emulsion films, the maximum density difference should not exceed 0.05 optical density units (as in the first procedure). For single-emulsion films, the maximum density difference between the halves cannot exceed 0.02 optical density units. Since single-emulsion film generally has a lower inherent contrast, it is vitally important to keep any additional fogging (which reduces contrast even further) to a minimum.

Leakage Testing and Processing Area Condition. While safelights are tested, a check for light leaks, other extraneous light sources (e.g., indicator lights on processors, duplicators, luminous dials on a clock), and processing area conditions usually also can be performed.

PROCEDURE

1. Turn on all white lights in the area surrounding the darkroom. Enter the darkroom, and shut off all safelights and overhead lights.
2. After eyes adapt to the dark (about 5 min), check for white light leaks, especially near the processor, darkroom doors, water pipes, ventilation ducts, and suspended ceiling tiles. Light leaks can cause artifacts and reduce image contrast.
3. Turn on the overhead lighting, and inspect the counter tops and processor feed tray for foreign objects, dampness, cleanliness, and sharp edges. These conditions can cause artifacts if not corrected.
4. Locate the reserve fixer and developer tanks. Check to ensure that they are properly ventilated and that the temperature of the area is within accepted limits. Excessive temperature can cause a deterioration of the processing solutions.
5. Locate the film storage area, and verify that the boxes of film are being stored vertically and under the proper temperature conditions. Also check the age of the film and the visibility of the expiration date. The oldest boxes of film should be positioned so that they will be used first. Artifacts can result if these conditions are not within proper parameters.
6. Correct any problems or deficiencies.

Film and Chemical Storage

Film should be stored at a temperature range between 55 and 75 °F (14–24 °C), whether in the darkroom (only open boxes of film, kept in the film bin), storage closet, or warehouse. Excessive heat can cause age fog, and too low of a temperature can lead to moisture condensation on the film, resulting in artifacts. Humidity also must be controlled (30–60% relative humidity), especially with film in which the moisture-proof inner seal has been opened. As previously mentioned, static artifacts can appear if the air is too dry. Premature aging of the film, condensation, and films sticking together could be a problem in high-humidity conditions. Film can be stored in a refrigerator or freezer to prolong the shelf life, provided the inner seal is unopened. If kept in a freezer at 0 °F or below, the deterioration or aging process stops and the expiration date can be extended for any time that the film was in the freezer. After removal, a 24-h warm-up period is required before the inner seal can be opened and the film used. This is to prevent condensation and the associated artifacts from appearing on the film.

Chemicals should be stored in a well-ventilated area with a temperature range between 40° and 85 °F (5–30 °C). The temperature should not exceed 70 °F (21 °C) for a prolonged period. The area should be darkened or have minimal lighting because the developer solution can degrade if exposed to bright light. It is best not to store film and chemicals near each other because film chemistry contains quantities of potassium, a percentage of which is in the form of potassium-40, which is a naturally occurring radioactive isotope that can fog film over time. Most film manufacturers recommend that background radiation not exceed 7 microroentgens (µR)/h. Levels near large quantities of processing chemicals can reach 12 µR/h. Most manufacturers of film and processing chemicals give a 12-month expiration date on the basis of an ambient temperature of 68 °F (20 °C).

VIEWBOX QUALITY CONTROL

Viewbox Illuminators

Most diagnostic images are transparencies and therefore require an illuminator to view the final image. Proper functioning of the **viewbox illuminator** is essential in maintaining image quality because it has a direct effect on the contrast. Over time, heat from the fluorescent bulb inside can discolor the plastic front of the viewbox. Dirt and dust can form on both the inside and outside of the plastic viewing surface, as well as the outside surface of the fluorescent bulb. This can reduce light output by as much as 10% per year, and the image contrast is decreased. For this reason, the bulbs should be changed every 2 years (especially viewboxes used in mammography), even though the typical fluorescent bulb has a rated life of 7500–9000 hours. With multiple viewboxes, replace all lamps at the same time, with bulbs of the same manufacturer, production lot, and color temperature to maintain consistency. All viewboxes should be cleaned weekly with an antistatic, nonabrasive cleaner, and the intensity of all viewboxes within the department should be checked for consistency. A viewbox quality control test should be performed on acceptance and then at least once a year (weekly for those used in mammography).

Viewbox Quality Control Test

The viewbox quality control test requires a screwdriver and either a photographic light meter or a 35-mm camera with a built-in light meter (Box 3-1, Fig. 3-7).

IMAGE DUPLICATING UNITS

Film duplicating units, or copiers, are standard pieces of equipment in diagnostic imaging darkrooms (Fig. 3-8). Because legal considerations make hospitals reluctant to release original images, copies are made so that patients can consult with specialty physicians without having to repeat the examinations. Most units emit **ultraviolet (UV)** light using special black light bulbs. UV light is more penetrating than visible light; thus, it can penetrate the darker areas of a processed image so the image can be duplicated. The copy film is single-emulsion film sensitive to UV light, so a standard safelight can be used. The emulsion side of the film should be placed against the original image during the duplication process. The emulsion of duplicating film is more unstable than conventional film because of latensification. This is because it has been preexposed by the manufacturer to the point of **solarization**, or image reversal. For this reason, large quantities should not be stockpiled. More information on solarization or image reversal can be found in Appendix A.

BOX 3-1 Photometry

The radiant energy that strikes or crosses a surface per unit of time or radiant energy emitted by a source per unit time is called *radiant flux* and is measured in watts (W). The watt is defined as the number of joules (J) of energy per second or 1 W = 1 J/s. Radiant flux, evaluated with respect to its capacity to evoke the sensation of brightness, is called *luminous flux*. The unit of luminous flux is the lumen and is affected by both the radiant flux and the wavelength (color) of the light (yellow can appear brighter than purple or violet, even with the same number of light photons in the beam). One standard candle radiates about 12.5 lumens. The luminous intensity of a light source is the amount of luminous flux per solid angle and is represented by the equation:

$$I = \frac{dF}{d\omega}$$

where I = Luminous intensity, dF = Luminous flux in lumens, and $d\omega$ = Solid angle in steradians, and where ω is equal to the area on the surface of a sphere divided by the square of the radius of that sphere. There are 12.5 steradians in one sphere. This value of lumens per steradian is also called the *candle*, or *candela* (cd), and is the official unit of luminous intensity. One candle or candela corresponds to 3.8×10^{15} photons per second being emitted from a light source through a cone like field of view.

The actual brightness of a particular area or source can be evaluated by one of two values, illuminance and luminance.

Illuminance

Illuminance is the amount of luminous flux incident per unit area, or the amount of light that falls on a given surface. It is not the amount of brightness of a light source, but rather the result of that light source in illuminating a particular area. For example, we are often more interested in the intensity of light falling on a surface than we are in the brightness of a light source. If you are reading, you are more concerned with the brightness of the page than in the brightness of a particular light bulb. The brightness of the page that you are reading is the illumination; the brightness of a particular light bulb is the luminance. The illumination that you obtain depends not only on how bright the bulb is (the luminance) but also on how far away it is (light intensity follows the inverse square law). Illuminance can be measured in units of lux (lumens per square millimeter) or foot-candles (ft-cd) (lumens per square foot). Conversion of foot-candles to lux can be accomplished by the following equation:

Lux = Foot-candles × 10.8 (because 1 ft-cd = 10.8 lux)

The illuminance of the interior of a typical home or office building from artificial light is approximately 1000 lux or 100 ft-cd. The light-localizing variable-aperture collimator must be able to illuminate a minimum of 15 ft-cd or 160 lux according to Food and Drug Administration guidelines (discussed in Chapter 7). Viewbox brightness can be measured with illuminance (because the light bulb is illuminating the acrylic plastic (Plexiglas) front), but luminance is more accepted. If illuminance is used, standard viewboxes will have a value of about 5000 lux, 500 ft-cd, or 13 EV. A photodetector that is covered with both a photometric filter and a cosine diffuser is required for the measurement of illuminance (see Fig. 3-7).

Luminance

Luminance is the luminous intensity per unit of projected area of source, or the amount of light that is emitted or scattered from a particular surface. In other words, luminance measures the brightness or intensity from a particular light source. Luminance is the preferred method of measuring viewbox brightness and is required for inspections according to the Mammography Quality Standards Act. Units that can measure luminance include candles or candela per square meter (also known as nit), candles per square centimeter, or candles per square foot. The range of human vision is from 6×10^{-6} nit to $10 \times 10 = 6$ nit. The optimum range is from about 1000 to 10,000 nit. The average viewbox for viewing film images has an average brightness level of 2000 nit, while a 36 W fluorescent tube has a brightness level of 8000 nit. Another set of units also can be used for measurement of luminance and is $1/\pi$ as great as those mentioned earlier. These units are the lambert, foot-lambert (often used to measure television and computer monitor brightness), and meter-lambert.

For conversion of nit to foot-lamberts, the following equation can be used:

1 lambert = $1/\pi$ cd/cm^2
1 foot – lambert = $1/\pi$cd/ft^2
1 meter – lambert = $1/\pi$cd/m^2

1 cd/m^2 (nit) = foot-lambert × 3.43
(because 1 foot-lambert = 3.43 nit)

For the luminance and illuminance units to be equated (because both can be used to measure viewbox brightness), 1 lux of illuminance may be thought of as the reflectance of a perfectly diffusing surface to 1 cd/m^2 (nit) of luminance (or 1 lux = 1 nit).

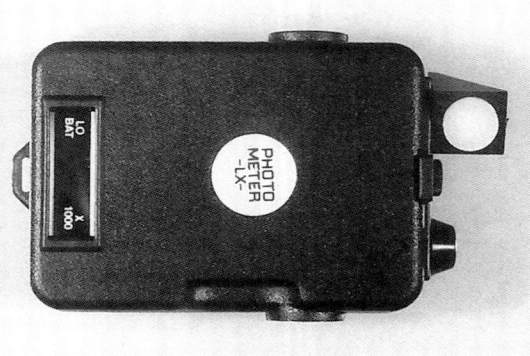

FIGURE 3-7 Photographic light meter (photometer) for viewbox evaluation. (*Courtesy Nuclear Associates, Carle Place, N.Y.*)

FIGURE 3-8 Duplicating unit for copying diagnostic images.

CHAPTER 3 Film/Screen Image Receptors, Darkrooms, and Viewing Conditions

PROCEDURE

1. Inspect the acrylic plastic (Plexiglas) front of the viewbox for discoloration, dust, and other artifacts. Clean or replace the acrylic plastic if necessary.

2. Unplug the viewbox, and remove the acrylic plastic front with the screwdriver. Inspect the fluorescent light bulb for proper wattage, cleanliness, and discoloration; clean or replace if necessary. When finished, replace the acrylic plastic front and screws.

3. Determine the brightness level. This procedure requires a basic understanding of the concepts of **photometry**, which is the study and measurement of light (see Box 3-1). To measure the brightness level of viewbox illuminators, use a photographic light meter (photometer) (see Fig. 3-7), which ideally can measure both **luminance** and illuminance. The American College of Radiology recommends measuring the luminance in **nit**. The aperture of the photometer should be nine inches away from the viewbox front when brightness is measured. This can vary slightly, depending on the manufacturer of the photometer (follow the manufacturer's instructions for your particular model). Make the first reading in the center viewbox. Conventional viewbox luminance should be at least 1500 nit, with 1700 nit being standard. Viewboxes used for viewing mammograms should have a luminance of about 3500 nit. If illuminance is used to measure brightness, the minimum illuminance should be 5000 lux or 500 **foot-candles** (ft-cd). The greater the brightness level of the viewbox, the greater the contrast observed in the viewed diagnostic image.

4. Determine viewbox uniformity. Once it has been determined that the viewbox has sufficient luminance (brightness level), then the uniformity of the brightness for each viewbox panel, each bank of viewboxes, and all viewbox banks within the entire radiology department must be determined. For an individual viewbox or a single-viewing panel (usually 14 × 17 inches) within a bank, mentally divide the viewing panel into quadrants. Hold the photometer nine inches away (or per manufacturer's instructions) from the center of each quadrant and record the luminance. Compare this value with the center reading obtained in Step 3. These readings should not deviate by more than ±10% of each other. To determine the uniformity of a single bank of viewboxes, hold a photometer nine inches away from the center of each individual viewbox within the bank, record the readings, and compare with each other. These readings should not vary by more than ±15% of each other. The uniformity of each bank of viewboxes found in the entire radiology department also should be determined. This can be accomplished by taking the average of the center readings from each bank of viewboxes in the radiology department and comparing them with each other. These values should be within ±20% of each other. If a photometer is unavailable, a photographic light meter or a 35-mm camera with a built-in light meter can be substituted (this cannot be accepted during Mammography Quality Standards Act inspections). A photometer can only measure illumination and not luminance. If the camera uses an exposure value (EV) scale to measure light intensity, set the film speed indicator to ASA 100. Place the camera lens in contact with the center of the viewbox front, look into the viewfinder, and record the reading. Repeat this procedure for each quadrant to verify viewbox uniformity. An EV of 13 indicates 500 ft-cd of illumination (the minimum acceptable value for a standard viewbox). An EV of 14 indicates twice as much light (or 1000 ft-cd), and an EV of 12 is one-half as much (250 ft-cd). If the light intensity is doubled, the maximum optical density that can be viewed is also doubled. For example, if 500 ft-cd can illuminate a maximum optical density of 2.5 on the image, then 1000 ft-cd can illuminate a maximum optical density of 2.8. Some cameras have a light meter that does not use an EV scale but instead indicates the shutter speed to use when taking the photograph and looking into the viewfinder. In this case, set the film speed indicator to ASA 64 and the shutter to f8. The denominator of the shutter speed indicated is the light intensity in foot-candles. For example, if the indicated shutter speed is 1/400 s, the light intensity is 400 ft-cd.

5. Measure the color temperature. The quality or spectrum of light that is emitted from a light source can be defined by its color temperature. This is the temperature at which a black body radiator emits light of a comparable color. A surface that absorbs all of the radiant energy that is incident on it would appear black and is called a *black body*. The color temperature is measured in degrees Kelvin (K) and expressed with a color temperature meter (available from scientific supply companies). Standard viewboxes should have color temperatures ranging from 5400 to 10,000 K. Most viewbox manufacturers prefer a rating of 6250 K.

6. Measure the ambient light conditions. The ambient light is the light level of the viewing room and the radiologist viewing area separate from the viewbox. This light must be less than that of the viewbox, or a decrease in contrast level is observed in the image. To survey this level, turn the illuminators off and place the meter or camera one foot away from the viewbox to record the reading. The maximum ambient room light should be 30 ft-cd (320 lux) or 8 EV. For mammographic viewing areas, the maximum ambient light should be 4.5 ft-cd (50 lux) or less (equivalent to a moonlit night). Ambient light can vary considerably in various areas of a hospital. Operating rooms typically have a range of 300–400 lux, emergency department rooms about 150–300 lux, and staff offices about 50–180 lux.

Most units have an exposure level switch to regulate the quality of the copy image. Film duplicators should faithfully copy optical densities of up to 2.5 from the original image. To verify this, make a copy of a sensitometer film, use a densitometer to measure each step, and compare with the original image. They should be the same or within an optical density of 0.02 and should be evaluated on a weekly basis. To check the contact between the copy film and the original during duplication, use a radiograph of a wire mesh screen (used to evaluate film/screen contact) and make a copy. The copy should demonstrate the same sharpness level of the mesh pattern throughout the image. This should be performed monthly.

Images obtained with a multiformat camera or a laser camera can be particularly difficult to duplicate because of its single emulsion. An image from a Society of Motion Picture and Television Engineers test pattern or AAPM TG 18-QC test pattern (see Chapter 9) should be produced from the camera and then duplicated with the copier. Optical density readings from the same areas of the copy and the original should be taken with a densitometer and compared. Again, they should be the same or within a value of 0.02.

FILM/SCREEN IMAGE RECEPTORS

Most of the images recorded during conventional analog radiography are obtained with film/screen combination image receptors. Thomas Edison developed intensifying screens in 1896, and Michael Pupin first used a film/screen combination in radiography that same year. The X-rays exiting the patient energize the phosphor crystals, and the result is the emission of light called **luminescence**. Luminescence can occur by one of two different processes, **fluorescence or phosphorescence**.

1. **Fluorescence** is the light of certain crystals emitted within 10^{-8} s after the crystals are exposed to radiation. This means that light is emitted promptly. This is the type of luminescence that is desired for use in intensifying screens.

2. **Phosphorescence** is the light of certain crystals emitted sometime after 10^{-8} s after the crystals' exposure to radiation, resulting in a delayed emission of light. This delayed emission of light is often called *afterglow* or *lag*. This is not desired for use in intensifying screens because the delayed emission of light fogs the film in the cassette before the radiographer can get it to the processor or daylight system. This type of luminescence is desired for the output phosphor of fluoroscopic image intensifiers and cathode-ray tube displays such as television and computer monitor screens.

The fluorescent light from the crystals in the intensifying screen is used to expose the film (rather than for X-ray interaction) and creates 95–98% of the optical density. This results in lower patient exposure (compared with a nonscreen exposure), because only a relatively small number of X-rays are necessary for the screens to emit a relatively large quantity of light. Proper application of intensifying screens is necessary to create adequate images. Because considerable variation can occur with the use of screens, proper quality control protocols should be in place. Several intensifying screen variables are discussed.

Intensifying Screen Speed

Intensifying screen speed refers to the amount of light emitted by the screen for a given amount of X-ray exposure. A screen that is designated as fast creates an increased amount of light compared with a screen designated as slow when both are exposed to identical kVp and mAs factors. Screen speed can be measured by intensification factor, relative name, or speed value.

Intensification Factor. The exposure required to create a certain optical density without a screen (direct exposure) is divided by the exposure required with a screen to create the same optical density, which determines the **intensification factor**.

$$\text{Intensification factor} = \frac{\text{Exposure without screens}}{\text{Exposure with screens}}$$

For example, if 100 mAs create an optical density of 1.0 on a direct exposure film and 5 mAs create the same optical density value with a film/screen combination, then that screen has an intensification factor of 20. The larger this value, the faster the speed of the screen.

Relative Speed Value. Relative speed is the most common method of designating screen speed and is used for all screens with rare earth phosphors. A mathematic number that is a multiple of 100 is used, with a larger number designating a faster speed. When one speed is changed to another, a change in mAs is required to maintain optical density. This can be calculated with the following equation:

$$\text{New mAs} = \frac{\text{Old mAs} \times \text{Old relative speed value}}{\text{New relative speed value}}$$

For example, if 10 mAs were used with a 100-speed screen, then 5 mAs would be used with a 200-speed screen.

Name of Screen. Older, non-rare earth screens use specific names such as *fast* or *slow* to designate screen speed. A listing of these older names, along with their relative speed values, is presented in Table 3-1.

Factors Affecting Screen Speed

Type of Phosphor Material. Many different phosphor materials have been used in screens since 1896. They are generally divided into two categories, rare earth and non-rare earth phosphors. The non-rare earth phosphors are the original type of screen material and emit light in the blue-violet portion of the color spectrum. Examples include calcium tungstate, barium strontium sulfate, and barium fluorochloride. The rare earth phosphors were developed in the early 1970s and are currently the most common type of intensifying screen material. The name *rare earth* is used because these materials possess atomic numbers ranging from 57 through 71 and are known as the *lanthanide*, or *rare earth*, series from the periodic table of elements. These materials possess a greater detective quantum efficiency (the ability to interact with X-rays) and a greater

TABLE 3-1	Older Names for Screen Speed
Name of Screen	**Relative Speed Value**
Ultra high or hi-plus	300
High or fast	200
Medium, par, or standard	100
Detail, slow, or high resolution	50
Ultra-detail	25

CHAPTER 3 Film/Screen Image Receptors, Darkrooms, and Viewing Conditions

conversion efficiency (the ability of screens to convert X-ray energy into light energy). The older calcium tungstate screens have a conversion efficiency of 4–5%, whereas the newer rare earth screens have values ranging from 15% to 25%. Thus, the rare earth phosphors are faster than the non-rare earth phosphors. Table 3-2 presents the more common rare earth phosphors and the color of light emitted.

The rare earth phosphors are mixed with materials called *activators* (the elements terbium, niobium, or thulium) that help determine the intensity and color of the emitted light.

Thickness of Phosphor Layer. A thicker layer of phosphor material causes the screen to emit more light because the extra material can absorb more X-rays. This decreases the resolution of the resulting image because of increased light diffraction or diffusion (Fig. 3-9). Rare earth screens generally demonstrate better resolution than non-rare earth screens because they have greater conversion efficiencies and therefore do not have to be placed in as thick a layer. The average range of phosphor thickness is from 150 to 300 µm.

Size of Phosphor Crystals. Using larger-sized phosphor crystals increases the speed of the screen by allowing more absorption of incident X-rays but decreases image resolution because of increased light diffusion. Crystals that are needle shaped help to minimize this effect.

Reflective Layer. When X-rays interact with the phosphor material of a screen, light is emitted isotropically (in all directions). Because the film is only on one side of the screen, light traveling away from the film is normally lost to the imaging process. Faster speed screens add a layer of titanium dioxide to reflect light back toward the film. This increases the speed but decreases the resolution because of the angle of the reflected light.

Light-Absorbing Dyes. Slower speed screens have light-absorbing dyes added to the phosphor layer to control reflected light (Fig. 3-10). This dye decreases speed but increases image resolution.

Ambient Temperature. When the ambient temperature of an intensifying screen increases significantly above room temperature (above 85 °F [30 °C]), the screen may function slower than usual. The higher temperature gives the phosphor crystal more kinetic energy. This additional energy does not cause more light to be emitted but, rather, increases the energy (and therefore the color) of the light emitted. Because the film may not be sensitive to this new color, the resulting radiograph appears underexposed.

Kilovolt (Peak) Selection. The phosphor material in a screen must interact with the X-ray photon for luminescence to occur. The greatest absorption of X-rays occurs when the X-ray photon energy and the binding energy of the K-shell electron are almost the same. This is called the *K-edge effect*. Because the kVp setting on the control panel regulates the X-ray photon energy and the phosphor material used controls the K-shell binding energy, care must be taken to match the kVp used in technique selection. For example, a dedicated mammography cassette usually has a lower K-edge value (15–20 kiloelectron volts [keV]), because lower kVp techniques are used. If one of these cassettes is used at 100 kVp instead, it functions much more slowly than if used at its proper kVp. Table 3-3 indicates the K-shell binding energies for different phosphor materials.

Quality Control Testing of Screen Speed

Quality control testing of screen speed should occur on acceptance and then yearly. First, one should evaluate whether similar cassettes marked with the same relative speed are the same using the following procedure.

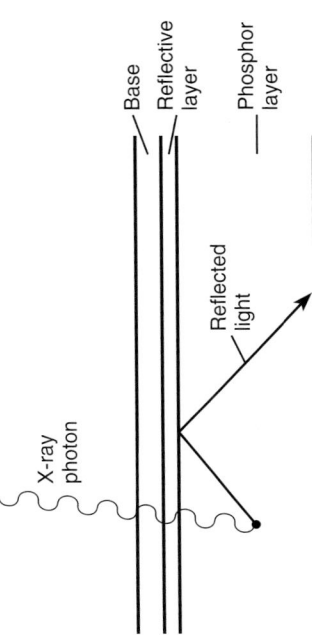

FIGURE 3-10 Reflected light within phosphor layer.

TABLE 3-2	Emission Color of Common Rare Earth Phosphors
Name of Screen	**Relative Speed Value**
Gadolinium oxysulfide	Green
Lanthanum oxysulfide	Green
Yttrium oxysulfide	Blue-green
Yttrium tantalate	Blue-green
Lanthanum oxybromide	Blue
Lutetium tantalate	Blue

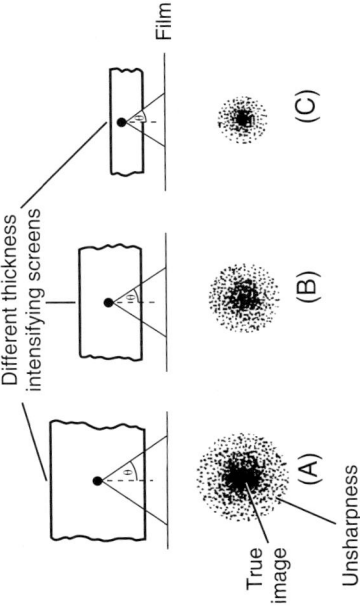

FIGURE 3-9 Effect of screen active layer on light diffusion and image sharpness.

CHAPTER 3 Film/Screen Image Receptors, Darkrooms, and Viewing Conditions

TABLE 3-3 K-Shell Binding Energies for Some Phosphor Materials

Element	Atomic number	K-Shell Binding Energy (keV)
Yttrium	39	17.5
Barium	56	37.4
Lanthanum	57	38.9
Gadolinium	64	50.2
Tungsten	74	69.5

PROCEDURE

1. Make an exposure of a step wedge or homogenous phantom onto an image receptor so the center of the image has an optical density of about 1.5.
2. Expose each image receptor to the same technical factors.
3. Process each radiograph, and take optical density readings of the same center area in each. If the image receptors are all the same relative speed, the optical density readings should not vary by more than a value of ±0.05.

Cassettes also should be evaluated to ensure that the screen speed is uniform throughout the entire surface. Intensifying screens should be uniform in speed throughout the entire surface of the screen itself. In other words, the speed in the center should be the same as the speed at the outer edges or anywhere else on the screen. During manufacturing processes, inconsistencies may occur in which the phosphor layer is applied more thickly at one portion of the screen than at another. In addition, during screen cleaning, excessive rubbing may remove more of the phosphor layer at one point than at another; therefore, a test of screen uniformity should be performed on acceptance and then yearly.

PROCEDURE

1. Make an exposure of a homogenous phantom onto an image receptor that yields an optical density of approximately 1.5.
2. Process the radiograph, and take optical density readings in the center and in each of the four quadrants of the image. These values should not vary by an optical density value of more than ±0.05. Any film/screen image receptors that exceed this limit should be removed from service.

Spectral Matching

Previously in this chapter, it is mentioned that various films are sensitive to specific colors of light and therefore require special colored safelights to illuminate the darkroom. Because intensifying screen phosphors emit blue, blue-green, or green light, the film used inside the cassette should be sensitive to the corresponding color.

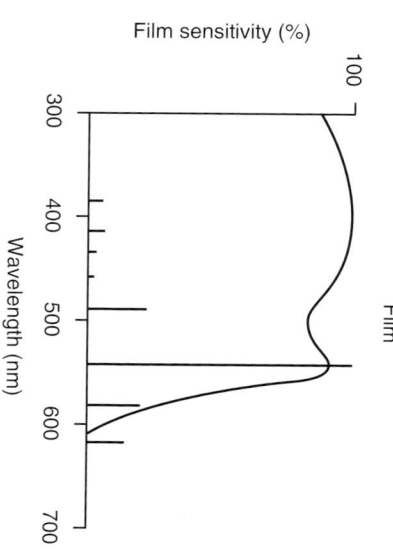

FIGURE 3-11 Broadband spectrum from non-rare earth phosphor.

This is known as **spectral matching**. Any blue-violet–emitting screen phosphor should be used with monochromatic blue-violet film, and green-emitting phosphors must be used with **orthochromatic** film. The non-rare earth screen phosphors tend to emit a broadband of light (Fig. 3-11), whereas rare earth phosphors emit specific colors of light, also known as *line emission* (Fig. 3-12).

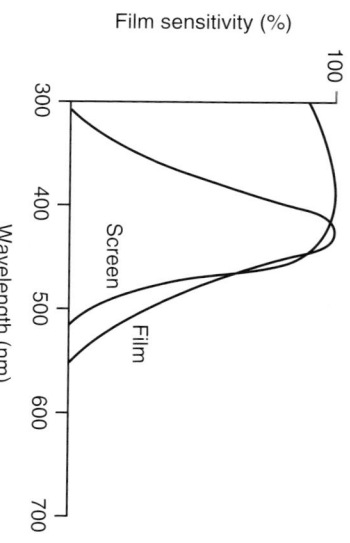

FIGURE 3-12 Line spectrum from rare earth screen phosphor.

Screen Resolution

Intensifying screens should be able to demonstrate clear images of patient anatomy so the proper diagnosis can be obtained. The ability of an imaging system to accurately display these images is known as *resolution*, of which there are two types, contrast resolution and spatial resolution.

Contrast Resolution. Contrast resolution is the ability of an imaging system to distinguish structures with similar X-ray transmission as separate entities (the term not only applies to intensifying screens but to all imaging systems including computed radiography [CR], digital radiography [DR], conventional and digital fluoroscopy, computed tomography, magnetic resonance imaging, and sonography). In other words, separate shades of gray (contrast) should appear so that one structure stands out from the other. Digital radiographic systems (both CR and DR) have superior contrast resolution to film/screen radiographic systems (discussed in Chapter 9).

Magnetic resonance imaging can demonstrate the best contrast resolution of all diagnostic imaging modalities. Contrast resolution is affected by the sensitivity of the image receptor (speed) and the amount of radiographic mottle (also called *noise*). If the radiographic mottle is increased, the contrast resolution decreases. The radiographic mottle is determined by film graininess (also called *random* or *stochastic noise*), the uniformity of the screen phosphor layer (also called *structured* or *nonstochastic noise*), and **quantum mottle** (also called *quantum noise*), which is the statistical fluctuation in the number of photons per unit area that contribute to image formation. The quantum noise that is perceived in the image is normally stated as a percentage and determined by the following equation:

$$\text{Quantum noise} = 100 \times \frac{\sigma}{N}$$

N is the mean number of photons per unit area, and σ is the standard deviation that measures the width of the distribution about that mean and is equal to the square root of N. For example, if a mean of 100 photons exposes a film, the σ is 10 and the quantum noise is 10%. If a mean of 100,000 photons exposes a film, the σ is 316 but the quantum noise is only 0.3%; therefore, as the total number of photons increases, the quantum noise perceived in the image decreases. The number of X-ray photons used to create a radiographic image is approximately $10^5/\text{mm}^2$ of image receptor. Care must be taken with very fast speed screens because lower mAs values are required. This decrease in the number of photons increases the quantum noise, which manifests as a blotchy appearance to the image and decreased contrast resolution. Contrast resolution is often measured with a value known as the **signal-to-noise ratio (SNR)**.

$$\text{SNR} = \text{Signal/Noise}$$

The signal in diagnostic imaging is the contrast, or gray scale, of the image. Because this value should be relatively large and the noise should be relatively small, a large SNR indicates high-contrast resolution. Increasing the SNR in film screen imaging can be accomplished by increasing the mAs (which can increase patient exposure and heat created in the X-ray tube), increasing the kVp (which can decrease radiographic contrast), increase phosphor layer thickness (which may degrade spatial resolution), or increase the X-ray attenuation capability of the phosphor material used in the screen. The SNR value is more commonly used when television and computerized images are described.

Contrast resolution also can be described using a value known as **contrast-to-noise ratio (CNR)**. As with the SNR, the CNR is defined as the contrast seen in the image, divided by the amount of noise existing in the image. Increasing the contrast and reducing image noise will increase the CNR and therefore improve image quality and increase the ability to detect a lesion (especially in mammographic images). Contrast can be improved by reducing the amount of scattered radiation, reducing all causes of fogging, or the use of a contrast agent. Reducing image noise can be obtained by reducing quantum mottle (accomplished by increasing the number of photons used to make the radiographic image) or by image postprocessing in digital imaging.

Digital imaging systems generally have superior contrast resolution to film/screen systems. Magnetic resonance imaging possesses the greatest contrast resolution capability of all current imaging modalities.

Spatial Resolution. **Spatial resolution** (also known as high-contrast resolution) is the ability of an imaging system to create separate images of closely spaced high-contrast (black-and-white) objects (as with contrast resolution, spatial resolution also applies to all imaging modalities). In other words, do the two objects appear sharp and clear, or do they blur together? This is determined by the amount of light diffusion that occurs between the screen and film, which is in turn affected by the screen thickness, phosphor crystal size, and film/screen contact. The most common method of measuring spatial resolution is to use a value known as *spatial frequency*. The unit of spatial frequency is the line pairs per millimeter (lp/mm) and is obtained with a resolution chart (Fig. 3-13). A line pair includes an opaque line and a radiolucent space. In the resolution chart, 1 lp/mm would have a 0.5 mm lead bar separated by 0.5 mm of radiolucent material. Two lp/mm would have 0.25 mm lead bars separated by 0.25 mm of radiolucent material and so on (see Table 3-4). The greater the lp/mm value, the smaller the object that can be imaged and the better the spatial resolution. The *limiting spatial resolution* (also known as the **Nyquist frequency**) is the maximum number of lp/mm that can be recorded by the imaging system. The resolving power of the unaided human eye

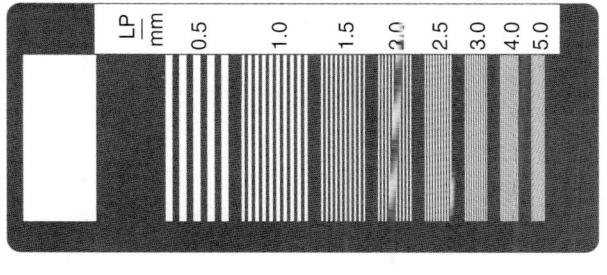

FIGURE 3-13 Line pairs per millimeter resolution chart.

CHAPTER 3 Film/Screen Image Receptors, Darkrooms, and Viewing Conditions

TABLE 3-4 Comparison of Spatial Resolution and Line Size

Spatial Resolution	Line or Space Width (mm)
1 lp/mm	0.5
2 lp/mm	0.25
3 lp/mm	0.167
4 lp/mm	0.125
5 lp/mm	0.10
6 lp/mm	0.083
7 lp/mm	0.071
8 lp/mm	0.063
9 lp/mm	0.056
10 lp/mm	0.050

is approximately 30 lp/mm when inspecting an image up close, and at normal reading distance (about 25 cm), it is about 5 lp/mm. Most film/screen systems cannot provide this level of spatial resolution. Non-screen film holders that were once used in radiography could yield up to 100 lp/mm (but at a price of extremely high radiation dose to the patient). Spatial resolution should be evaluated with a resolution chart upon acceptance and then yearly, using the following procedure:

PROCEDURE

1. Place each film/screen cassette tabletop in a radiographic room, and create an image of the resolution chart at 50 kVp, 40 inches SID, small focal spot, and mAs appropriate to create an optical density of about 1.5 in the center of the pattern.
2. Examine each image, and determine the spatial frequency. Record all readings in a log book or documentation form.
3. Compare readings to previous readings for each cassette. There should be no change from year to year. If the values did change, the screen should be replaced.

Other methods of measuring spatial resolution include point spread function (PSF), line spread function (LSF), edge spread function, and **modulation transfer function** (MTF).

Point Spread Function. Point spread function is a graph that is obtained with a pinhole camera and a microdensitometer. The pinhole camera creates a black dot in the center of a film, and a microdensitometer is used to take readings of this point. These values are plotted on a graph versus the distance from the center of the point, as shown in Fig. 3-14. The narrower the peak on the graph, the better the spatial resolution and quality of the image. The width of the peak (in millimeters) of the PSF graph can be measured to yield a numerical value to indicate spatial resolution (the smaller the number, the better the spatial resolution and vice versa). The width is usually measured at half the maximum value and is termed **full width-half maximum** (FWHM). The limiting

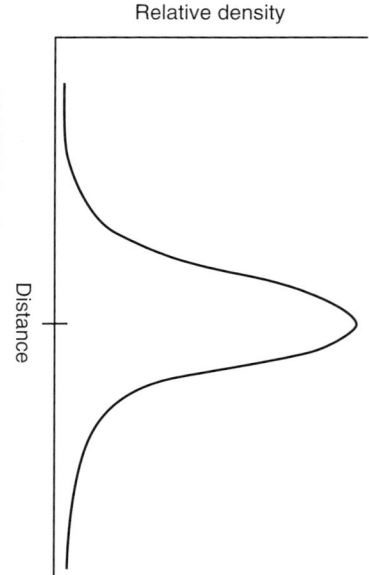

FIGURE 3-14 Point spread function graph.

spatial resolution in lp/mm may be estimated by using the following equation:

$$1/(2 \times \text{FWHM})$$

For example, if the PSF has an FWHM value of 0.1 mm, the limiting resolution would be 1/(2 × 0.1 mm) or 5 lp/mm.

Line Spread Function. Line spread function is a graph that is more accurate and easier to obtain than the PSF graph. It requires an aperture with a slit that is 10 μm wide instead of the pinhole camera. Density readings of the centerline are taken and plotted (Fig. 3-15). FWHM values also can be obtained from this graph and interpreted much the same way as discussed with point spread function.

Edge Spread Function. Edge spread function requires a sheet of lead to be placed on a cassette and exposed. Density readings are taken at the border between the black-and-white areas and plotted on a graph (Fig. 3-16).

Modulation Transfer Function. Modulation transfer function is a numeric value that is used to measure the spatial resolution and is obtained from the LSF graph with a mathematic process known as *Fourier transformation*. Just as a mathematic number (slope) can be obtained from a linear graph, Fourier transformation can obtain a number from a curve. This number ranges

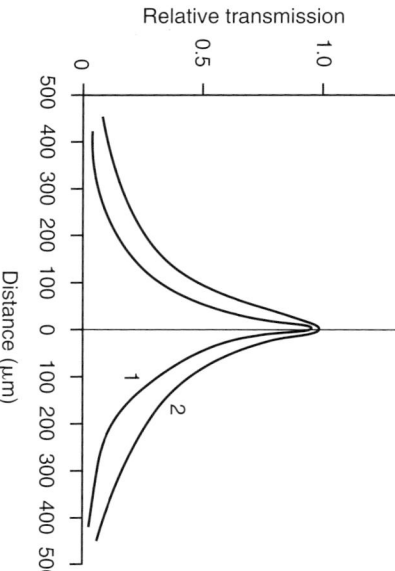

FIGURE 3-15 Line spread function graph.

CHAPTER 3 Film/Screen Image Receptors, Darkrooms, and Viewing Conditions

from 0 to 1 (0–100%), with 1 being the maximum spatial frequency. An easier way to think of MTF is demonstrated by the following equation:

$$MTF = \frac{\text{Information recorded in an image}}{\text{Information available in the part}}$$

If all of the patient information is recorded in the image, a value of 1 is obtained. For example, an MTF value of 0.5 indicates that 50% of the patient's anatomy is recorded. The total MTF of an imaging system is obtained by combining all of the component MTF values.

$$MTF_{total} = MTF_1 \times MTF_2 \times MTF_3, \text{ and so on}$$

For example, if a film can demonstrate 80% of the patient anatomy on an image (MTF = 0.8) and a screen can demonstrate 70% (MTF = 0.7), the total system MTF equals 0.8×0.7, or 0.56. A Weiner spectrum graph is sometimes used to demonstrate the relationship of MTF and spatial frequency (Fig. 3-17).

The resolution test tool (see Fig. 3-13) can be imaged with a cassette on acceptance and then yearly to evaluate any variation. One variable that can affect resolution is the film/screen contact. Because poor film/screen contact increases light diffusion, (Fig. 3-18) and therefore decreases resolution, a wire mesh test should be performed at least annually (more often with larger cassette sizes because they are more prone to develop poor contact) (Fig. 3-19).

PROCEDURE

1. Expose the wire mesh test tool that is placed on the cassette front, using exposure factors of 50 kVp and 5 mAs tabletop.
2. Process the film, and evaluate the resulting image. Areas of poor contact appear as localized blurring (see Fig. 3-19). Bent or warped cassettes, warped screens, and foreign objects inside the cassette are the most common causes of poor film/screen contact.

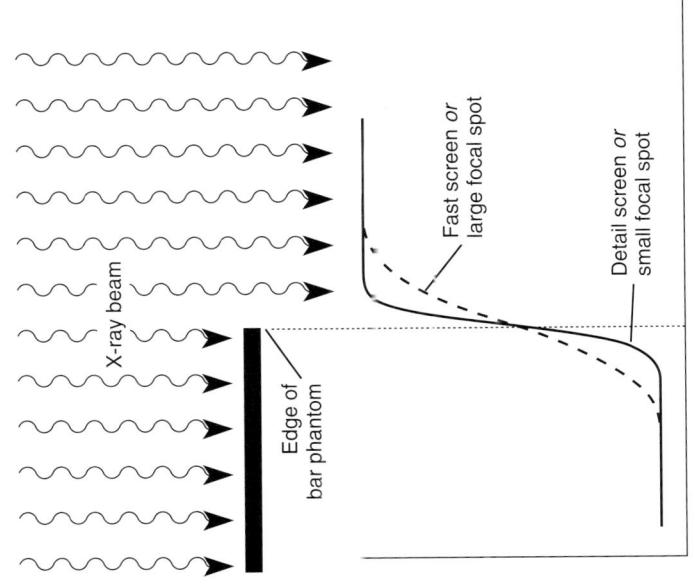

FIGURE 3-16 Edge spread function graph.

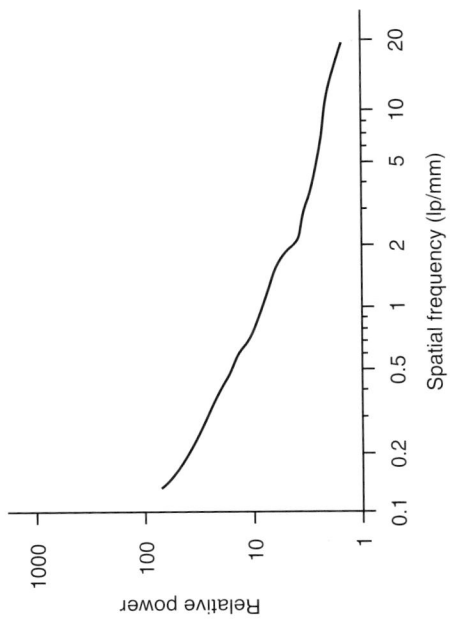

FIGURE 3-17 Weiner spectrum indicating the modulation transfer function.

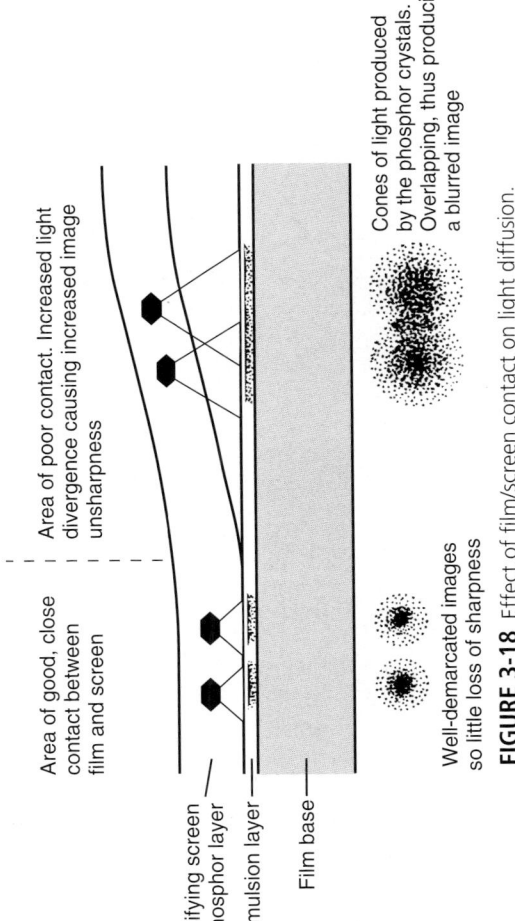

FIGURE 3-18 Effect of film/screen contact on light diffusion.

Screen Condition

Cassettes containing intensifying screens must function as designed in order to create optimum radiographic images. Errors to avoid include improper film position within the cassette, poor film/screen contact, and uneven closure of the cassette. Intensifying screens also must be free of dirt, stains, and defects to properly image anatomic structures. A regular schedule (at least every 6 months) of screen cleaning with an antistatic solution should be standard department policy because artifacts can mimic certain pathologic conditions. The end of the day is usually the best time to clean cassettes because of decreased demand for their use. An ultraviolet (UV) lamp can be used in the darkroom to examine the surface condition of the screens (Fig. 3-20). Be sure to remove the film from the cassette before turning on the UV lamp. The following is an accepted procedure for cleaning intensifying screens.

PROCEDURE

1. Choose a clean location to clean screens and cassettes. Wipe the outside of cassettes, and clean the countertop before cleaning screens.
2. Moisten a lint-free wipe with a small amount of commercially available screen cleaner and antistatic solution. A mild soap and water solution or a 70% solution of isopropyl alcohol may be used as an alternative (check with your screen manufacturer to see if this is acceptable), but a screen cleaner and antistatic solution must be used afterward.
3. Clean and dry the screen. Be sure to avoid excessive pressure or rubbing on the screen surface.
4. Use a second lint-free wipe to clean the frame and inside cover (for single-screen cassettes).
5. Stand the cassettes on edge to dry.
6. Once the screen and cassette cover are dry, inspect them for any particles of dust. Use a UV light if necessary. If they are clean, reload with fresh film. For mammography cassettes, the screen surface should be carefully brushed with an antistatic brush and then inspected before loading with fresh film. This is discussed more completely in Chapter 11.

FIGURE 3-19 Wire mesh image.

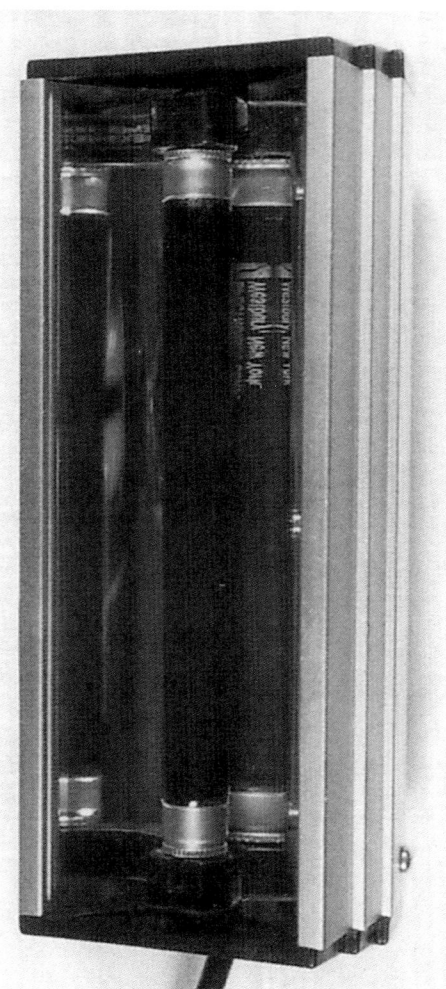

FIGURE 3-20 Ultraviolet lamp for inspecting intensifying screens. (Courtesy Nuclear Associates, Carle Place, N.Y.)

SUMMARY

Maintaining proper darkroom conditions and procedures is essential to achieving the desired film-based radiographic image. These images also must be displayed with the use of proper viewing conditions for optimum diagnostic capability. Quality control procedures must also be performed for film/screen image receptors and film-based image duplicator units. All radiographers also should have knowledge of image receptor factors such as spatial resolution, contrast resolution, signal-to-noise ratio, etc., as these factors are also important in discussing image quality with digital image receptors.

CHAPTER 3 Film/Screen Image Receptors, Darkrooms, and Viewing Conditions

Refer to the Evolve website at https://evolve.elsevier.com for Student Experiments 3.1: Darkroom Fog Check and Viewbox Illuminations and 3.2: Measurement of Spatial Frequency.

REVIEW QUESTIONS

1. Which of the following is the main reason to prohibit food and drink in a film darkroom?
   a. Avoid contamination of processor solutions
   b. Prevent artifacts
   c. Prevent pressure marks on the film
   d. Prevent static artifacts

2. Which of the following terms best describes the amount of light that is emitted from or scattered by a surface?
   a. Photometry
   b. Luminance
   c. Illuminance
   d. Optical density

3. Which of the following names a device that can be used to measure darkroom humidity levels?
   a. Sensitometer
   b. Densitometer
   c. Hydrometer
   d. Psychrometer

4. Proper darkroom ventilation should include _____ room changes of air per hour.
   a. 3 to 5
   b. 6 to 8
   c. 8 to 10
   d. 10 to 12

5. Which of the following terms refers to the amount of light emitted by a screen for a given amount of X-ray exposure?
   a. Speed
   b. Sensitivity
   c. Lag
   d. Resolution

6. Which of the following terms best describes the ability of a screen material to convert X-ray energy into light energy?
   a. Screen speed
   b. Quantum detection efficiency (QDE)
   c. Conversion efficiency
   d. Resolution

7. Why should boxes of film and containers of developer solution not be stored near each other?
   a. Developer contains naturally occurring radioactive material.
   b. Pressure marks can occur on the film.
   c. Static electricity is more common.
   d. None of the above is correct.

8. Photometric readings from each quadrant of a single viewbox panel should not vary by more than ± _____ %.
   a. 2
   b. 5
   c. 10
   d. 20

9. Which of the following terms is the unit most commonly used to measure luminance?
   a. Lux
   b. Nit
   c. Foot-candle
   d. Lumen

10. Which of the following terms best describes the ability of an imaging system to create separate images of closely spaced high-contrast objects?
    a. Screen speed
    b. Spatial resolution
    c. Contrast resolution
    d. Quantum mottle

CHAPTER 4
Film Processing

KEY TERMS

Agitation
Archival quality
Developer
Fixer
Flood replenishment
Hyporetention
Latent image
Manifest image
Oxidation/reduction reaction
Synergism
Volume replenishment

OBJECTIVES

At the completion of this chapter, the reader should be able to do the following:

- Describe the main differences between manual and automatic film processing
- List the main components of the developer and fixer solutions, and state the function of each component
- Explain the proper mixing procedure for developer and fixer concentrate solutions
- State the chemical safety procedures for the safe handling of processing chemicals as described by the Occupational Safety and Health Administration (OSHA)
- Describe the basic tests for determining the archival quality of processed images
- List the six main systems of automatic film processors and state the function of each system
- Describe the methods of installing film processors in a darkroom

OUTLINE

Manual and Automatic Film Processing
Manual Processing
Automatic Processing
Processing Chemicals
Developer
   Developer Components
   Developer Activity
   Developer Mixing Procedure
Fixer
   Fixer Ingredients
   Fixer Mixing Procedure
Washing
Chemical Safety

Automatic Processor Main Systems
Transport System
   Roller Subsystem
   Transport Rack Subsystem
   Drive Subsystem
Temperature Control System
   Water-Controlled System
   Thermostatically Controlled System
Circulation System
Replenishment System
   Volume Replenishment
   Flood Replenishment
Drying System
Electrical System
Types of Automatic Processors
Processor Size
   Floor-Size Processor
   Intermediate-Size Processor
   Tabletop-Size Processor
Processor Location
   Totally Inside
   Bulk Inside
   Bulk Outside
   Totally Outside

Summary

After a film has been exposed to radiation, the image it contains is still invisible to the human eye and is called a **latent image**. For the film to be processed by various solutions that change the latent image to a visible one, and also preserves or **manifest image**, the silver contained in the film must be changed from an ionized state (Ag^+) to a neutral, or reduced, state ($Ag^°$), in which the silver turns black. This conversion requires the film to be processed by various solutions that change the latent image to a visible one, and also preserves the image for permanent storage. The two basic methods of film processing are manual and automatic.

MANUAL AND AUTOMATIC FILM PROCESSING

Manual Processing

During the manual processing method, film is moved manually from one solution to the next until processing is complete. This method requires more labor and time, and is more prone to variations than automatic processing. For this reason, manual processing is seldom done in diagnostic imaging today. For film to be processed manually, several steps are required after the films are hung on special hangers.

1. *Wetting agent.* The wetting agent is a chemical that loosens the emulsion so subsequent solutions can reach all parts of the emulsion uniformly, which reduces development time. This step is optional because developer ingredients also soften the emulsion. If a wetting agent is used, the film should remain in the solution for about 15 seconds.

2. *Developer.* The developer solution converts the latent image to the visible image; therefore, this is the most important processing chemical. The film remains in the developer for 3 to 5 minutes, depending on the temperature of the solution.

3. *Stop bath or water rinse.* The stop bath or water rinse step stops the development process and removes excess developer from the film. A stop bath is a 1% solution of acetic acid that neutralizes the developer chemically (because it is an alkaline solution) and requires only 5 to 10 seconds of film immersion time. A water rinse relies on water to remove the excess developer and requires about 30 seconds of film immersion.

4. *Fixer.* The fixer solution removes the unexposed and undeveloped silver halide crystals from the film emulsion, and also hardens the emulsion so the film can be stored permanently. The time of fixation varies with solution temperature, but the general rule for manual fixation is use of the following equation:

Fixing time = Cleaning time + Hardening time

The clearing time is the time necessary for the fixer to clear away the unexposed and undeveloped silver halide crystals, which should be accomplished within 5 minutes. The hardening time is the time it takes the emulsion to harden properly and is usually equal to the clearing time. Therefore, a film that requires 5 minutes to clear requires another 5 minutes to harden, resulting in a total fixing time of 10 minutes.

5. *Washing.* Excess fixer must be removed from film before it is allowed to dry or the fixer components crystallize on the film surface, a process known as **hyporetention**. This white, powdery residue can impair the diagnostic quality of the final image and must be avoided. An example of an image with hyporetention is shown in Chapter 10. This step may take as long as 20 minutes.

6. *Drying.* Drying prepares the film for viewing and storage, and it is accomplished either by using an electric dryer, which works in less than a minute, or by exposing the film to room air while the film is mounted on a special hanger. The air exposure method may require an hour or more to complete.

Automatic Processing

Automatic processing requires an electromechanical device called an *automatic film processor*. This processor transports the film from one solution to the next without any manual labor except for placing the film into the device. Automatic processing shortens the overall processing time, increases the number of films that can be processed during a given period, and ensures less variability of overall film quality than manually processed films because processing time, solution temperature, and chemical replenishment are controlled automatically. The disadvantages of automatic processing include greater capital and maintenance costs, increased chemical fog resulting from greater processing temperatures, and transport problems that can damage or destroy images during processing. In a diagnostic imaging department that has not converted to digital imaging, the advantages of automatic processing versus manual processing far outweigh the disadvantages, and automatic film processing is virtually exclusive.

PROCESSING CHEMICALS

Developer

As mentioned previously, the **developer** is the most important processing solution; it converts the latent image to a manifest image. This process is accomplished by the developer solution, which carries out an **oxidation/reduction reaction**, or *redox*. When a chemical is oxidized (broken down), it releases electrons. These electrons are then available to convert another compound into a more simplified, or reduced, state (hence the term *oxidation/reduction reaction*). During film processing, the developer solution ingredients are oxidized and the silver halide crystals are reduced to black metallic silver. This chemical reaction can be summarized by the following equations that occur at different times during oxidation reduction.

The first occurs during exposure to radiation:

$$Ag^+ + Br^- + \text{radiation} \rightarrow Ag^\circ + Br^- + Ag^\circ$$
$$\text{(five atoms, latent image)}$$

The second occurs during immersion in developer:

$$Ag^+ + \text{developer} + Ag^\circ \text{ (five atoms, latent image)} \rightarrow$$
$$Ag^\circ \text{ } (10^8 \text{ atoms, visible image}) + \text{oxidized developer}$$

Developer Components. Developer is composed of developing or reducing agents, preservatives, accelerators or activators, restrainers, regulators, antifoggants or

54   CHAPTER 4 Film Processing

starters, hardeners, solvents, and sequestering agents. All these components act on the film.

Developing or Reducing Agents.
Developing or reducing agents carry out the oxidation/reduction reaction that converts the latent image to a manifest image. Two different reducing agents are used in standard developer solutions: phenidone and hydroquinone.

Phenidone. Phenidone (Elon or Metol in manual developing) is fast acting and produces image optical densities of as much as 1.2. It is responsible for the minimum diameter (D_{min}) and speed indicators used during sensitometric testing (described in Chapter 5).

Hydroquinone. Because hydroquinone acts more slowly than phenidone, the developmental process is completed so image optical densities greater than 1.2 are visualized. Hydroquinone is responsible for the maximum diameter (D_{max}) and for contrast indicators used in sensitometric testing. These indicators are the first variables to show an indication of developer failure, because hydroquinone is the processing chemical most sensitive to changes in temperature, concentration, pH, and exposure to light and heavy metals. Hydroquinone levels should be maintained in the range 20 to 25 g/L.

The overall optical density is created by the synergistic action of the two reducing agents. *Synergism* means the action of the two agents working together is greater than the sum of each agent working independently. **Synergism** is also known as *superadditivity* (Fig. 4-1).

Preservative. The preservative, or antioxidant, protects the hydroquinone from both aerial oxidation (chemical reaction with air) and internal oxidation (chemical reaction with other developer ingredients). If the hydroquinone is oxidized, there is a decrease in the D_{max} and contrast indicators during a sensitometric test, along with a loss of the shoulder on the H and D curve. Oxidized developer causes the developer solution to turn from a clear, brown liquid to one that is dark and muddy. If strongly oxidized, the solution also has the odor of ammonia, because this is a by-product of the oxidation chemical reaction. Most developer replenishment tanks have a floating lid inside the tank in addition to the main lid on the outside to minimize contact with the outside air. The chemicals sodium sulfite, potassium sulfite, and cycon can be used as developer solution preservatives.

Accelerator, Activator, or Buffering Agent.
The accelerator, activator, or buffering agent has two functions: to soften and swell the emulsion so reducing agents can work on all the emulsion, and to provide an alkaline medium for the reducing agents. The developing agents must exist in an alkaline medium to have the free electrons available to reduce the silver to $Ag^°$.

An indicator known as *potential hydrogen*, or *pH*, is used to measure the alkalinity of a solution, and it refers to the exponential (p) value of hydrogen ions (H^+) available for a reaction. Those chemicals with high hydrogen potential (H^+) are called *acids*; those with a high alkaline or hydroxide potential (OH^-)—and, therefore, a low hydrogen potential—are called *bases*. The pH scale ranges from 0 to 7 (acids) and from 7 to 14 (bases) (Fig. 4-2). This scale is based on the concentration of positively charged hydrogen ions (H^+), measured in moles per liter. For example, a pH of 4 means a particular solution contains one-ten thousandth (10^{-4}) of a mole of hydrogen ions per liter. For this value to be converted to pH, the negative exponent (−4) is changed to a positive number (4). A solution with an H^+ concentration of one-ten millionth (10^{-7}) moles per liter has a pH of 7, and so on. Because the pH scale is logarithmic in nature, a change of one whole number on the pH scale can represent a 10-fold change from the previous concentration. A pH of 1 denotes 10 times more H^+ ions than a pH of 2; a pH of 3 has 10 times fewer H^+ ions than a pH of 2, and so on. Pure water is neutral and has a pH of 7. Fixer is an acidic solution; therefore, care must be taken

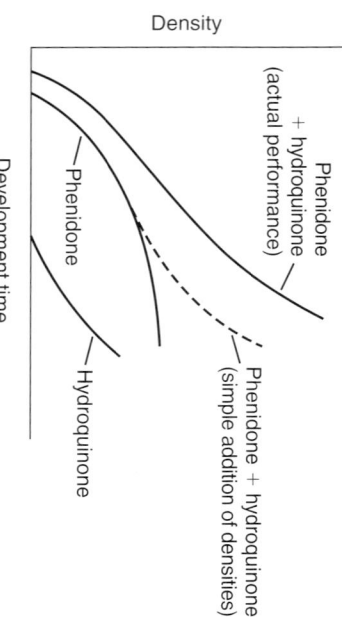

FIGURE 4-1 Graph demonstrating the superadditivity effect of phenidone and hydroquinone.

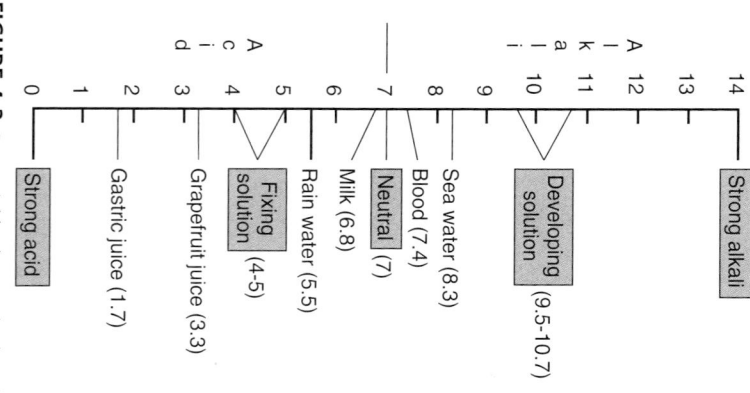

FIGURE 4-2 Potential hydrogen (pH) scale.

not to add it to developer solutions, because only 0.1% contamination deteriorates the developer activity enough to compromise image quality. Chemicals that can be used as accelerators include sodium carbonate, sodium hydroxide, potassium carbonate, and potassium hydroxide.

Restrainer, Regulator, Antifoggant, or Starter. The restrainer (regulator, antifoggant, or starter) holds back or restrains, the action of the developing agents so they reduce only the silver halide crystals exposed to radiation. The chemical used in most brands of developer is potassium bromide in the form of K^+ Br^-, which is similar chemically to Ag^+ Br^-. If the reducing agents become too active, they attack the potassium bromide instead of the silver halide. Potassium iodide can also be used as the restrainer. Overdiluting or underreplenishing can reduce the levels of restrainer and increase the speed indicator during a sensitometric test.

Hardener. When a film enters the warm developer solution, the gelatin emulsion begins to soften and swell, which causes the film to stick to the rollers of an automatic film processor. Therefore, developer manufacturers add a weak hardener (a stronger one is present in fixer solutions) to control emulsion swelling and stickiness. If the amount of hardener is depleted because of underreplenishment, wet films, transport problems, and films that have not been cleared of undeveloped silver halide may result. The chemical agent used as a hardener is glutaraldehyde.

Solvent. The previously mentioned ingredients are mixed with a solvent to form developer solution. The most common and readily available solvent is water. The water should be drinkable and have the following characteristics: filtration to particles less than 40 µm, dissolved solids less than 250 parts per million (ppm), a pH of 6.5 to 8.5, a hardness of 40 to 150 ppm, heavy metals less than 0.1 ppm, chloride less than 25 ppm, and sulfate less than 200 ppm.

Sequestering Agent. Much of the developer used in hospital darkrooms is shipped in concentrated form and then mixed with tap water at the clinical site. Because impurities (e.g., calcium ions, metals such as iron and copper) can be found in tap water, many manufacturers add a sequestering agent called *ethylenediamine tetraacetic acid* (*EDTA*) or *edetate* to prevent impurities from interfering with the developer chemicals. EDTA is an oily substance that causes calcium and other mineral contaminants to stick together and dissipate to the bottom of the processing tanks. EDTA also helps form stable chemical complexes with metallic ions.

Developer Activity. How well a developer functions is called *developer activity*, and it is governed by the following five factors: solution temperature, immersion time, solution concentration, type of chemicals used, and solution pH.

Solution Temperature. The greater the solution temperature (Fig. 4-3), the more active the developing agents become, especially hydroquinone. A warmer solution temperature will increase the optical density of the resulting image and vice versa. If the temperature decreases to less than 60 °F (15.5 °C), the hydroquinone stops working, which causes the resulting images to decrease in optical density and contrast. At temperatures greater than 75 °F (24 °C), the developing agents become increasingly active, which increases the optical density of subsequent images. The optimum temperature range for developer solution is 68 to 72 °F (20 to 22.2 °C). However, automatic processing solutions may range from 85 to 105 °F (29.4 to 40.5 °C) to process images more rapidly.

Immersion Time. The greater the length of time in the solution, or immersion time (Fig. 4-4), the greater the optical densities recorded on the processed image and vice versa. The reason for this is the developing agents are in contact with the silver ions for a longer period and can reduce more silver ions to metallic silver.

Solution Concentration. Solution concentration refers to the percentage of water versus other chemicals in the solution and is measured by specific gravity (the density of a liquid compared with water). An instrument called a *hydrometer* measures specific gravity, which ranges from 1.07 to 1.10 in typical developer solutions. The specific gravity should not vary by 14 ± 0.004 from the manufacturer's specifications. This is discussed in more detail in Chapter 5.

Type of Chemicals Used. Developer solutions that contain elon or metol behave differently from those that contain phenidone. The DuPont Cronex HSD system uses an acid developer solution to process the film, and therefore it behaves quite differently from conventional developer solutions.

Solution pH. The developer solution should maintain a pH between 10 and 11.5 and should not vary by more than ±0.1 from the manufacturer's specifications. Excessive pH increases the optical density of a processed image or causes increased oxidation, whereas a pH value that is too low decreases the optical density of any resulting image.

Over time, the developer becomes exhausted and requires replenishment. Reasons for this replenishment include the following:

- Significant quantities of developer are consumed during the development process.
- The liberating of bromide and hydrogen bromide acid into the developer during development can lower the pH and cause a decrease in activity. These bromide levels should be maintained in the range 4–8 g/L to maintain proper pH.
- Aerial and internal oxidation begins as soon as the solution is mixed and developing agents are consumed.
- A certain volume of developer solution is removed by the film's emulsion each time a film is fed into the processor. The squeegee action of the crossover rack helps minimize this effect.

Developer Mixing Procedure.
Developer solution is usually available in two forms: as a premix or as a concentrate.

Premix or Ready-Mix. As the name implies, a premix or ready-mix solution has all the ingredients combined with the solvent so no mixing is required at the clinical site. The solutions are usually delivered in 5- or 10-gallon containers and are poured directly into the replenishment tanks. The disadvantages of this method include a relatively short shelf life (from 2 weeks to 3 months) and greater cost (about 40% more than the concentrate). Therefore, large quantities should not be stockpiled, and frequent deliveries must be made.

Concentrate. The main ingredients of the solution may also be shipped to the clinical site in a concentrated form and are mixed with water at the clinical site. This form is less convenient, but the cost is reduced significantly. The concentrate kit usually comes in three parts. Part 1 contains the hydroquinone, preservative, and accelerator and has a pH between 11 and 12. Part 2 contains the phenidone and restrainer and has a pH of 3. Part 3 contains the hardener and has a pH of 3.

When solution from the concentrate is mixed, the proper amount of water should be present in the tank, and then each solution is added in the proper order. Large quantities of chemicals should be mixed electrically with a commercially available system. These systems use a propeller type of variable-speed mixer. The speed must be regulated, because excessive speed introduces unwanted air into the chemicals, which can oxidize the developer. These systems are not practical for facilities that use only a small volume of developer each week. Fresh chemistry should last 2 weeks and then be discarded. Concentrate lasts 1 year when stored at room temperature and away from direct sunlight. Excessive agitation (shaking of the bottles) during mixture and storage should be avoided, because this may cause a decomposition of the chemicals, resulting in reduced activity of the solution.

Fixer
Fixer solutions remove all the unexposed and undeveloped silver halide crystals from the film. Thus, the image is cleared. They are also responsible for halting

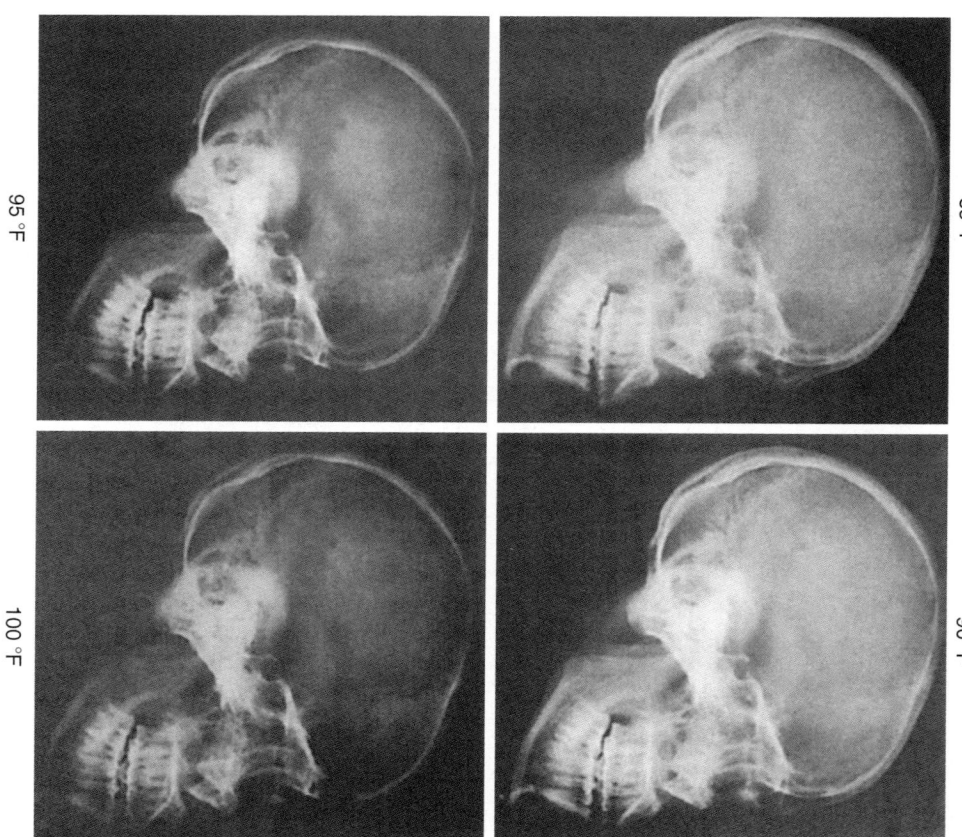

FIGURE 4-3 Radiographs showing the effect of solution temperature on optical density and contrast.

CHAPTER 4 Film Processing

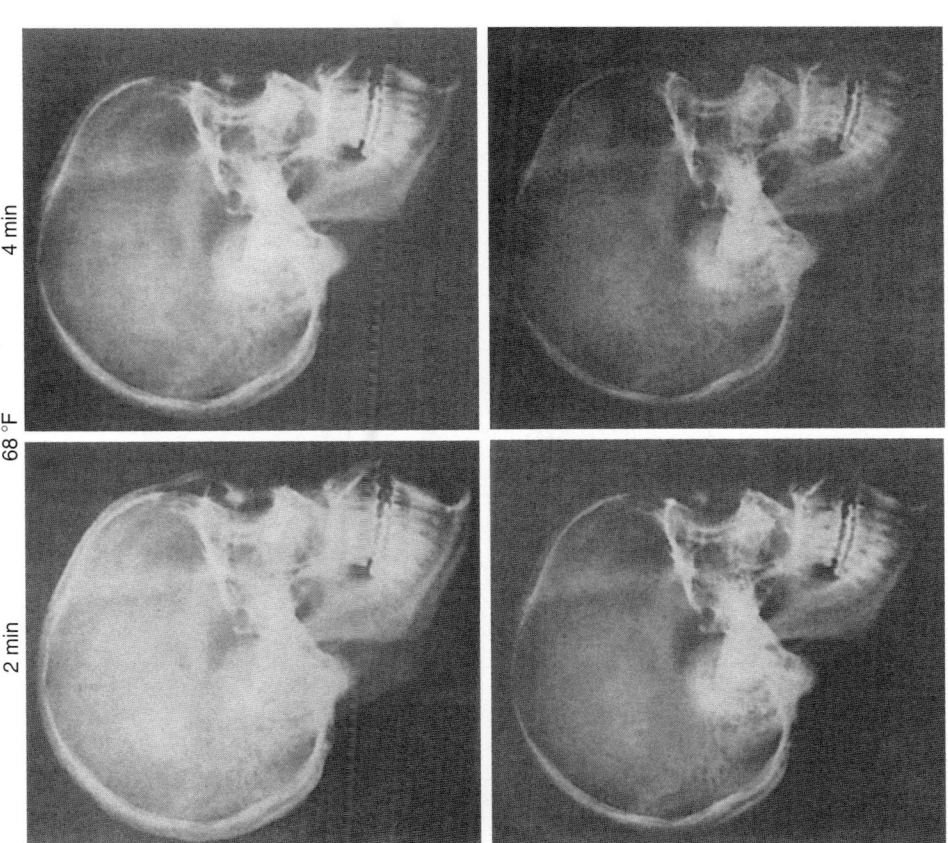

FIGURE 4-4 Radiographs showing the effect of developer time on optical density and contrast.

the development process and hardening the emulsion for permanent storage.

Fixer Ingredients. Fixers are composed of the following six components: fixing agent, preservative, hardener or tanning agent, acidifier, sequestering agent, and solvent.

Fixing Agent, Clearing Agent, or Hypo. The fixing agent (clearing agent or hypo) removes the unexposed and undeveloped silver halide crystals from the film. The chemical ammonium thiosulfate is used in most modern fixing solutions (sodium thiosulfate has been used in manual solutions). *Hypo* is a common name for thiosulfate compounds. It picks up unexposed silver atoms from the silver halide crystal to form ammonium thio-silver-sulfate. The fixing process is summarized by the following equation:

$$2AgX + Na_2S_2O_3 \rightarrow Ag_2S_2O_3 + 2NaX$$

where X designates the halide used in the film emulsion (either bromide or iodide).

The action of this agent is controlled by dilution, replenishment, and the use of a recirculating electrolytic silver recovery unit (discussed in Chapter 6).

The effectiveness of the fixing agent is evaluated by a clearing time test.

PROCEDURE

1. Take a strip of undeveloped green film and dip it into the fixer solution. Use a stopwatch to measure the clearing time.
2. Film should clear in 10 seconds at room temperature and in less than 7 seconds at 90 °F (32 °C). If it does not, the fixing agents are not working properly and the problem may be the result of improper mixing (usually too much water), a pH that is too high, or expired solution. To correct this problem, dispose of the fixer, clean out the replenishment tank, and refill it with fresh solution. It is recommended that the clearing time test be performed again on the new solution to be sure it is functioning according to accepted levels.

Preservative. The chemical sodium sulfite dissolves the silver out of the ammonium thio-silver-sulfate, and it is returned or recycled back to ammonium thiosulfate. In this way, sulfite is available to clear more of the undeveloped silver from the film. It can be depleted by excess developer carry-in, underreplenishment, and the use of recirculating electrolytic silver recovery units, which deplete sodium sulfite. The concentration of this chemical should be maintained in a range 15 to 50 g/L.

CHAPTER 4 Film Processing

Hardener or Tanning Agent. For the film to be stored permanently, the emulsion must be hardened to keep the image from fading or being scratched during handling. This process is called *tanning*. Potassium alum, chrome alum, and aluminum chloride are the more common chemicals used as fixer hardeners. When these materials combine with the gelatin proteins to form complex molecules, "hardened" emulsion results. These agents also help reduce water absorption during washing, and drying time is reduced.

Acidifier, Activator, or Buffer. The acidifier, activator, or buffer has two functions: neutralizing any developer remaining in the emulsion and providing an acid medium for the fixing agent. Just as the developing agents need an alkaline medium in which to function, the fixing agent can dissolve undeveloped silver only in an acidic solution. The acid allows the fixing agent to diffuse into the emulsion, which allows the necessary contact with the undeveloped silver ions to be made. Fixer pH should be maintained at a level between 4 and 4.5 and should not vary more than ±0.1 from the manufacturer's specifications. Chemicals that help maintain pH are commonly known as *buffers*. Both acetic acid and sulfuric acid can be used as the acidifier.

Sequestering Agent. Sequestering agents help prevent the development of aluminum hydroxide, which forms as the developer solution is carried into the fixer. Because aluminum hydroxide is an alkaline compound, its formation results in an increase in fixer pH. Carboxylic acids, boric acids, or borate salts may be used as sequestering agents in fixer solutions.

Solvent. Water is used as the solvent in which to suspend the other chemicals. The same standards listed for the developer solvent—water—also apply to the fixer. The concentration of fixer is measured by specific gravity and may range from 1.077 to 1.11. The specific gravity should not vary by more than ±0.004 from the manufacturer's specifications.

Fixer Mixing Procedure. The fixer solution may be purchased in either ready-mixed or concentrated form. The ready-mix may cost as much as 20% more but has the same convenience as ready-mixed developer. The concentrate must be mixed with water and usually comes in two parts. Part 1 contains the ammonium thiosulfate, preservative, and acidifier; part 2 contains the hardener in a strong acidic solution.

As with developer, one starts with water in the tank and mixes large quantities with a commercial mixing unit. It is recommended the fixer be mixed before the developer because inadvertent splashing of fixer could contaminate the developer.

Washing

Washing is important for the **archival quality** of the film because it removes the fixer from the film emulsion before drying. If hyporetention is allowed to take place, the reaction of the thiosulfate with the silver in the emulsion produces Ag$_2$S, or silver sulfide, which can stain the image from pale yellow to dark brown. By law, films must be archived 5 years; groups such as the military require an archival time of 40 years after death, separation, or retirement. Commercial test kits are available to measure the amount of hyporetention (Fig. 4-5). One type of test kit involves the use of a specialized test strip that is placed in contact with a processed film after a drop of solution is applied to its surface, and the test strip changes color. An accompanying color guide then allows the matching of the color on the strip to the appropriate value on the guide, which then indicates the amount of hyporetention.

Another type of hyporetention test kit involves placing a drop of hypo test solution on a film and then judging the color of the resulting stain. The hypo test solution is a mixture of silver nitrate, acetic acid, and water, and it must remain in a dark container because it is light sensitive. When a drop of this solution is applied to a processed film, it causes a chemical reaction with any fixer that still remains. The result is a brown stain. The more fixer that remains on the film, the darker this stain becomes. A test strip containing different-color stains is supplied with the solution test kit and is then used to indicate the exact level of hyporetention. The solution is applied to a processed film in the darkroom and is allowed to stand for 2 minutes. After 2 minutes, the excess solution is blotted (not wiped) and the film is taken to the lightroom area for comparison with the test strip. The American National Standards Institute (ANSI) suggests the amount of hyporetention not exceed 2 µg/cm^2 for radiographic film images and 5 µg/cm^2 for mammographic film images. These ANSI tests should

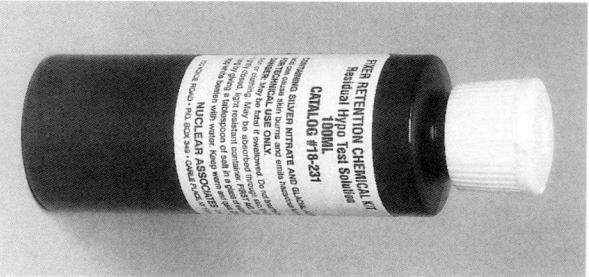

FIGURE 4-5 Hyporetention kit for evaluating residual fixer in processed films. (*Courtesy Nuclear Associates, Carle Place, N.Y.*)

be performed at least semiannually (every 6 months) for radiographic images (preferably every 3 months) and must be performed quarterly (every 3 months) for mammographic images. If the level of hyporetention exceeds these values, determine whether the wash tank has the correct amount of water present (there should be a level mark on the side of the tank). If amount of water is sufficient, then check the water flow rate to ensure it is set to the processor manufacturer's standard.

The water used in washing should have the following characteristics: hardness of 40 to 150 ppm, pH of 6.5 to 8.5, dissolved solids less than 250 ppm, and a specific gravity of 1. Washing time should be at least 50% to 100% of the developer time, and the temperature should be about 5 °F (3 °C) less than the developer temperature to help trigger the heater thermostat in the automatic processor. The water flow rate should be at a rate of 1 to 3 gal/min for removal of hyporetention, proper agitation, and prevention of algae and bioslime. If this is a problem, a few milliliters of laundry bleach (5% sodium hypochlorite) may be added to the wash tank at shutdown.

Chemical Safety

Because OSHA considers the darkroom a scientific laboratory, it has several safety requirements in place, including the implementation of hazard communication standards and the use of personal protective equipment (PPE).

- Hazard communication standards were established by OSHA to ensure that both employers and employees have knowledge of all workplace chemical hazards, in addition to the appropriate protection procedures from these hazards. One important tool to help diagnostic imaging departments comply with these standards is the Material Safety Data Sheet (MSDS), which should be displayed for all chemical compounds (i.e., processing solutions) used by employees (Fig. 4-6). These forms must be kept on file for each hazardous chemical compound and must be readily accessible to all employees. They also must contain the potentially toxic chemical agents to which a worker may be exposed, the chemical and physical characteristics, precautionary and control measures for the chemical, primary routes of chemical entry, and limits of exposure to the chemical. They also should contain basic warnings concerning the product, such as any possible health effects from exposure and any emergency treatment information. The MSDS also must contain the preparation date of the chemical, and the name and address of the manufacturer. Each MSDS uses a rating scale to indicate the hazard level of various chemicals. A level 1 rating indicates a slight hazard, level 2 is a moderate hazard, level 3 is a serious hazard, and level 4 is a severe hazard. The MSDS also must indicate the category of chemical hazard. OSHA categorizes hazardous chemicals as being either a physical hazard or a health hazard. Chemicals that are a physical hazard are those that can cause either a physical injury or a burn. Examples include compressed gases (such as oxygen), oxidizers (such as chlorine bleach), combustible liquids (such as gasoline or kerosene), and flammable materials (such as cleaning solvents). Chemicals that can cause acute or chronic health effects such as irritants, corrosives, sensitizers, and carcinogens are categorized as health hazards. Processing solutions are considered health hazards. An MSDS should be included with each shipment of processing solution. If not, one can be obtained by contacting the manufacturer. OSHA's hazard communication standards also include information on hazard evaluation, the proper labeling of containers, the maintaining of lists of chemicals used by the facility, and employee training, which were discussed in Chapter 1.

- OSHA developed PPE standards to ensure that employees have proper protection from workplace hazards. These standards include selecting the appropriate PPE, training employees in the proper use of the PPE, maintaining the PPE in a safe and sanitary condition, and replacing the PPE when it becomes damaged or defective. Safety equipment such as eye protection (preferably full-face or nonvented goggles) must be available to personnel who handle, mix, transport, or use processing chemicals. The equipment must meet or exceed the requirements of ANSI Standard Z87.1-1989, "American National Standard Practice for Occupational and Educational Eye and Face Protection." In case of failure or nonuse of the PPE, an eyewash station should be located prominently in the area where chemicals are in use. Should any amount of processing solution come in contact with the eye, the employee should wash the eye copiously and contact a physician immediately. For protection of the rest of the body, chemically resistant aprons composed of neoprene (chemically resistant) or similar material should be provided. In addition, shower facilities should be available to remove any chemical that has come in contact with the skin. For hand protection, gloves made of neoprene or a similar material should be available for employees who handle processing solutions. OSHA's PPE standards require gloves whenever employees' hands are exposed to potential absorption of harmful substances (such as processing solutions). Training programs for personnel also must be established, and attendance of participants documented. Only trained personnel should perform mixing, cleaning, or maintenance work.

The Environmental Protection Agency (EPA) also has regulations concerning the use and disposal of processing chemicals. The EPA-SARA Title III (Superfund

CHAPTER 4 Film Processing

Amendments and Reauthorization Act of 1986) requires all users of developer solution to report the quantity used. The Resource Conservation and Recovery Act of 1987 governs waste management practices and limits liquid waste containing silver to a level of no more than 5 mg/L, or 5 ppm, which limits the amount of used processing chemicals and wash tank water that can be placed in public sewers and private septic systems before a special permit is required. Waste management may also come under the jurisdiction of the Clean Water Act of 1977, which is a 1977 amendment to the federal Water Pollution Control Act of 1972, which set the basic structure for

IDENTITY (As Used on Label and List)	Note: Blank spaces are not permitted. If any item is not applicable, or no information is available, the space must be marked to indicate that.

Section I

Manufacturer's Name	Emergency Telephone Number
Address (Number, Street, City, State, and ZIP Code)	Telephone Number for Information
	Date Prepared
	Signature of Preparer (optional)

Section II - Hazardous Ingredients/Identity Information

Hazardous Components (Specific Chemical Identity; Common Name(s))	OSHA PEL	ACGIH TLV	Other Limits Recommended	% (optional)

Section III - Physical/Chemical Characteristics

Boiling Point		Specific Gravity (H_2O = 1)	
Vapor Pressure (mm Hg)		Melting Point	
Vapor Density (AIR = 1)		Evaporation Rate (Butyl Acetate = 1)	
Solubility in Water			
Appearance and Odor			

FIGURE 4-6 Material Safety Data Sheet components. OSHA, Occupational Safety and Health Administration; ACGIH TLV, American Conference of Governmental Industrial Hygienists threshold limit values; PEL, permissible exposure limits; LEL, lower exposure limit; UEL, upper exposure limit; NTP, nucleoside triphosphates; IARC, International Agency for Research on Cancer.

Continued

CHAPTER 4 Film Processing

Section IV - Fire and Explosion Hazard Data

Flash Point (Method Used)	Flammable Limits	LEL	UEL

Extinguishing Media

Special Fire Fighting Procedures

Unusual Fire and Explosion Hazards

(Reproduce locally) OSHA 174, Sept. 1985

Section V - Reactivity Data

Stability	Unstable	Conditions to Avoid
	Stable	

Incompatibility *(Materials to Avoid)*

Hazardous Decomposition or Byproducts

Hazardous Polymerization	May Occur	Conditions to Avoid
	Will Not Occur	

Section VI - Health Hazard Data

Route(s) of Entry:	Inhalation?	Skin?	Ingestion?

Health Hazards *(Acute and Chronic)*

Carcinogenicity:	NTP?	IARC Monographs?	OSHA Regulated?

Signs and Symptoms of Exposure

Medical Conditions Generally Aggravated by Exposure

Emergency and First Aid Procedures

FIGURE 4-6, cont'd

CHAPTER 4 Film Processing

Section VII - Precautions for Safe Handling and Use

Steps to Be Taken in Case Material is Released or Spilled	
Waste Disposal Method	
Precautions to Be taken in Handling and Storing	
Other Precautions	

Section VIII - Control Measures

Respiratory Proctection (Specify Type)			
Ventilation	Local Exhaust		Special
	Mechanical (General)		Other
Protective Gloves		Eye Protection	
Other Protective Clothing or Equipment			
Work/Hygienic Practices			

FIGURE 4-6, cont'd

*U.S.G.P.O.: 1986 - 491 - 529/45775

regulating discharge of pollutants to water in the United States. The Act prohibits the discharge of pollutants into any surface water unless strict standards are in place and a special National Pollution Discharge Elimination System (NPDES) permit has been filed with the EPA. Any medical facility that discharges directly to any surface water must have an NPDES permit. The EPA describes a local wastewater treatment facility as a publicly owned treatment works (POTW), which must also have an NPDES permit. If the wastewater from the diagnostic imaging department is discharged to the local POTW and it has a silver concentration of 5 ppm or more, and more than 15 kg/month is being discharged, the facility must submit a one-time written notification to the local POTW, the EPA, and the state hazardous waste authority. The discarding or recovery of silver is discussed more in Chapter 6. Material with a pH between 5.5 and 10 can be disposed of safely down the drain; all three parts of the concentrated developer and both parts of concentrated fixer are disqualified. A shipment of scrap film, a silver-laden fixer, and silver recovery cartridges from the clinical site to a refiner or treatment plant also require a special permit from the EPA or the Department of Transportation or both.

The developer solution is considered the most dangerous processing chemical because of its high alkalinity, which makes it especially dangerous to the eyes (hence OSHA's requirement for eye protection) and skin. A main component of film emulsion is gelatin (a form of collagen), which is an organic form of protein that is broken down by chemicals with a high pH. Because human soft tissue contains collagen, the skin and eyes are at risk if contact is made with developer. Hydroquinone can be absorbed through the skin and is corrosive to the eyes and nasal membranes. Glutaraldehyde is a tanning agent (made to harden collagen-based material) and, therefore, is a skin irritant. Wearing eye protection, rubber gloves, and an apron should always be standard operating procedure when pouring or mixing developer. Fixer is a strong acid that can burn the eyes and irritate the skin. As with developer, proper safety apparel should be worn when pouring and mixing fixer. Wash immediately any skin that has been in contact with processing solutions.

CHAPTER 4 Film Processing

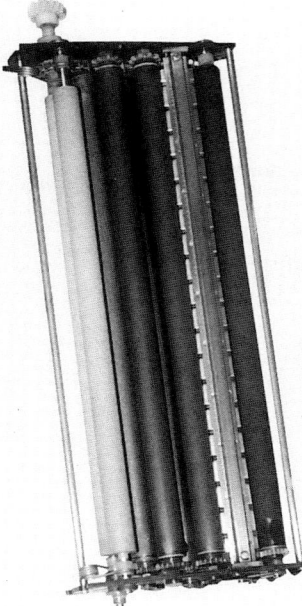

FIGURE 4-7 Entrance rollers for automatic film processor.

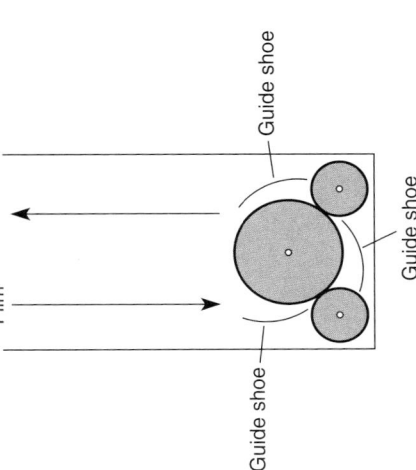

FIGURE 4-8 Transport rollers for automatic film processor.

AUTOMATIC PROCESSOR MAIN SYSTEMS

All automatic film processors have six main systems: transport, temperature control, circulation, replenishment, drying, and electrical.

Transport System

The transport system is responsible for transporting the film through the various steps in processing and for controlling development and total processing times. This system also plays a minor role in solution agitation and concentration. It is the largest and most complex system in an automatic processor. Because it has many moving parts, it is also the system most likely to break down. The transport system is made up of three smaller subsystems: the roller subsystem, the transport rack subsystem, and the drive subsystem.

Roller Subsystem. The rollers are responsible for "grabbing" the film and transporting it through the various stages of processing. They also provide a squeegee action that helps prevent too much solution carryover. There are three main types of rollers:

- *Entrance rollers* are primarily serrated rollers made of rubberized plastic, which enables these rollers to grip the film better as it enters the processor (Fig. 4-7).
- *Transport,* or *planetary, rollers* are responsible for the transportation of film and they often have a diameter of 1 inch. They usually are mounted in pairs, either staggered or directly opposite each other (Fig. 4-8).
- *Master,* or *solar, rollers* are larger rollers, with a 3-inch diameter. These rollers are found at the bottom of each solution tank, where the film must bend and turn back upward.

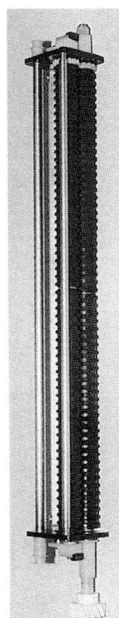

FIGURE 4-9 Vertical rack assembly.

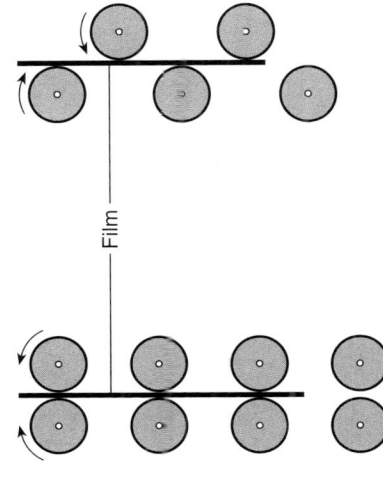

FIGURE 4-10 Turnaround rack assembly.

- Rollers can be made of acrylic plastic (Plexiglas), stainless steel, polyester plastic, rubberized plastic, and phenolic resin. The phenolic rollers are orange-brown and wooden. Care must be taken when cleaning phenolic rollers (no abrasive pads). Because these rollers are made of relatively soft material that can be scratched, liquid can be absorbed into the roller and warping can occur. For these reasons, rollers made of phenolic resin are usually found in the dryer section.

Transport Rack Subsystem. The transport rack subsystem is the rack or frame that contains the rollers, guide shoes, and associated hardware. There are four types of transport racks:

- *Entrance rack.* The entrance rack contains the entrance rollers, guide shoes, and a microswitch to activate the replenishment system (in volume replenishment systems) (see Fig. 4-7).
- *Vertical or deep racks.* Vertical or deep racks contain the transport rollers that transport the film into or up out of the tank (Fig. 4-9). Side plates and tie bars hold the rollers in place. The side plates and tie bars can expand and contract over time and may cause misalignment.
- *Turnaround rack.* The turnaround rack is found at the bottom of the tank and it contains a master roller, transport rollers, and two to three guide shoes (Fig. 4-10).

- *Crossover rack.* Crossover racks move from developer to fixer, fixer to wash tank, and wash tank-to-dryer transition. The crossover rack for the wash tank-to-dryer transition is often called a *squeegee rack* because it helps to remove water from the film, and faster drying occurs. Usually, these racks contain a master roller, transport rollers, and two guide shoes, but they can vary from manufacturer to manufacturer. These racks are not in solution and therefore must be cleaned before use because chemical residue can crystallize on the rollers during downtime. If the processor is on standby for longer than 2 hours, then the crossover racks should be cleaned before use.

Drive Subsystem. The drive subsystem is the portion of the transport system that supplies the mechanical energy to move the film (Fig. 4-11). This subsystem includes the following:

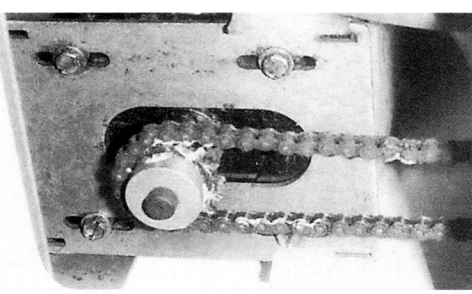

FIGURE 4-11 Drive system.

- *Drive motor.* The drive motor is a 1/20- to 1/8-hp electric motor that runs at 1725 to 1750 rpm.
- *Main drive chain.* The main drive chain is a no. 25 chain that attaches the drive motor to the gear system (similar to a bicycle chain). It is located on the side of the deep racks.
- *Gear reduction mechanism.* The gear reduction mechanism is a series of gears of different sizes that reduce the speed to between 10 rpm and 20 rpm.
- *Gears.* Gears transfer the mechanical energy from the motor to the rollers. The two types of gears are "drive" gears, which normally are attached to the ends of the rollers, and "worm" gears, which are located on the main drive shaft and are used to power the drive gears (Fig. 4-12). The gears can be made of plastic or metal.
- *Main drive shaft.* The main drive shaft connects the gear reduction mechanism to the drive gears with a system of worm gears.

Gears out of solution may be coated lightly with grease. Sprockets and chains out of solution require a light coating of oil, but care must be taken to avoid getting

petroleum-based products in chemical solutions or on rollers. In the dryer section, lubricants must be avoided; therefore, the gears must be kept clean to minimize friction.

The average transport system speed for a 90-second processor is about 60 inches of film per minute.

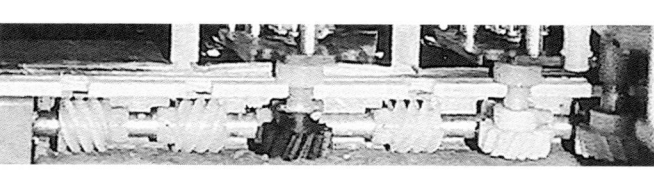

FIGURE 4-12 Worm and drive gears.

Temperature Control System

The temperature control system is also called the *tempering system* and it regulates the temperature of each solution. The two basic types of this system currently in use are water-controlled systems and thermostatically controlled systems.

Water-Controlled System. The water-controlled system is often called a *warm-water processor*. It uses the wash water temperature to regulate the solution temperature by circulating the water around the outside of the stainless steel processing tanks. This method requires a large supply of hot water and a mixing valve to regulate water temperature (Fig. 4-13).

Thermostatically Controlled System. Processors with a thermostatically controlled system are often called *cold-water processors* because they require only cold wash water to enter the unit. These systems use either an electronic heater for each tank or a heat exchanger, with a thermostat to regulate the system. The heat exchanger is a thin-wall stainless steel tube located at the bottom of each tank (Fig. 4-14). When a heat exchanger is used, the dryer air is used to heat the solutions in each tank. Because the dryer air temperature can exceed 120 °F (49 °C), the cooler wash water is pumped through the heat exchanger tube to keep the solution temperature in the proper range (typically 85 to 95 °F or 29 to 35 °C). This system is much more practical than

CHAPTER 4 Film Processing

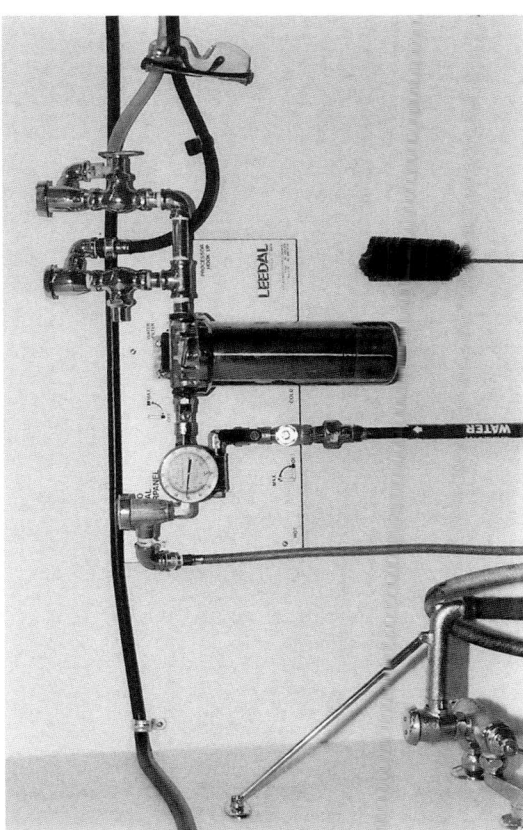

FIGURE 4-13 Mixing valve for warm-water automatic processors.

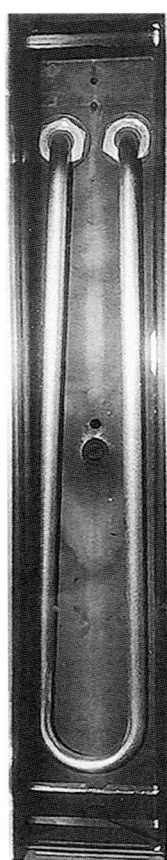

FIGURE 4-14 Heat exchanger located at the bottom of the water tank in a thermostatically controlled temperature system.

the others because it does not require the large hot-water heater and associated utility cost to maintain the supply necessary for the water-controlled system. For this reason, most of the newer processors are of this type. Regardless of the type of temperature control system used, the system must maintain the developer temperature to within ±0.5 °F (0.3 °C) of the manufacturer's specifications.

Circulation System

The circulation system is also referred to as the *recirculation and filtration system*. It uses a series of pumps to circulate the solution continuously in each tank and serves the following functions:

- *Ensures complete chemistry mixing.* During processor downtime, chemicals inside the tanks may begin to separate, with the water rising to the top and the chemicals dissipating to the bottom (a condition known as *stratification*). Swirling of the solutions by the circulation system ensures uniform concentration.
- *Provides uniform temperature.* Because the heating or heat-exchanging elements are typically on the bottom of the tank, uneven regions of temperature can develop unless the solutions are being circulated continuously.
- *Provides the equivalent of agitation performed in manual processing.*

During manual film processing, the halide ions that have been separated from the silver leave the emulsion in the form of bromine gas, which can cause a layer of bubbles to form on the outside surface of the film. This layer may block developing agents from reaching the inner portion of the emulsion, and areas of uneven development called *streaking* occur. **Agitation** in manual processing involves "jiggling" the film every 30 seconds to shake this layer of bubbles on the film. With the developer swirling over the surface of the film in an automatic processor, the layer of bubbles is removed in much the same way as agitation in manual processing.

A 25-μm filter is often located in the developer loop of this system to remove gelatin and other impurities that become dissolved in the developer during processing (Fig. 4-15). This filter must be replaced periodically as part of processor maintenance. Most manufacturers recommend

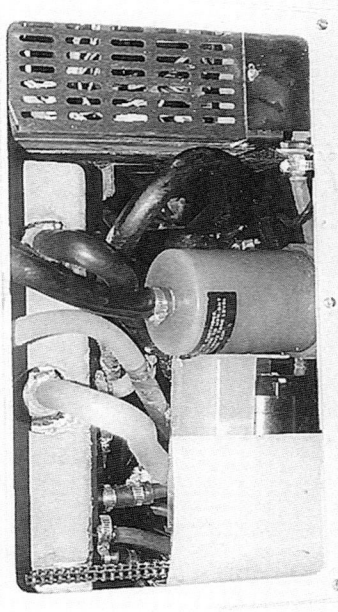

FIGURE 4-15 Developer circulation system filter.

replacement of this filter on a monthly basis or after the processing of 5000 films. A filter is not required for the fixer portion of this system. The circulation rate of this system is roughly 3 to 5 gal/min for the developer tank and 1 to 3 gal/min for the fixer. Failure of this system usually results in uneven development of the resulting image.

Replenishment System

The replenishment system is also called the *regeneration system* and it is responsible for replenishing processor solutions. It consists of a series of pumps, plastic tubing, and plastic storage tanks. The plastic tubing linking the replenishment solution storage tanks to the processor should be inspected periodically because it may become pinched or twisted, which blocks the flow of fresh solution (resulting in underreplenishment). The two different types of replenishment systems available in film processors are volume replenishment and flood replenishment.

Volume Replenishment. With the volume replenishment system, the most common type of replenishment system, a volume of chemicals is replaced for each film that is fed into the processor. A microswitch is placed usually at either end of the entrance rack that senses the film and then activates the system so the size of the film controls the amount of replenishment that takes place.

The average replenishment rates for this system are as follows:

- *Developer:* 4 to 5 mL/in of film, or roughly 60 to 70 mL/sheet of 14 × 17-inch film (35 × 43 cm)
- *Fixer:* 6 to 8 mL/in, or roughly 100 to 110 mL/sheet of 14 × 17-inch film

The volume replenishment system is used for relatively busy processors that process at least 25 to 50 sheets of 14 × 17-inch film or the equivalent per 8-hour workday.

Flood Replenishment. Flood replenishment is also called *timed replenishment* or *standby replenishment* and is used for processors that are not in constant use or that process less than 25 to 50 sheets of 14 × 17-inch film or equivalent per day. With the low volume of patient films processed per day, there may be a considerable gap in time between films entering the processor, which allows the developer solution inside the automatic processor to become oxidized, and subsequent films are underdeveloped. This situation prompts the radiographer either to increase technical factors (the result is a greater patient dose) or to increase the replenishment rate of a volume replenishment system (the results are greater department costs). With a flood replenishment system, the replenishment is controlled by a timer, which replenishes the solutions periodically, regardless of the number of films processed. This system was developed by Donald E. Titus of the Eastman Kodak Company. The replenishment pump should operate for approximately 20 seconds every 5 minutes and deliver about 65 mL of each solution. These variables maintain a total replenishment rate of 780 mL/h. All developer in the processing tank should be replaced every 16 working hours.

Most processors include a replenishment rate indicator, so monitoring is easy. In the case of other types of processors, special test paper is available for testing certain concentrations in the developer and fixer.

For developer, the special test paper estimates the levels of bromide ions dissolved in the solution. Stable developer should have a bromide level of about 6 g/L. Levels greater than 8 g/L indicate underreplenishment, which can cause underdevelopment and lead to a lack of optical density and contrast of the resulting image. Underreplenishment is caused most often by a pinched or blocked replenishment line, pump failure, microswitch failure, or failure of the timer circuit during flood replenishment. Levels less than 4 g/L indicate overreplenishment, which can result in overdevelopment that causes increased optical density and fogging. Overreplenishment is caused most often by a microswitch that fails to shut off or a pump that does not shut off.

Fixer replenishment can be estimated with silver estimating paper, which estimates the dissolved silver content in the solution. Normal fixer contains about 4 to 6 g/L (0.4–0.6 troy oz/gal). Levels greater than 8 g/L indicate underreplenishment (which causes a lack of clearing and a possible lack of hardening in the resulting film), whereas levels less than 4 g/L indicate overreplenishment, which does not affect film quality adversely but does waste fixer (and therefore money).

Drying System

The dryer system consists of two or three heating units between 1500 W and 2500 W that are used to dry the film. The system draws at least 10 A of electric current, which means the system consumes 60% to 80% of the electrical power going into the processor. A hot-air blower moves the air at a rate between 100 ft³/min and 300 ft³/min over the film. A series of air fins and air tubes are used to direct the air onto the film (Fig. 4-16). These fins and tubes must be kept clean for maximum efficiency. Most automatic processors also require an exhaust tube (which is similar to one found on a clothes dryer) to empty the hot air out of the processing area. This air can have a temperature exceeding 100 °F (37.8 °C) and relative humidity values between 25% and 100%, which are not conducive to proper film storage.

Electrical System

The electrical system consists of a solid-state circuit board or microprocessor that distributes electrical power to the other systems. In some newer processors, the microprocessor can be accessed to disclose quality control information such as solution temperature and replenishment rate. It usually handles 4 to 5 kW/h and

CHAPTER 4 Film Processing

between 15 A and 25 A of current. This system requires periodic replacement because of the heat, humidity, and corrosive environment inside of the processor.

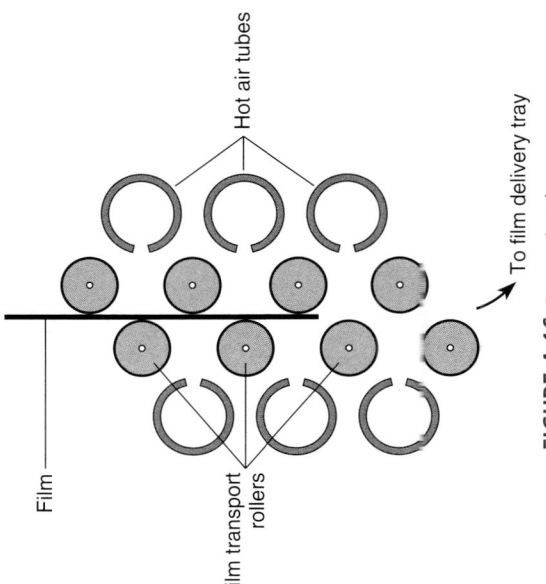

FIGURE 4-16 Dryer air tubes.

TYPES OF AUTOMATIC PROCESSORS

Automatic processors are of several types and they usually are named according to the time it takes to process the film completely, often called the *dry-to-drop time*.

- *Seven minutes*: the original Kodak automatic processor from the 1950s; processes about 100 films/h
- *Three minutes*: also called a *double-capacity processor* because it processes 200 films/h
- *Ninety seconds*: also called a *fast-access processor* because the film is available in 90 seconds and the processor has a capacity of 300 films/h. This was developed by Kodak in the mid 1960s and it is still the most commonly used film processor.
- *Sixty seconds*: a newer type of processor that can process up to 350 films/h
- *Forty-five seconds*: the newest type of processor; requires special film and chemistry to function properly

Many newer processors come with a variable-speed option so that processing time can be varied according to the type of film used. In other words, the radiographer may select a 90-second processing time, a 180-second processing time, and so on. An example of this is the "extended processing" used in mammography, which increases normal processing time to increase the film contrast. This is covered more completely in Chapter 11. Some processors also have a stand-by option that is useful for low-volume facilities. The drive system and dryer blower are shut off and the water flow rate is reduced, but the chemical and the dryer temperatures are maintained. This activity occurs when 2 minutes pass without a film entering the unit.

Processor Size

Automatic film processors come in three basic sizes according to the number of films processed during a given period: the floor-size processor, the intermediate-size processor, and the tabletop-size processor.

Floor-Size Processor. The floor-size processor is the largest processor and, as its name implies, it sits on the floor of the darkroom or lightroom. It has heavy-duty rollers, gears, and a drive motor so it can handle a high volume of operation. This size processor is found primarily in the main radiology department of hospitals.

Intermediate-Size Processor. The intermediate-size processor is a smaller version of the floor-size processor and usually sits on four support legs. It is about the size of a single laundry sink. This processor costs less than the floor-size model and is often found in physicians' offices and clinics, and in specialized areas of hospitals, such as surgery.

Tabletop-Size Processor. The tabletop-size processor is the smallest and least expensive processor. It is designed for low-volume operation, such as in a mobile facility, and is small enough to fit on the countertop of a darkroom.

Processor Location

A processor can be installed in the darkroom in one of four methods: totally inside, bulk inside, bulk outside, or totally outside.

Totally Inside. With totally inside installation, the processor is completely inside the darkroom, and noise, heat, and humidity are generated. Therefore, this is the least desirable method of installation. An advantage of this method, however, is easy retrieval of film that has jammed in the processor because it can be removed in safe lighting.

Bulk Inside. With bulk inside installation, most of the processor is inside the darkroom and only the drop tray is on the outside. This method minimizes the heat and noise in the darkroom but still allows easy retrieval of jammed film.

Bulk Outside. Bulk outside installation places the feed tray inside the darkroom but all other components outside. This method eliminates the heat, noise, and humidity inside the darkroom but makes retrieval of films more difficult because they must be removed in white light.

The minimum space on all sides of the processor must be 24 inches, to allow for servicing.

Totally Outside. Daylight processing systems and processors are designed to eliminate the need for a darkroom, so they are located totally outside any darkroom area. They are discussed in detail in Chapter 5.

SUMMARY

Even though most hospitals have switched to digital radiographic image acquisition, many (along with most smaller clinics and physician offices) have not and,

CHAPTER 4 Film Processing

therefore, require film/screen systems. For radiographers working in nondigital imaging departments, a basic understanding of film processing and automatic processing systems is essential for the performance of the quality control activities discussed in Chapter 5.

Refer to the Evolve Website at https://evolve.elsevier.com for Student Experiments 4.1: Hyporetention Test and 4.2: Automatic Processor Inspection.

REVIEW QUESTIONS

1. When mixing developer solution from concentrate, which part should be placed into the tank first?
   a. Part A
   b. Part B
   c. Part C
   d. Water

2. What would cause an ammonia-like odor in a darkroom?
   a. Contamination of the fixer by the developer
   b. Oxidation of the developer
   c. Improper mixing of the developer
   d. Overreplenishment of the developer

3. In an automatic processor, which of the following is not considered part of the three principal subsystems of the film transport system?
   a. Microswitch
   b. Rollers
   c. Transport racks
   d. Drive motor

4. According to ANSI standards, the maximum amount of hyporetention allowed is _____ µg/cm^3.
   a. 2
   b. 5
   c. 8
   d. 10

5. If the developer temperature is set at 96 °F, then the wash water temperature should be set at _____ °F.
   a. 86
   b. 91
   c. 96
   d. 101

6. Which processing chemical is responsible for creating optical densities greater than 1.2 on a diagnostic image?
   a. Phenidone
   b. Hydroquinone
   c. Elon
   d. Metol

7. Which system of the automatic processor consumes the greatest amount of electrical power?
   a. Transport
   b. Replenishment
   c. Circulation
   d. Dryer

8. Which of the following is located at the bottom of each processing tank?
   a. Entrance rack
   b. Vertical rack
   c. Turnaround rack
   d. Crossover rack

9. Which of the following materials are used in the construction of an entrance roller?
   a. Acrylic plastic (Plexiglas)
   b. Stainless steel
   c. Polyester
   d. Rubberized plastic

10. Hydrogen ions (H$^+$) that constitute one-ten thousandth of a molar of a liquid would have which of the following pH values?
    a. 2
    b. 4
    c. 6
    d. 8

CHAPTER 5

Processor Quality Control

KEY TERMS

Base + fog
Bromide drag
Chemical activity
Contrast indicator
Daylight systems
Densitometer
Flow meters
Hydrometer
Incident light
Locational effect
Sensitometer
Sensitometry
Speed indicator
Time-of-day variability
Transmitted light

OBJECTIVES

At the completion of this chapter, the reader should be able to do the following:

- Understand the importance of a processor quality control program in diagnostic imaging
- List the main components of a processor quality control program in diagnostic imaging
- Describe the factors that affect chemical activity
- Indicate the proper processor cleaning procedures
- Describe the basic types of processor maintenance and appropriate maintenance procedures
- Perform sensitometric tests to monitor processor function and chemical activity performance
- Describe the importance of quality control in daylight systems

OUTLINE

Chemical Activity
Solution Temperature
Processing Time
Replenishment Rate
Solution pH
Specific Gravity and Proper Mixing
Processor Cleaning Procedures
   Daily
   Monthly
   Quarterly
   Yearly
Processor Maintenance
Scheduled Maintenance
Preventive Maintenance
Nonscheduled Maintenance
   Daily at Startup
   Daily During Operation
   Daily at Shutdown
   Weekly
   Monthly
   Quarterly
   Yearly
Processor Monitoring
Sensitometer
Densitometer
Control Chart
Quality Control Film
Characteristic Curve
Processor Troubleshooting
Daylight Systems
Summary

The most important part of a quality management program in departments using film/screen image receptors is the quality control of the film processor, resulting primarily from the large degree of variability that can occur with processing systems. Daily monitoring of processor operation and function is required to keep these variables from degrading the image quality. There are four components to a processor quality control program: chemical activity, cleaning procedures, maintenance, and monitoring.

CHEMICAL ACTIVITY

As mentioned in Chapter 4, chemical activity refers to how well the processing chemicals are functioning. Many

FIGURE 5-1 Digital thermometer for monitoring solution temperatures. (Courtesy Gammex/RMI, Middleton, WI.)

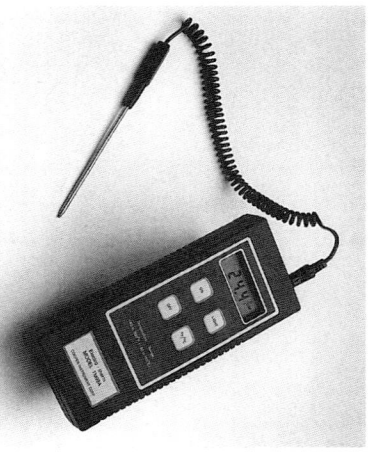

variables affect chemical activity, including the solution temperature, processing time, replenishment rate, solution pH, and specific gravity and proper mixing.

Solution Temperature

Variations in developer temperature can affect image contrast, optical density, and the visibility of recorded details significantly. Therefore, developer temperature should not vary by more than ±0.5 °F (0.3 °C) from the manufacturer's recommendations. It should be monitored at the beginning of the workday and then periodically throughout the day. Many film processors have either an analog thermometer or a light-emitting diode indicator of solution temperature built into the front panel. If this is unavailable, a digital thermometer with a remote probe (Fig. 5-1) is the best instrument to monitor solution temperature because it is the most accurate and works quickly. A glass, alcohol-filled thermometer is an adequate alternative. A mercury thermometer should never be used because mercury is a toxic substance, and it poses a difficult and potentially hazardous cleanup problem in the event of breakage. Mercury can also sensitize film, even in small quantities. The accuracy of any built-in thermometer should be checked monthly with a digital thermometer and should be within ±0.5 °F (0.3 °C).

Fixer activity is not as temperature sensitive as developer activity, but the temperature should be maintained within ±5 °F (3 °C) of the developer temperature to avoid reticulation marks (discussed in Chapter 10) and to clear the film properly. Wash water temperature should be the same as that of the fixer to complete washing.

To check the solution temperatures, place the probe in each tank, starting with the developer. Be sure the probe is clean to avoid contamination. Next, check the wash water temperature and then the fixer temperature. Afterward, rinse the probe with water so it is ready for the next inspection.

Processing Time

Variations in developer time can have the same effect on image quality as solution temperature. Therefore,

developer time should be maintained to within ±2% to 3% of the manufacturer's specifications. As mentioned in Chapter 4, the transport system is responsible for maintaining processing time. Most of this system is made up of moving parts (and experiences the most wear and tear of any system), so it is subject to the most variability and breakdown. Processing time should be checked daily at the beginning of each workday (or more often if a malfunction is suspected), and can be determined with a stopwatch or digital timer. To establish developer time, feed the film into the processor with the top open. When the leading edge of the film enters the solution, start the timer; when the leading edge first emerges from the solution, stop the timer. For a 90-second processor, the time should be between 18 and 22 seconds, with a margin of error of roughly 0.5 second. Total processing time is evaluated using a stopwatch to measure the time when the leading edge of the film enters the processor to when it begins to appear in the drop section; then, compare that time with the manufacturer's specification. For help with this procedure, a time-in-solution test tool is available (Fig. 5-2). The tool consists of a strip of clear film base with two white tape strips that form the letter T. A black line is drawn about halfway on the first strip as a "get ready" line to alert the person performing the test to prepare to start the stopwatch. Timing begins when the cross of the T enters the solution.

Replenishment Rate

As film is processed during the course of the workday, the processing solutions are being depleted. If they are not replenished adequately, a decrease in image contrast and optical density occurs. Excessive replenishment has the opposite effect. Most film processors have replenishment rate **flow meters** that indicate the replenishment rate for each solution. The values indicated should be within ±5% of the manufacturer's specification for the type of replenishment system in use (volume replenishment versus flood replenishment, described in Chapter 4. The amount of replenishment also should be within 5% of these values. A stopwatch and a graduated cylinder can be used to verify replenishment rate and flow meter accuracy. With the top of the processor open, an 8 × 10-inch (20 × 25-cm) film should be

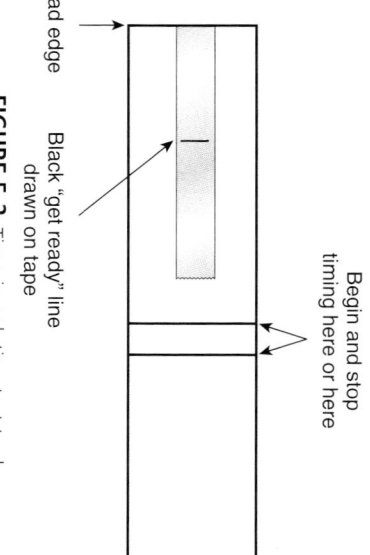

FIGURE 5-2 Time-in-solution test tool.

fed into the processor lengthwise. The graduated cylinder should be placed under the opening of the replenisher line so the fresh solution pumps directly into the cylinder. When the film passes through the entrance rack, the replenishing pump shuts off, stopping the flow of solution. When this happens, the volume of solution in millimeters should be divided by 10 to get the milliliter-per-inch value (or divided by 25 to obtain milliliters per centimeters) and then compared with the manufacturer's values.

Solution pH

Most developer solutions must function in a pH range between 10 and 11.5 to convert the latent image to a visible image. A developer pH that is too low (caused by underreplenishment or contamination) decreases image contrast and optical density, whereas excessive pH has the opposite effect. Fixer solutions should maintain a pH between 4 and 4.5 for proper clearing. Although not as critical as the other factors affecting chemical activity, pH should be checked daily to avoid potential problems. A digital pH meter is recommended for evaluating pH because of its accuracy. If one is not available, litmus paper or similar commercially available test strips are an inexpensive alternative. The strips are dipped into the solution and they change color to indicate the pH value. Care should be taken (by wearing rubber gloves) not to get processing chemicals on one's skin when using this method.

Specific Gravity and Proper Mixing

Processing chemicals must be mixed to the manufacturer's concentration specifications to function within operating parameters. The easiest method to evaluate solution concentration is to measure the specific gravity.

$$\text{Specific gravity} = \frac{\text{Density of X liquid}}{\text{Density of water in equal amount}}$$

A **hydrometer** is the instrument used to measure specific gravity. It resembles a large glass thermometer (Fig. 5-3). When placed in a liquid, the hydrometer sinks to a certain depth in the solution, and the level of the liquid indicates the specific gravity on the stem of the hydrometer. Measure the developer first, then rinse the hydrometer with water and measure the fixer. Developer specific gravity should be in the range 1.07 to 1.1 and should not vary by more than ±0.004 from the manufacturer's specifications. Fixer solutions should be in the range 1.077 to 1.11 and should not vary by more than ±0.004 from the manufacturer's specifications.

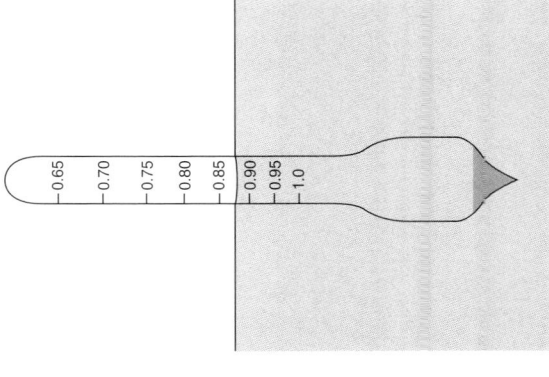

FIGURE 5-3 A floating hydrometer is used to measure specific gravity. In this particular instance, the specific gravity indicated by the hydrometer is 0.87 g/cm^3.

Daily

These procedures should be performed daily at startup.

PROCEDURE

1. Open the top of the processor to determine whether the crossover racks were removed the previous night (which should be the case, as shown later in this section). Use of the processor may have been necessary during the night on an emergency basis. If the racks are present, remove the splash guards and crossover racks and rinse them with water. Be sure the rollers and guide shoes are free of dirt, debris, gelatin, or crystallized processing chemicals. Use a soft sponge or plastic cleaning pad for cleaning; avoid using steel wool pads or other metallic scrubbers. Turn the rollers by hand so all surfaces can be reached.
2. Remove the deep transport racks from each solution and rinse with water. Take care not to drip one solution into another—especially the fixer into the developer—when lifting the racks out of the solution tanks. Remove stubborn dirt or residue with a soft sponge or plastic scrubber. Inspect the rollers and gears for any obvious defects. Replace the racks back into the solutions carefully while avoiding contamination.
3. Activate the transport system and observe the rollers and gears for asymmetry, rotation, and hesitation during operation. Replace the crossover racks and again observe the rollers and gears during operation. Replace any defective parts (especially gears and roller tension springs) and be sure all mounting screws are tightened.
4. Observe the level of processing solutions to be sure that they are within 1 mm of specified levels. Activate the replenisher pump or add fresh solution from the storage tank if the level is low.
5. After shutdown, remove the crossover racks and store them adjacent to the processor (if practical) to minimize the formation of chemical residue. Raise the top of the processor so that a 2- to 4-inch gap exists to allow chemical fumes to escape and to avoid condensation of chemicals onto the various processor components.

PROCESSOR CLEANING PROCEDURES

Processors that are dirty—the most common cause of processor breakdown—cannot function according to established parameters. Therefore, proper cleaning procedures should be performed daily, monthly, quarterly, and yearly.

The procedure just mentioned normally requires 15 to 20 minutes daily to complete and can add several years to the life expectancy of the processor in addition to eliminating most processor artifacts.

Monthly

PROCEDURE

1. Drain all processing tanks and wash the inside with water. Use a soft sponge or plastic scrubber to remove stubborn dirt or residue.
2. Rinse all tanks with water and refill them with the proper amount of chemical solution. The developer solution must be "seasoned" before any films can be processed, because typical replenisher solution is too concentrated. Seasoning involves adding starter solution, which is stabilized potassium bromide. This addition raises the bromide level to between 4 g/l and 8 g/l, which is the normal level for developer solution while processing films. Fresh developer replenisher used to refill the tank has levels far less than this, which can increase the fog level of the film. The amount of starter solution required is about 100 ml/gal solution.

Quarterly

PROCEDURE

1. Drain, wash, and rinse all replenishment tanks with water. Be especially careful to remove the oxidized developer from the sides of the developer replenisher tank.
2. Refill tanks with fresh solution and check the specific gravity with a hydrometer.

Yearly

Replenisher and circulation system pumps and tubing can experience a buildup of dirt and chemical residue that can reduce the efficiency of these systems; therefore, some manufacturers suggest the use of a system cleaner to reduce these deposits. The developer system cleaner has an acidic pH level to counteract the alkaline developer, whereas the fixer system cleaner has an alkaline pH to counteract the acidic fixer. Remove the transport racks before a system cleaner is used, because phenolic and soft rubber rollers can absorb the cleaner and contaminate future processing solutions slowly. Most system cleaners are either chlorine based (which can break down hydroquinone) or sulfamic based (which also breaks down hydroquinone and dissolves metallic silver). Take great care to flush systems with water to remove residual cleaner. Some manufacturers do not recommend the use of a system cleaner in their processors because of the risk of contamination, so it is best to check with a technical representative.

PROCESSOR MAINTENANCE

Poorly maintained processors (in addition to dirty ones) cannot function according to established parameters and can degrade image quality. They also can lead to premature replacement of the processor, which is a large capital expense ($5000 to $50,000). A film processor should last for at least 10,000 hours of operation or a minimum of 5 years. Therefore; a proper maintenance schedule must be maintained by the diagnostic imaging department to ensure continued satisfactory operation of the film processor. Keep a log of any maintenance procedures to document care. There are three types of processor maintenance: scheduled, preventive, and nonscheduled.

Scheduled Maintenance

Scheduled maintenance includes procedures that are performed daily, weekly, and monthly. For automatic film processors, scheduled maintenance includes proper lubrication of moving parts; observation of all moving parts; replacement of filters in the water and developer circulation system; adjustment or replacement of tension springs, pulleys, and gears; and correction of any mechanical problems.

Preventive Maintenance

Preventive maintenance is a planned program that details specific parts of the processor to be replaced regularly. Items such as gears and rollers should be replaced after a certain number of hours of operation.

Nonscheduled Maintenance

Nonscheduled maintenance is required when a system failure occurs. The need for this type of maintenance can be minimized by proper cleaning of the processor, along with performing scheduled and preventive maintenance procedures.

Suggested Scheduled Maintenance Procedures

A processor maintenance schedule should include maintenance procedures daily at startup; daily during operation; daily at shutdown; and weekly, monthly, quarterly, and yearly.

Daily at Startup.

PROCEDURE

1. Follow the daily cleaning procedures listed earlier in this chapter.
2. Make sure the processor feed tray and darkroom countertops are clean.
3. Feed four 14 × 17-inch (35 × 43-cm) green, unprocessed films into the processor to clean the rollers of any residual matter and to assess transport system operation. Do not use preprocessed radiographs because they may contain residual fixer and have a hardened emulsion, which causes extra stress on the transport system. Any residual fixer also may contaminate the developer solution.

CHAPTER 5 Processor Quality Control

Daily During Operation.

PROCEDURE

1. Assess any changes in the normal operation of the processor, including noise level, vibration, odors, indicator buzzer, and film feeding characteristics.
2. Shut down the unit after 2 hours if no films have been processed (unless the system is equipped with a stand-by option). If the unit has been shut down for 30 minutes or longer, run another 14 × 17-inch piece of green film through the system to clean the rollers.

Daily at Shutdown.

PROCEDURE

1. Follow the cleaning procedures for shutdown listed previously (item 5 in the section on daily processor maintenance).
2. Note any obvious problems or changes in the unit such as abnormal odors or residues.

Weekly.

PROCEDURE

1. Use a thermometer to evaluate the solution temperature and dryer thermostats for accuracy. Compare the value on the thermostat with the value indicated on the thermometer. Solution temperatures must be maintained at previously mentioned parameters. The dryer thermostat should be accurate to within ±5 °F (3 °C).
2. Evaluate replenishment rates for accuracy using the previously mentioned procedure.
3. Lubricate the main driveshaft bearings, motor, and drive chain with motor oil.
4. Inspect replenishment system microswitches on the entrance rack for proper operation on units equipped with volume replenishment.
5. For units equipped with flood replenishment, drain the developer tank, rinse it with water, and fill it with fresh solution.
6. Inspect and service the silver reclamation unit (discussed in Chapter 6).

Monthly.

PROCEDURE

1. Follow the monthly cleaning procedures listed earlier in this chapter.
2. Use a large bottlebrush to remove and clean all dryer air tubes.
3. Replace the filter in the developer circulation. This filter removes dissolved gelatin and other impurities larger than 75 μm from the developer. Before installing the filter, soak it in fresh developer solution to remove any air from the system.
4. Replace the water filters if the flow rate decreases by more than 10% of the accepted amount.
5. Flush the floor drain with a commercial drain cleaner.
6. Perform a safelight test (see Chapter 3).

Quarterly.

PROCEDURE

1. Follow the quarterly cleaning procedure listed earlier.
2. Inspect all transport racks, rollers, gears, and guide shoes for wear or malfunction.
3. Check the integrity of all electrical connections and remove any dirt or corrosion.
4. Perform a hyporetention test on processed films using an American National Standards Institute test kit (see Chapter 4) to evaluate the archival quality of images.

Yearly.

PROCEDURE

1. Disassemble each transport rack and replace worn rollers, gears, or mounting springs.
2. Disassemble the drive motor and gearbox, lubricate the internal components, and replace worn parts.
3. Disassemble all replenishment and circulation system pump heads and replace worn parts, including rubber diaphragms and seals.
4. Replace the tubing in the circulation and replenishment system with one-eighth-inch clear polyvinyl chloride tubing. Install new clamps to mitigate the corrosive environment in the processor.

PROCESSOR MONITORING

Processor monitoring is accomplished with the performance of daily sensitometric tests that evaluate the performance of both the processor systems and processing chemicals. **Sensitometry** measures the relationship between the intensity of radiation absorbed by the film and the optical density produced. Two British amateur photographers, F. Hurter and U. Driffield, developed the current system of comparing these quantities (hence the Hurter and Driffield curve, which demonstrates film contrast). The following equipment is required to perform sensitometric tests: a sensitometer, a **densitometer**, either a control chart or graph paper, and quality control film.

Sensitometer

The **sensitometer** is an instrument designed to expose a reproducible, uniform, optical step-wedge pattern onto a film (Fig. 5-4). It contains a controlled-intensity light source with a standardized optical step-wedge image (also called a *step tablet*). These patterns are available in 11- and 21-step versions (Fig. 5-5). The 11-step pattern increases the optical density by a factor of two (100%) between each step. The 21-step pattern increases optical density by a factor of 1.41 (41%) between each step and is more useful in sensitometric tests. A radiograph taken with an aluminum

74 CHAPTER 5 Processor Quality Control

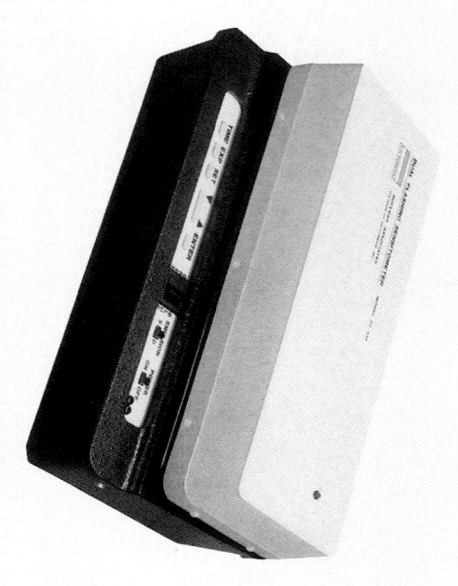

FIGURE 5-4 Sensitometer. (Courtesy Gammex/RMI, Middleton, WI.)

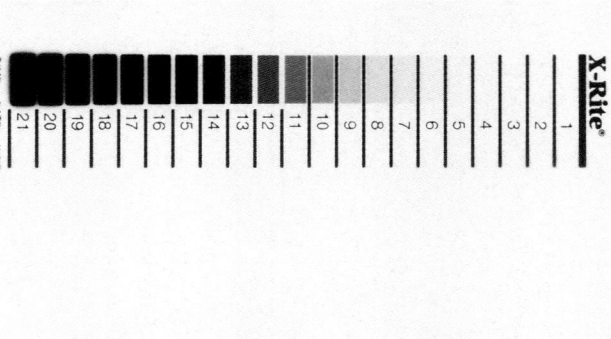

FIGURE 5-5 Twenty-one-step sensitometry film image. (Courtesy Nuclear Associates, Carle Place, NY.)

step wedge or penetrometer should not be used in processor sensitometric tests because X-ray generators are subject to too much variation from day to day, and the origin of any differences in radiographic images cannot be determined (i.e., the problem could be with the processor or with the X-ray generator). The controlled light source of the sensitometer eliminates these variations.

Most sensitometers have settings that allow the selection of blue-violet light emission or green light emission to match the spectral response of the film being tested. They also should have an option for exposing single-emulsion film or double-emulsion (duplitized) film. These settings must be selected properly to match the type of film to be used. Sensitometers remain fairly consistent in their operation until the light bulb burns out. The main concern for quality control technologists is to make sure the exposure window of the sensitometer (where the light exposes the film) is kept clean—free of dirt and dust. Do not touch these windows or wipe them with any type of cloth or gauze pad because they are fragile. Instead, purchase a can of compressed air (which is free of moisture and therefore prevents condensation) from a photographic supply store and use it to remove any dirt or debris.

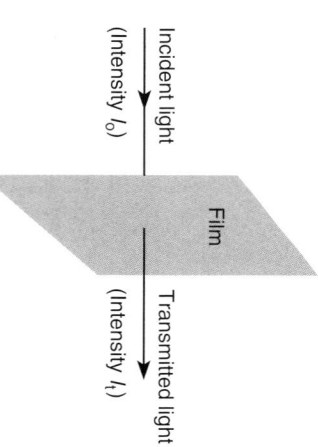

FIGURE 5-7 Diagram of incident and transmitted light. I_o, original intensity; I_t, transmitted intensity.

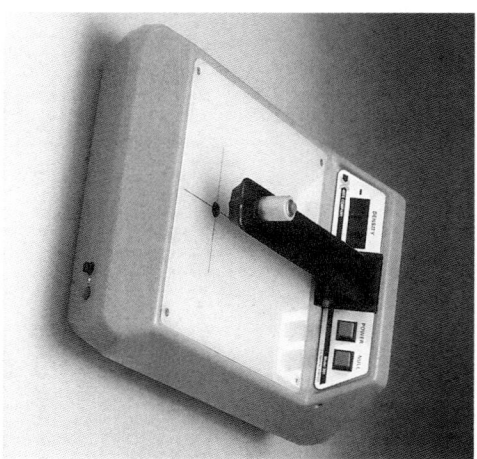

FIGURE 5-6 Densitometer, which is used to measure of optical density. (Courtesy Gammex/RMI, Middleton, WI.)

Densitometer

The densitometer, also known as *a transmission densitometer*, measures the optical density of a portion of an image using a 0- to 4-point scale (Fig. 5-6). It is a photographic light meter that measures the amount of light transmitted (**transmitted light**) through a portion of film and compares it with the original amount of light incident on the film (Fig. 5-7). A value of 0 to 4 points is then calculated with the following equation:

$$\text{Optical density} = \log_{10}\frac{\text{Incident light}}{\text{Transmitted light}} \text{ or } \log_{10}\frac{I_i}{I_t}$$

CHAPTER 5 Processor Quality Control

If the transmitted light were 10% of the incident light, the optical density would be 1 because the equation would be the following:

$$\text{Optical density} = \log_{10} \frac{100}{10}$$

Because the **incident light** is the full amount of light striking the film, it has a relative value of 100%. The $\log_{10}$ symbol (meaning log to the base 10) in the equation asks the question: Ten to what power equals the number in the equation? Because 100 divided by 10 equals 10, the $\log_{10}$ of the number 10 is 1 ($10^1 = 10$); therefore, if only 1% of the incident light is transmitted through the film, that portion of the image has an optical density of 2, because $100/1 = 100$ and $10^2 = 100$. A difference in the optical density scale of 0.3 is equivalent to a difference of two times in the amount of light transmission through the film because $10^{0.3} = 2$. This means that an optical density of 1.3 is twice as dark as an optical density of 1, and so on. The anatomic structures displayed on a diagnostic image usually have optical density values ranging from approximately 0.25 to 2.5 when measured with a densitometer; this is known as the *diagnostic range*. Optical densities outside this range do not contain diagnostic information when viewed on a standard viewbox illuminator.

Control Chart

A control chart is a graph that has predetermined upper and lower thresholds indicated (see Chapter 2) and is used to plot the data obtained during the sensitometric test (Fig. 5-8). Most control charts are designed to have these data recorded each day, for an entire month.

PROCEDURE

1. Place an 8 × 10-inch (20 × 25-cm) sheet of unexposed film in the sensitometer and expose it according to the manufacturer's instructions.
2. Feed the exposed film into the processor as soon as possible. Avoid variability by keeping the time between the exposure of the sensitometer film and the processing consistent. Be sure to feed the film into the processor correctly (see "Locational effect" discussed in the following list). This helps avoid the following variables:
   - **Bromide drag**, also called *bromide flow* or *directional effect*, is caused by the release of halide ions by the emulsion during development and their subsequent coating of the trailing areas of the film, which decreases the optical density of these areas. To minimize this effect, feed the least-dense end of the sensitometric strip first, with the long axis of the wedge pattern parallel to the entrance rollers. The steplike image created by the sensitometer is usually created at the edge of one side of the film, along the 10-inch (25-cm) dimension, as shown in Fig. 5-5. The opposite side of the film is unexposed and should be fed into the processor first to reduce the number of halide ions that are "dragged" over the remainder of the film.
   - **Locational effect** results from a difference in the location of the test film insertion into the processor. To minimize this effect, always try to insert the film on the same side of the feed tray each time a sensitometric test is performed.
   - **Time-of-day variability** is important because chemical activity and processing system parameters can vary considerably throughout the course of the workday. Therefore, sensitometric test films should always be processed at the same time each day, preferably early in the morning, after the processor has reached optimum operating levels.
3. After the film is processed, optical density readings of each of the 21 steps and the clear portion of the image should be measured with a densitometer and recorded. After the first day, when the operating parameters of the processor are established, it is not necessary to measure all 21 steps for succeeding days' test films.
4. From these optical density readings, the following indicators of processor performance are established:
   - *Base + fog*. Often abbreviated B + F, **base + fog** is the optical density of the clear portion of the image and is the result of the blue tint added to the base of the film and any black metallic silver grains that were created by aging of the film or background radiation exposure. The B + F value for most film ranges from 0.1 to 0.2 and should never exceed 0.25. When the accepted operating level is established, it should never vary by more than an optical density value of ±0.05 for dual-emulsion films and 0.03 for single-emulsion films during subsequent days' sensitometric test films. An above-normal developer temperature, an above-normal developing time, overreplenishment, contaminated solution, improper film or solution storage conditions, improper safelights, an incorrect starter solution in the developer, and fogged film can increase the B + F value above accepted limits.
   - **Speed indicator** or *mid-density point* (MD). MD is a measure of the amount of exposure energy necessary to produce an optical density of one greater than the B + F. After the B + F is determined, find the step with an optical density closest to one greater than this value. The value of this step is always measured and recorded as the speed indicator, regardless of the value obtained. For example, if the B + F is 0.2 on the first day, and step 8 of the sensitometry image yields an optical density of 1.2 on the same day, then the optical density of step 8 is always used to determine the speed indicator for all future days' tests. This value should not vary by an optical density of ±0.15 from the accepted operating level. Increased developer temperature, increased replenishment, overreplenishment, excessive concentration of developer or replenisher (usually resulting from developer mixed incorrectly; not enough water is added to the concentrate), no starter solution in fresh developer, or a contaminated solution can increase this value above established limits. A reversal decreases the speed indicator below accepted limits.
   - *Minimum density* (D_{min}) or *low density* (LD). D_{min}, or LD, is the optical density of the step closest to 0.25 greater than the B + F, which approximates the low end of the diagnostic range of optical densities. Again, after this indicator is established, the same step is used in future days' testing, regardless of the optical density reading. The optical density of this step should not vary by more than ±0.05 for dual-emulsion films and 0.03 for single-emulsion films from the accepted operating level during any future test. The optical density value of this indicator is created primarily by the action of phenidone, which is less sensitive to variability than hydroquinone. Essentially, the same factors affecting the B + F indicator also affect D_{min}.
   - *Maximum density* (D_{max}) or *high density* (HD). D_{max}, or HD, is the optical density of the step closest to two greater than the B + F, which is close to the upper value of the diagnostic density range. This value should stay within ±0.15 from the

Continued

CHAPTER 5 Processor Quality Control

PROCEDURE—cont'd

accepted operating level. This optical density value is created primarily by hydroquinone, which is more sensitive to variability than phenidone. An increase in developer time, temperature, or pH; overreplenishment; or overconcentration of developer solution can increase this value above the upper limit and vice versa.

- *Contrast indicator* or *relative density difference* (DD). Because contrast is defined as the difference among optical densities on the processed image, a **contrast indicator** can be obtained by calculating the difference between the D_{max} and D_{min} values during each day's sensitometry test. When the accepted operating level is determined initially, it should not vary by more than ±0.15 during any subsequent tests. Increased developer temperature or developer time, overreplenishment, or overconcentration of developer solution can increase the contrast indicator above the upper limit. A decrease below the lower limit occurs if the given factors are decreased.

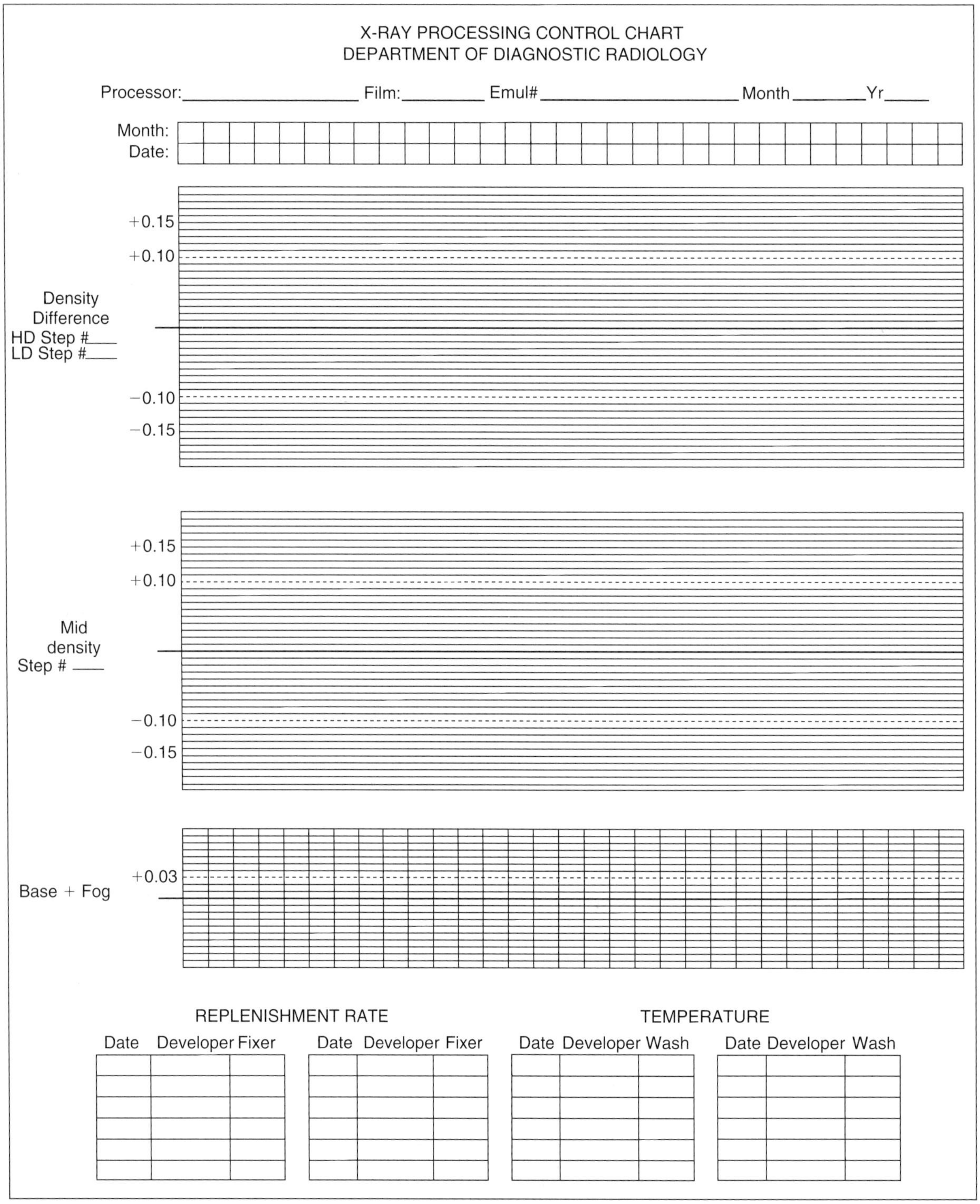

FIGURE 5-8 Processor control chart.

CHAPTER 5 Processor Quality Control

Before sensitometric tests are performed, ensure the processor is clean and functioning properly; that fresh, properly mixed chemicals are available; and that a safelight test has been performed with satisfactory results. The processor also should be in operation for at least 20 minutes so that the temperatures are at optimal levels.

After all the previously mentioned values are determined, they should be plotted on a control chart (see Fig. 5-8). This chart helps monitor chemical activity and processor performance, and documents the quality control activities for accreditation or government agencies. Because control charts have data plotted for an entire month, any trends in processor performance may appear and need to be addressed. The minimum number of data points in one direction that constitutes a trend that should be investigated is five for general radiography and three for mammographic processors. A processor quality control documentation form and daily sensitometric test form are included on the accompanying Evolve website. If a processor quality control program has not been implemented previously, the accepted operating level or base control number for each indicator has to be established. This established operating level is the value plotted at the center line of the control chart for each indicator. To establish the accepted operating level for each indicator, establish the control box of film (see the later discussion on quality control film) and expose a sheet of film with a sensitometer for 5 consecutive days. Determine the B + F, MD, and DD for each day. At the end of the fifth day, average the B + F, MD, and DD values for all 5 days. These averages are the accepted operating levels or base control numbers used on the control chart.

CHARACTERISTIC CURVE

In addition to the control chart, many diagnostic imaging departments may also benefit from the daily creation of a characteristic curve (also known as the *sensitometric curve*, *Hurter & Driffield curve*, *H & D curve*, or *D log E curve*) to monitor processor performance. Because the characteristic curve demonstrates film contrast, changes in the curve from day to day can indicate problems in the processing solutions or processor system performance. The characteristic curve also demonstrates B + F and film speed or sensitivity (Fig. 5-10).

PROCEDURE

1. Remove a sheet of 8 × 10-inch (20 × 25-cm) film from the film bin and expose it with a sensitometer. Process the film.
2. Using a densitometer, take optical density readings of each step of the 11- or 21-step pattern.
3. On a sheet of graph paper, plot the optical density of each step on the y-axis and the step number (beginning with the least-dense step) on the x-axis. Connect the points on the graph. The resulting curve should have the characteristic S or sigmoidal shape (see Fig. 5-10).
4. Calculate the average gradient (slope) of the straight-line portion of the curve using the optical density points of 0.25 and two greater than the B + F. This yields the contrast indicator of DD. The speed indicator or MD step also should be plotted as the step closest to one more than the B + F. These values should not vary by more than ±0.15 from the established value. More information on characteristic curves is available in Appendix A.

PROCESSOR TROUBLESHOOTING

As mentioned earlier in this chapter, an automatic film processor is subject to considerable variability during the course of operation, resulting in visible changes in image quality. The troubleshooting guide in Table 5-1 identifies specific processor problems, conditions, or both, and details the necessary corrective action.

DAYLIGHT SYSTEMS

Many diagnostic imaging departments have eliminated traditional darkrooms in favor of **daylight systems**, which

Quality Control Film

When a processor quality control program is implemented, a fresh box of film should be selected and dedicated to sensitometric testing only. This box of film is known as the *control box* and should be labeled clearly and stored under ideal conditions (e.g., no light, ionizing radiation, or chemical fumes). When all but a few sheets of film in the control box have been used, a crossover procedure to a new box of control film should be performed to minimize any variation that may occur from one batch of film to another (Fig. 5-9).

PROCEDURE

1. Expose and process five films from the old and new boxes of film with a sensitometer. Do this at the same time, processing the films one after the other. Be sure to identify which five films are from the old box and which five are from the new box.
2. From each film, determine the B + F, MD value, and DD indicators as described previously. Determine an average of these values for the old box of film and the new box of film (see Fig. 5-9).
3. Determine the difference between the boxes of film by subtracting the average of the old box of film from the average of the new box of film.
4. Determine the new operating level for each indicator (B + F, MD, or DD) to be used as the accepted value by taking the original operating level (the accepted value of each indicator used for the original box of film) and adding to it the difference between the boxes determined in step 3. In other words, the new indicator operating level equals the original operating level plus the difference.

CHAPTER 5 Processor Quality Control

CROSSOVER WORKSHEET

Site _____ Date _____
Film type _____ Technologist _____

New Emulsion #					Old Emulsion #				
Film #	Low Density (LD) Step #	Mid Density (MD) Step #	High Density (HD) Step #	B+F	Film #	Low Density (LD) Step #	Mid Density (MD) Step #	High Density (HD) Step #	B+F
1					1				
2					2				
3					3				
4					4				
5					5				
Average					Average				

Average Density Difference: DD = HD − LD = _____   Average Density Difference: DD = HD − LD = _____

MD difference between new and old film (New MD − Old MD)
DD difference between new and old film (New DD − Old DD)
B+F difference between new and old film (New − Old)

	MD	DD	B+F
Old operating levels			
Difference between new and old film			
New operating levels			

CROSSOVER WORKSHEET EXAMPLE

New Emulsion #	24578				Old Emulsion #	23456			
Film #	Low Density (LD) Step #10	Mid Density (MD) Step #11	High Density (HD) Step #13	B+F	Film #	Low Density (LD) Step #10	Mid Density (MD) Step #11	High Density (HD) Step #13	B+F
1	0.49	1.25	2.39	0.18	1	0.46	1.27	2.33	0.17
2	0.50	1.23	2.43	0.18	2	0.48	1.30	2.30	0.17
3	0.49	1.26	2.40	0.17	3	0.46	1.27	2.28	0.18
4	0.53	1.28	2.41	0.18	4	0.48	1.28	2.32	0.17
5	0.49	1.28	2.43	0.18	5	0.47	1.31	2.35	0.18
Average	0.50	1.26	2.41	0.18	Average	0.47	1.29	2.31	0.17

Average Density Difference: DD = HD − LD = 1.91   Average Density Difference: DD = HD − LD = 1.84

MD difference between new and old film (New MD − Old MD)   −0.03
DD difference between new and old film (New DD − Old DD)   +0.07
B+F difference between new and old film (New − Old)   +0.01

	MD	DD	B+F
Old operating levels	1.34	1.90	0.17
Difference between new and old film	−0.03	+0.07	+0.01
New operating levels	1.31	1.97	0.18

FIGURE 5-9 Cross-over worksheet for determining new operating levels.

load cassettes automatically with fresh sheets of film and unload exposed cassettes directly into a processor (Fig. 5-11). Because the film is loaded and unloaded from the cassette mechanically, a regular maintenance program is essential for continued proper operation. This program includes cleaning and lubrication of moving parts and replacement of parts as needed. Excessive dirt or dust in the loading section of these systems may enter the cassettes, causing artifacts to appear on subsequent images. It also may result in excessive friction between the sheets of film and the inside of the cassette. Improper loading may occur, and films may become stuck inside the system. Keep the cassette-unloading section of these systems clean and free of dirt so films unload properly and do not become stuck in the unit (white light exposure may ruin any image present).

Create separate areas for loaded and unloaded cassettes and label them clearly. Clean, maintain, and monitor the processing section the same way as conventional film processors. When performing sensitometric tests, create a sensitometry image in a darkroom area as discussed previously. Then, place the film manually into a cassette (obviously, in the darkroom) and unload it into the system so it can be processed by the daylight system's automatic film processor. At this point, the indicators of processor performance (e.g., B + F or D_{min}) are determined. Maintain temperature and humidity in the area where the daylight system is in use according to the manufacturer's specifications, because high humidity results in films sticking together and jamming inside the unit. Humidity that is too low could result in static artifacts on the resulting images.

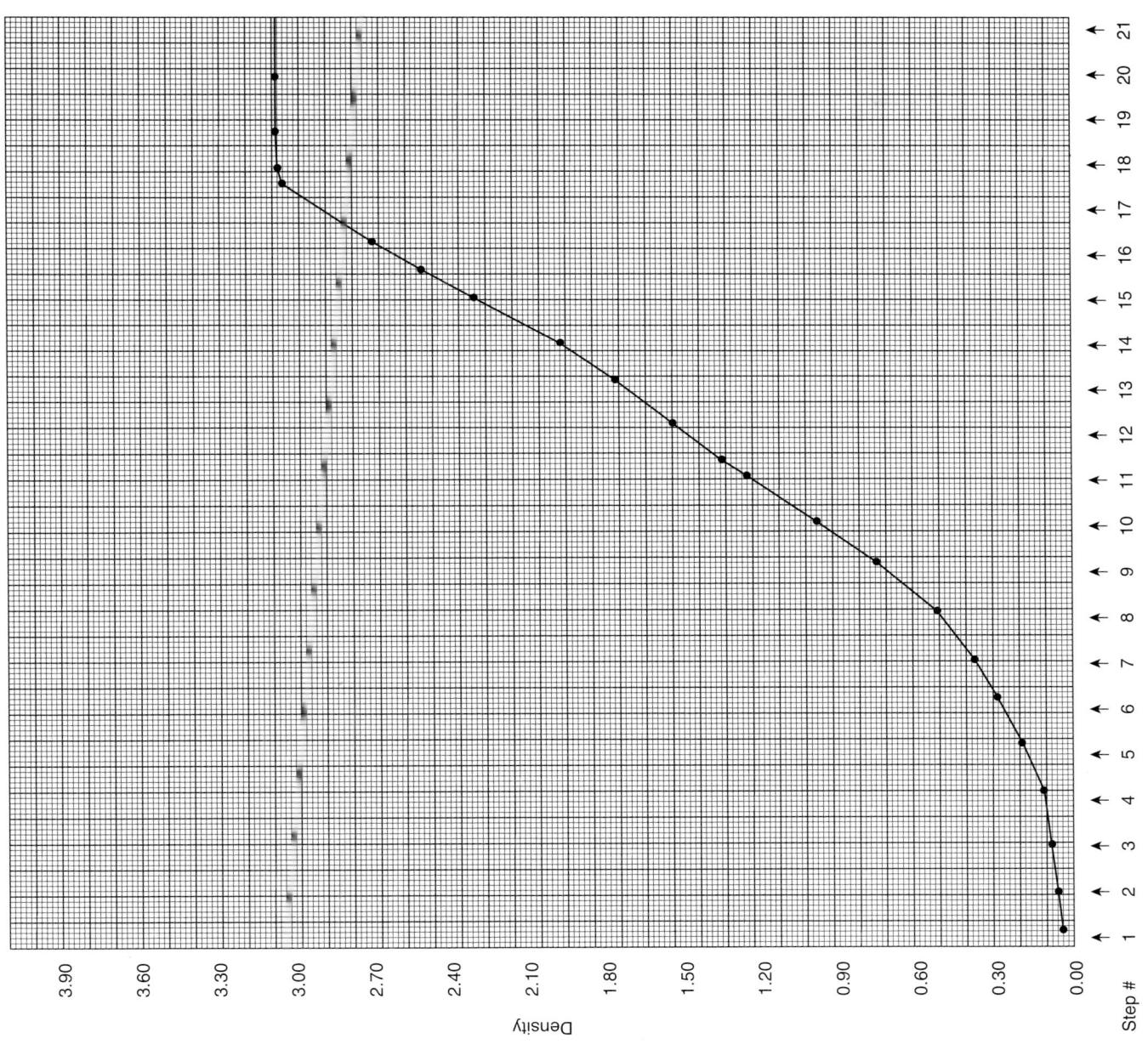

FIGURE 5-10 Sample plotting of a characteristic curve.

CHAPTER 5 Processor Quality Control

TABLE 5-1 | Processor Control Chart Troubleshooting Guide

Processor Problem	Trend in Graph	Image Appearance	Corrective Action
Unsafe darkroom	Sharp increase in B + F with a sudden decrease in the contrast indicator but no change in developer temperature	Increased fog level	Check safelight filter, check for light leaks, check film type and safelight type, check film storage conditions
Developer temperature too high	Sharp increase in speed and contrast indicators, with a smaller increase in B + F	Excessive optical density	Check incoming water temperature or developer thermostat setting
Developer temperature too low	Slight decrease in B + F, with sharp drops in speed and contrast indicators	Optical density too low	Check incoming water temperature or developer thermostat setting
Developer concentration or pH too high	Sharp increase in speed and contrast indicators, with a smaller increase in B + F	Excessive optical density	Check replenishment rates, mix fresh solutions, or both
Developer concentration or pH too low	Sharp increase in speed and contrast indicators, with a smaller increase in B + F	Optical density too low	Check replenishment rates, mix fresh solutions, or both
Underreplenishment	Gradual decline in contrast and speed indicators, with normal values for B + F	Decreased fog level and overall decrease in optical density	Check replenishment rates
Overreplenishment	Increase in B + F level and speed indicator, with a decrease in contrast indicator temperature	Increased fog level and decrease in image contrast	Check replenishment rates
Oxidized developer	Slight increase in B + F with a decrease in speed and contrast indicators	Loss of image contrast	Drain developer tank and mix fresh solution; add correct amount of starter solution

B + F, base + fog.

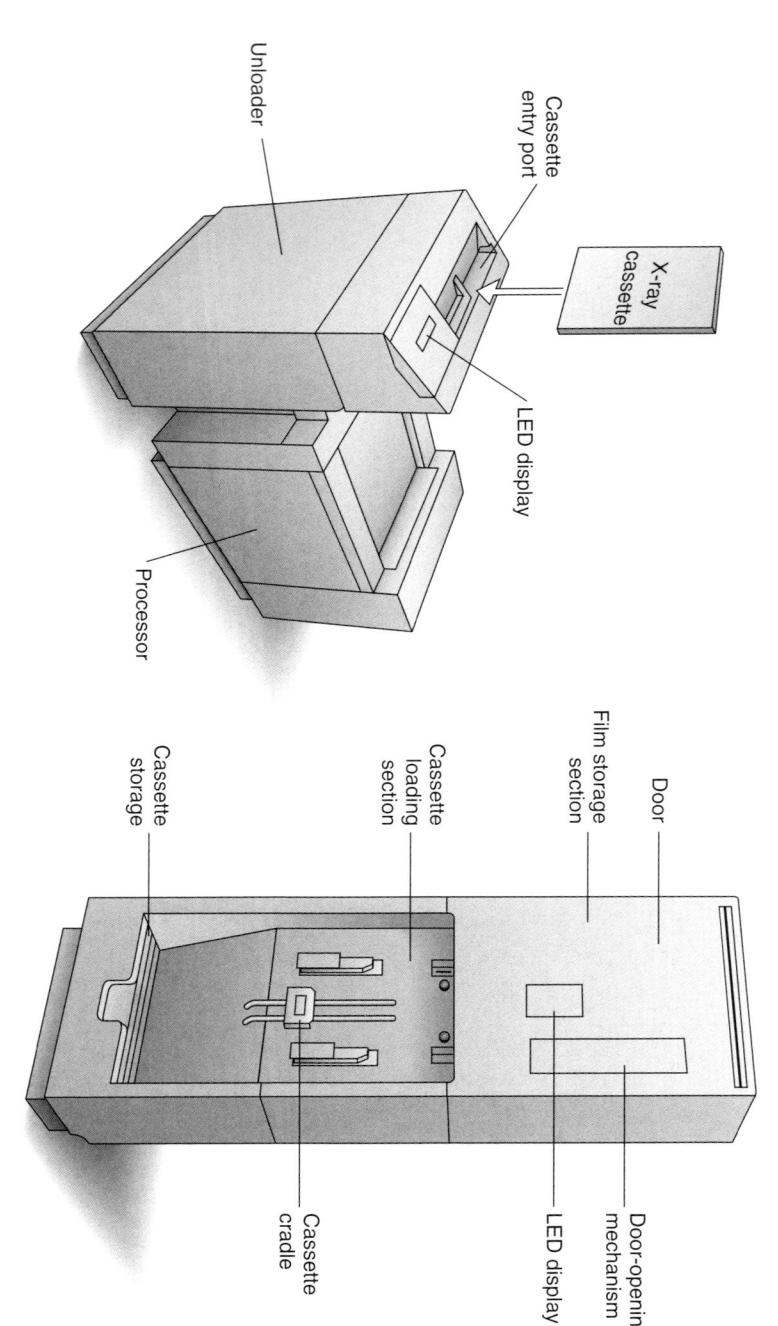

FIGURE 5-11 Daylight systems. LED, light-emitting diode.

CHAPTER 5 Processor Quality Control

SUMMARY

An established processor quality control program should reduce image variability to a minimum, which should also reduce the number of repeat images required and maintain the acceptable level of image quality established by the facility.

Refer to the Evolve website at https://evolve.elsevier.com for Student Experiments 5.1: Quality Control of Mechanized Processors and 5.2: Daily Processor Quality Control.

REVIEW QUESTIONS

1. What is the margin of error for the specific gravity of processing solutions?
   a. 0.002
   b. 0.004
   c. 0.006
   d. 0.1

2. Which of the following cannot be determined by an H and D curve or a processor control chart?
   a. Film sensitivity
   b. Film contrast
   c. Recorded detail
   d. B + F

3. What type of film does the presence of bromide drag produce?
   a. Overdeveloped
   b. Underdeveloped
   c. Underfixed
   d. Overfixed

4. When is the best time to process sensitometric films?
   a. Morning, after the processor is warmed up
   b. Late morning or midday, after the peak-demand period
   c. Late afternoon, during the low-demand period
   d. Evening, during the lowest-demand period

5. Which of the following terms best describes a device designed to give precise, reproducible, and graded light exposures to a film?
   a. Densitometer
   b. Photometer
   c. Sensitometer
   d. Penetrometer

6. Which of the following values is the maximum variation allowed for the contrast indicator in daily sensitometric films?
   a. ±0.01
   b. ±0.05
   c. ±0.15
   d. ±0.2

7. Which of the following characteristics explains why daily quality control activities are usually required for film processing systems?
   a. High degree of complexity
   b. High degree of variability
   c. High degree of consistency
   d. None of the above

8. Which of the following will have the greatest effect in causing the processor control limits to exceed accepted values?
   a. Dryer temperature too low
   b. Amount of water flow too high
   c. Increased replenishment rates
   d. Fluctuation in developer temperature

9. How often should sensitometric testing be performed on automatic film processors?
   a. Weekly
   b. Daily
   c. Monthly
   d. Semiannually

10. Which of the following terms defines the relationship between the intensity of radiation absorbed by the film and the optical density produced?
    a. Densitometry
    b. Dosimetry
    c. Sensitometry
    d. Sensitivity

CHAPTER 6
Silver Recovery

KEY TERMS

Agitation
Archival film
Avoirdupois oz
Channeling
Chemical precipitation
Dwell time
Electrolysis
Green film
Metallic replacement
Recirculating electrolytic unit
Scrap exposed film
Sulfurization
Terminal electrolytic unit
Troy oz

OBJECTIVES

At the completion of this chapter, the reader should be able to do the following:

- Describe the role of silver recovery in diagnostic imaging
- List the reasons for silver recovery in diagnostic imaging
- Describe the methods of recovering silver from processing solutions
- List the factors that affect the efficiency of silver reclamation devices
- Describe the methods of recovering silver from film

OUTLINE

Justification for Silver Recovery
  Worldwide Supply of Silver
  Monetary Return to the Diagnostic Imaging Department
  Federal and State Pollution Laws
Silver Recovery from Processing
  Chemicals
  Metallic Replacement
    Steel Wool Cartridge
    Iron-Impregnated Foam Cartridge
  Electrolytic Silver Recovery
    Terminal Electrolytic System
    Recirculating Electrolytic System
  Direct Sale of Used Fixer
  Chemical Precipitation
  Ion Exchange or Resin Systems
Silver Recovery from Film
  Green Film
  Scrap Exposed Film
  Archival Film
Summary

Before the digital revolution in diagnostic imaging, the recovery of silver from film and film processing was a standard practice in most hospitals and medical centers for more than 40 years. In 1967, the federal government lifted previous regulations governing the sale of silver, which escalated the price and therefore increased the demand on worldwide markets. Since digital imaging became the norm in diagnostic imaging, the use of silver in the photographic industry (which was the largest single user of silver worldwide in 1980, consuming approximately 30% of the total used) has decreased to only 5.5% worldwide. Film used in diagnostic imaging, which is estimated to be roughly one-half of all photographic film, is included in this amount. Approximately 58 million troy oz of silver is used in the photographic film worldwide each year. The total worldwide consumption of silver is approximately 1 billion troy oz. A **troy oz** is a unit for measuring precious metals such as silver. There are 14.58 troy oz in 16 **avoirdupois oz**, or standard ounces.

The largest industrial consumer of silver is the electronics industry, which uses approximately 44% of all silver. Silver conducts electricity better than most substances, and it also resists oxidation and rusting. For this reason, most electronic devices, from the smallest electronic watches to the space shuttle, contain some quantity of silver.

The sterlingware industry consumes approximately 22% of all silver. Pure silver is relatively soft (much like lead) and is mixed with copper to create sterling silver. In general, 925 parts of pure silver are mixed with 75 parts of copper to make sterling silver.

Some medical uses of silver (other than film) include the construction of metal prostheses used in repairing broken bones or replacing joints, and the 1% solution of silver nitrate sometimes put into the eyes of newborns by physicians to prevent infection.

Other uses of silver include water treatment filters, in which silver is used as a bactericide, and the catalytic converters of some automobiles. The federal government stopped minting silver coins for general circulation in 1964 but still issues special-edition or commemorative coins on a limited basis.

JUSTIFICATION FOR SILVER RECOVERY

The three basic reasons for a diagnostic imaging department to institute a silver recovery program are the dwindling worldwide supply of silver, monetary return to the diagnostic imaging department, and compliance with federal and state pollution laws.

Worldwide Supply of Silver

The current worldwide shortage of silver is the result of little silver being mined because of low prices and high refining costs. Political instability in countries where silver is abundant also contributes to this shortage. Currently, more than 120 million troy oz of silver is consumed than produced annually in the United States. At this rate, current silver supplies may not last through this century. Even with the advent of digital cameras (used by the general public) and digital imaging for diagnostic purposes, the demand for silver in film still exceeds the supply. The economic downturn in 2008 led to a dramatic increase in the price of silver; as of the writing of this text, the price is approximately double the 2008 rate of $15/troy oz. The photographic industry can recover approximately one-half of what is required annually, but eventually a serious shortfall will exist. Because diagnostic imaging constitutes a significant portion of the photographic use of silver, efforts to recover as much silver as possible are the responsibility of all diagnostic imaging department managers. Of the imaging departments that are still film based, it is estimated that 10% to 20% of all hospitals and 30% to 40% of all doctors' offices and clinics do not have silver recovery protocols in place.

Monetary Return to the Diagnostic Imaging Department

Money obtained from silver recovery procedures can be returned to the diagnostic imaging department to help offset the cost of processing supplies, materials, and equipment. Many studies have demonstrated that about 10% of the purchase price of film can be recovered through proper silver reclamation procedures. Therefore, if a department spends $50,000 annually for film, then about $5000 can be returned to the department's budget to help offset costs.

When silver reclaimed from processing chemistry or films is sold, bids should be solicited from several dealers so the best price can be negotiated. Familiarity with the current market prices according to the *Wall Street Journal* or similar business publications and websites is also helpful. It is also better to sell only once a year so that a higher volume price is obtained, and shipping and handling costs are reduced.

Federal and State Pollution Laws

The continual replenishment of chemical solutions used in film processors means that used solutions are disposed of in some manner. Used fixer and wash water contain silver in some form, which is a toxic heavy metal and therefore subject to strict pollution guidelines by the Environmental Protection Agency (EPA) and many state regulations. California has particularly strict pollution guidelines. Some of the important federal pollution laws are described in Box 6-1.

BOX 6-1 Important Federal Pollution Laws

Water Pollution Control Act of 1972
The Water Pollution Control Act of 1972 bans the placement of toxic substances in public waterways and sewer systems.

Resources Conservation/Hazardous Waste Act of 1976
The Resources Conservation/Hazardous Waste Act of 1976 requires available devices be used to remove toxic substances from waste water.

Clean Water Act of 1984
The Clean Water Act of 1984 amends the previous law (Clean Water Act of 1977), in that it requires the best available methods to be used to remove toxic substances from waste water. Silver is classified as a "priority pollutant" under this law, and the Act prohibits the discharge of these pollutants into surface waters.

Resource Conservation and Recovery Act of 1987
The Resource Conservation and Recovery Act of 1987 contains many guidelines affecting film processing and silver recovery methods, including the following:

1. The Act limits liquid waste to a level of no more than 5 mg/L or 5 parts per million (ppm) of silver. Used fixer and wash water may exceed this amount. Silver is considered a "characteristic hazardous material" under this law (Environmental Protection Agency (EPA) Hazardous Waste Number D011). Solid wastes containing 5 ppm or more of silver also are given the same classification. This may include processed and unprocessed radiographic film.
2. Special permits are required to dump more than 27 gallons of waste per month into public sewers. For private septic systems, a permit from the National Pollutant Discharge Elimination System and/or the EPA is required.
3. Shipping manifests are required to ship material such as silver recovery cartridges, scrap film, silver flake, or silver-laden fixer. The manifest forms required are EPA Forms 8700-12 and 8700-22.

A silver recovery system is required for most hospitals to remove silver from used processing solutions to meet the requirements of these laws. Some states and municipalities require that used wash water also be collected and disposed of through approved disposal companies because about 5% of the silver may be carried into the wash water. Silver recovery in a diagnostic imaging department can occur in processing solutions and film.

SILVER RECOVERY FROM PROCESSING CHEMICALS

One function of the fixer solution is to remove the unexposed and undeveloped silver halide crystals from the film. These crystals are suspended in the solution and eliminated with the used fixer by the replenishment system. Silver may accumulate at a rate of 100 mg/m² of film processed. This dissolved silver averages about 50% of the silver that was on the film originally and can be recovered by a variety of methods.

Metallic Replacement

The metallic replacement method is sometimes called the *displacement method* and it is the simplest and least expensive method a diagnostic imaging department can use to recover silver. It is the most widely used method of silver recovery from processing chemicals. The metallic replacement system incorporates a plastic bucket that is also referred to as a canister or cartridge (Fig. 6-1). These canisters are available in a variety of sizes, including 3.5, 5 (most popular in diagnostic imaging), 7.5, and 10 gallons, depending on the amount of film processed per month. Inside the canister is iron in some form, which reacts chemically with the acid and silver ions in the fixer through ion exchange (an oxidation-reduction reaction). When the acid in the fixer oxidizes the iron, electrons are released and used by the silver ions to form metallic silver. The more active iron ions replace the less active silver ions, which remain in the canister as the ions are picked up and washed out in the used fixer, hence the name **metallic replacement** (Figs. 6-2 and 6-3). The metallic replacement process is summarized by the following equation:

$$2Ag(S_2O_3)_2^{-3} + Fe^0 \rightarrow 2Ag^0 + Fe^{+2} + 4S_2O_3^{-2}$$

The two types of iron cartridges that can be used inside the canister are the steel wool cartridge and the iron-impregnated foam cartridge.

Steel Wool Cartridge. Because the primary component of steel is iron, packing the inside of the cartridge with steel wool yields a large surface area in which metallic replacement can occur. One pound of steel wool can collect 3 to 4 lb of silver. This is the more common type of cartridge insert because of its lower cost, but it is subject to three potential problems: channeling, rusting, and drain stoppage.

Channeling. Channeling occurs when an intermittent or low volume of fixer is used or when a fixer that is too acidic is used. In these situations, the fixer concentrates in almost a straight path, or channel, into and out of the cartridge, rather than moving uniformly throughout the steel wool. Because the solution comes in contact with very little steel wool, not much silver is reclaimed. Channeling can be avoided by filling the cartridge with fixer or water at the time of installation and allowing the fixer to dissipate throughout the cartridge as it enters.

Rusting. Iron exposed to moisture and air undergoes a chemical reaction that forms iron oxide, or rust. The

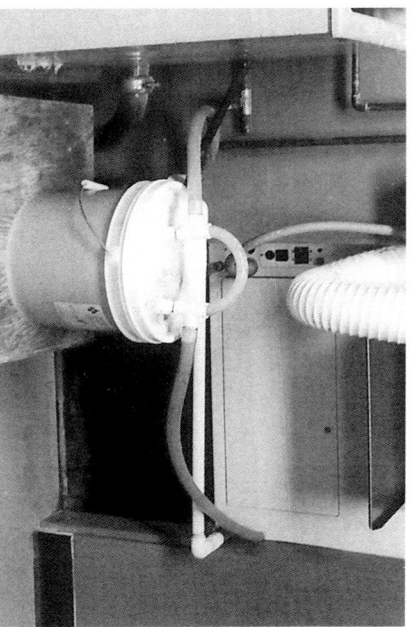

FIGURE 6-1 Metallic replacement silver recovery unit.

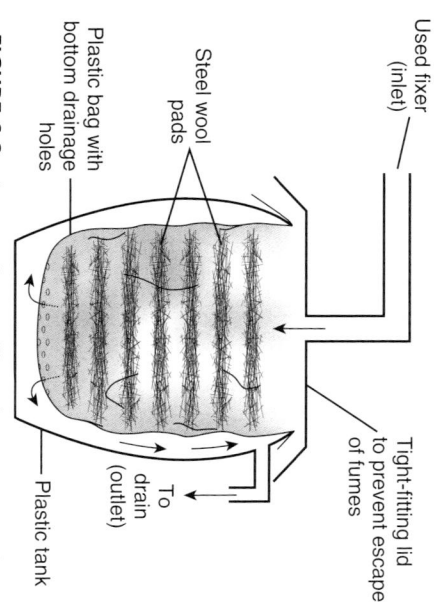

FIGURE 6-2 Diagram of a metallic replacement cartridge.

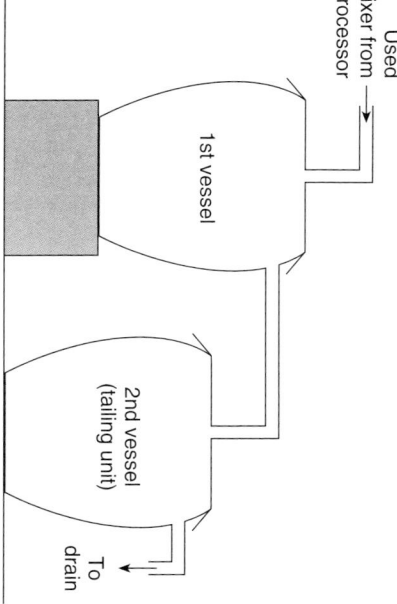

FIGURE 6-3 "Piggybacking" or "tailing" of metallic replacement units.

rust forms a barrier between the silver ions and the iron ions that prevents the metallic process from occurring or, at the very least, reduces the efficiency of the unit. Rusting occurs with units that are used infrequently.

Drain Stoppage. As the steel wool is dissolved by the acid present in the fixer, iron ions may be deposited on the inside of the drainage pipes, which can cause obstruction. A commercial drain cleaner composed of sodium bisulfate is used monthly, as mentioned in Chapter 5, to prevent this buildup.

Iron-Impregnated Foam Cartridge. An iron-impregnated foam cartridge uses fine iron powder impregnated in a tightly wound piece of plastic foam, similar to a plastic sponge. This design helps minimize channeling and rusting because the foam distributes the fixer more evenly. The suspended iron powder also provides 50% more surface area, so the efficiency of the unit is increased. The advantages and disadvantages of the metallic replacement method are discussed in Boxes 6-2 and 6-3.

Electrolytic Silver Recovery

The electrolytic silver recovery method is based on electrolysis, or electroplating, and uses an electric current to reclaim the silver (Fig. 6-4). Because unexposed, undeveloped silver halide is removed from the film by the fixer, the suspended silver is in the form of a positive ion (Ag$^+$), which means it is attracted to a metal electrode that has a negative charge (cathode). As these Ag$^+$ ions come in contact with the metal cathode, the silver collects in a layer that can be removed at a later time. The chemical reaction occurring at the cathode is summarized by the following equation:

$$Ag(S_2O_3)_2^{-3} + e^- \rightarrow Ag^0 + 2(S_2O_3)^{-2}$$

The cathodes in the electrolytic recovery units are usually made of stainless steel and are either drum shaped (Fig. 6-5) or disk shaped. For best results, the solution requires agitation so the silver ions are distributed evenly over the cathode surface. This is accomplished by rotating the cathode with a stationary anode or by a

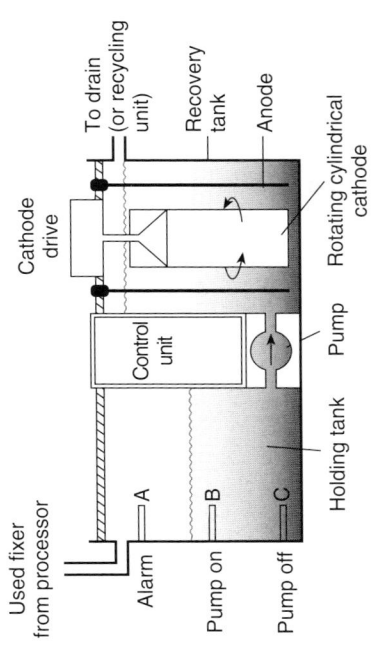

FIGURE 6-4 Diagram of an electrolytic silver recovery unit.

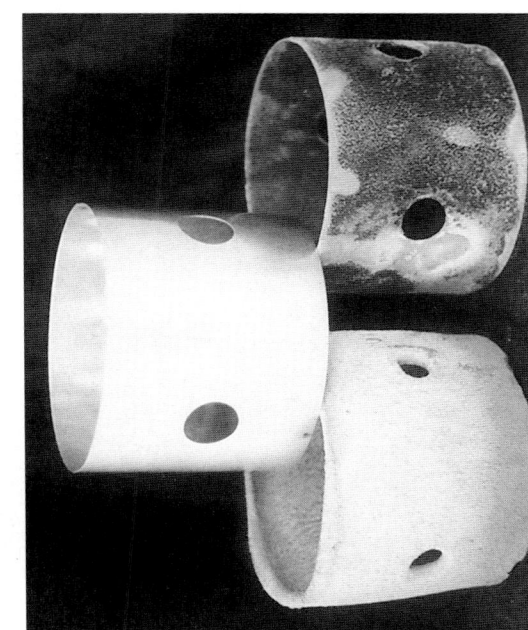

FIGURE 6-5 Cathodes from an electrolytic silver recovery unit. The top cathode is clean and unused. The left cathode contains more than 20 lb of silver flake after the correct amperage has been used. The right cathode contains silver that has been "burned" by an amperage setting that is too high.

BOX 6-2 Advantages of the Metallic Replacement Method

- Operating costs are not incurred because no electric current is used.
- Initial expense is low. These units can be purchased in bulk and stockpiled, and the cost per unit can be reduced even further. The average service life of a metallic replacement cartridge is 6 months. After this time, it must be replaced because most of the iron is gone.
- No moving parts or electrical connections are needed, so the unit requires very little maintenance.
- The units have a relatively high efficiency rating because as much as 95% of the recoverable silver is usually removed.

BOX 6-3 Disadvantages of the Metallic Replacement Method

- The units are not as efficient as the other methods discussed in this chapter. The cartridges operate at 100% efficiency for the first quarter of their life only, after which they operate at about 25% efficiency for the remaining life of the cartridge. A second unit can be connected to the primary unit to increase efficiency. This is known as *piggybacking* or *tailing* (see Fig. 6-3).
- The silver recovered is in the form of silver sludge, which is about 30% to 50% silver and 50% to 70% iron oxide. After the elapsed time of use has occurred, the unit is disconnected and the contents of the canister are sold to a silver dealer. Silver refiners charge a handling fee to process the silver from this sludge, which reduces the amount of money returned to the department.
- The unit must be replaced with a new one each time it is expended in the recovery cycle.
- Payment for the silver recovered is delayed until after processing the sludge because the amount of actual silver content in the sludge is not known until this time.

stationary cathode with rotating anodes. Another design that is available keeps the cathode and anode stationary and uses a self-contained pump to swirl the solution. Systems are available that recover 3 troy oz of silver or more per hour at 98% efficiency. The purity level of the silver ranges from 92% to 98%. The cathodes are removed periodically and the silver is stripped off. The silver-laden cathodes can be replaced immediately with cathodes that are clean so that only a minimal interruption in film processing occurs. When the silver-laden cathodes are cleaned (usually by scraping them with a screwdriver or paint scraper), they are reused at a later date. The anodes are also cleaned at this time because they may develop a layer of sulfate, which reduces efficiency. The chemical reaction that takes place at the anode of an electrolytic silver recovery unit is summarized by the following equation:

$$SO_3^{-2} + H_2O \rightarrow SO_4^{-2} + 2H^+ + 2e^-$$

The silver removed from the cathode is in the form of silver flake (Fig. 6-6), and its color ranges from cream or a light color to black. Silver flake that is cream or a light color reflects maximum purity. The darker the flake, the less pure the silver that has been recovered. An amperage control switch located on the unit regulates the amount of charge on the cathode to control the color and purity of the recovered silver flakes. The amount of this current is usually around 8 A for most systems. If the flake is too dark, too much amperage is being used and it is "burning" the silver. Too much amperage also causes the fixing agent to be converted to sulfide, which results in a foul-smelling (like rotten eggs), yellow-brown deposit of sulfur on the cathode. This process is known as *sulfating* or *sulfurization*. If the silver flake coating is very light or

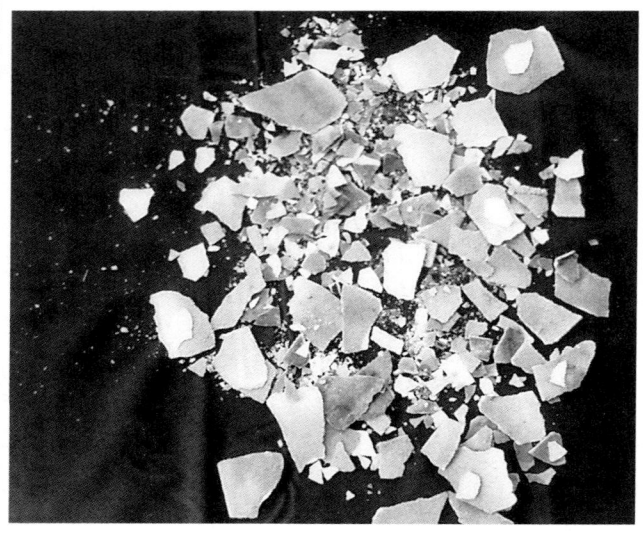

FIGURE 6-6 Silver flake that has been removed from a cathode after the correct amperage has been used.

silver, the amperage is too low. A computerized timer and current selector available on some models of electrolytic silver reclaimers adjust the current according to the time of day or use.

The two types of electrolytic silver recovery units are the terminal electrolytic system and the recirculating electrolytic system.

Terminal Electrolytic System. The terminal electrolytic unit is connected to the fixer overflow line from the processor replenishment system. When this unit recovers the silver, the used fixer is flushed down the drain. Most processor manufacturers recommend this type of electrolytic unit.

Recirculating Electrolytic System. The recirculating electrolytic unit (sometimes referred to as an *inline electrolytic unit*) is designed to recover silver from used fixer and then recirculate the fixer back into the processor. In general, this process does not conserve much fixer, because electrolysis destroys the preservative in the fixer. Fixer replenishment is decreased by no more than 20%. The main advantage of this method is that the overall concentration of silver in the fixer tank is decreased; therefore, the amount of silver transported into the wash water through the fixer is decreased, and the wash water may have a low enough silver content to avoid the thresholds of certain pollution standards. Most film manufacturers do not recommend using a recirculating electrolytic system because of the decreased archival quality of the processed films. The advantages and disadvantages of electrolytic silver recovery methods are discussed in Boxes 6-4 and 6-5.

Direct Sale of Used Fixer. Roughly 0.5 to 0.8 troy oz of silver is in each gallon of used fixer. In small-volume facilities (<10 gal/week), metallic replacement or electrolytic units may not be practical. In this case, used fixer can be collected in storage drums and sold to a refiner who reclaims the silver from the solution. The advantages of this method are that no capital outlay for equipment is required by the facility and no pollutants other than the used developer and wash water are discharged into a sewer system. The disadvantages are that considerable

---

BOX 6-4 Advantages of Electrolytic Silver Recovery

- Electrolytic silver recovery is more efficient than metallic replacement, without the problems of channeling, rusting, or drain stoppage.
- The silver recovered is in the form of silver flake, which is 92% to 98% pure, as opposed to sludge, which is 30% to 50% pure.
- Payment for the silver can be received on delivery of the flake to the refiner because the content is immediately apparent.
- Shipping costs of materials to the refiner are minimal.
- The system produces no new pollutants (as opposed to the sludge produced by metallic replacement).
- The system is reusable because the cathodes can be cleaned and reused.

handling or storage and a fee for the pickup and hauling of the solution (as much as $2-$6/gal of used solution) may be required, and the profit margin from the sale of the silver may be reduced.

Chemical Precipitation

Chemical precipitation is the oldest form of silver recovery. Using this method, the mixing of compounds such as sodium sulfite and zinc chloride with used fixer can cause a chemical reaction that results in the silver precipitating, or sinking, to the bottom of the tank or drum, where it can be removed. This method is fairly efficient, but it has many disadvantages including the following:

- The chemicals used are hazardous and require special precautions.
- Toxic fumes such as chlorine gas and hydrogen are created by the chemical reaction.
- A large drum or vat with adequate space is required.
- The process is labor intensive, which reduces the profit margin.

Because of these disadvantages, this method should not be attempted by diagnostic facilities; it should be carried out by licensed silver refiners or commercial photographic laboratories only. The silver in fixer sold directly to a silver refiner is usually reclaimed in this fashion.

Ion Exchange or Resin Systems

Ion exchange or resin systems use resin particles treated with an acid to give them a negative ionic charge. This system is similar to the resin system of a water softener found in many homes. The silver (Ag^+) is attracted to the negative charge in the resin, where it remains. A regeneration cycle is used to release the silver from the resin. This method requires a large amount of space (because of the resin columns) and is labor intensive (for the regeneration cycle). The resin can be regenerated only for so many cycles and then it must be replaced. The old resin column can be sent to a silver refiner for further recovery of silver. This method is best used for recovering silver from the used wash water (the acid in the fixer may mimic the regeneration cycle), and it can reduce the amount of silver in the wash water to as little as 0.1 to 0.5 ppm. Box 6-6 lists factors affecting silver recovery from processing solutions.

SILVER RECOVERY FROM FILM

As mentioned earlier, 50% of the silver is dissolved in the fixer, which means the other 50% remains on the film. For images not of diagnostic quality (which are not kept in patient files), the sheets of film can be stored in a bin and then sold to a silver refiner. Film of this nature is sometimes referred to as *pete*. A price per pound is negotiated for the film and the money paid to the facility. The three basic categories of film that hospitals and medical centers can release for sale are green film, scrap exposed film, and archival film.

BOX 6-5 Disadvantages of Electrolytic Silver Recovery

- A greater capital cost for equipment is incurred as opposed to metallic replacement. These units begin at about $250, and larger units cost several thousand dollars. Metallic replacement canisters cost vary considerably in price, but usually average about $25.
- An operating cost exists for these units because of the electricity consumed during operation.
- Special electrical or plumbing connections may be required in the processing area.
- Periodic monitoring and servicing of the equipment are required. Most units call for at least monthly monitoring and servicing, including checking the current level and flake color of the silver deposited on the cathode, to ensure maximum efficiency. The efficiency of silver recovery is estimated with special silver paper that changes color to indicate the silver content of the fixer that has passed through the unit. These test papers are usually accurate to within ±10% of the actual silver content. The amount of silver measured in the fixer should not exceed the values specified by the manufacturer. Otherwise, the current value must be changed or the cathode cleaned.

BOX 6-6 Factors Affecting the Efficiency of Silver Recovery from Processing Solutions

Dwell time: Dwell time is the time the fixer remains within the recovery device. The longer the dwell time, the greater the efficiency.

Agitation: Agitation helps distribute the silver ions throughout the device, thereby increasing its efficiency.

Surface area: An increase in the surface area of the recovery device increases the efficiency of silver recovery.

Solution temperature: If the solution temperature exceeds 95 °F (35 °C), the efficiency of the system decreases because of the increased kinetic energy of the silver ions.

Fixer pH: Silver recovery must take place in an acidic solution to release the silver ions; therefore, the fixer pH must be kept to less than 5.

Amperage: Amperage applies to electrolytic units only. The amperage must be kept to an optimal range to achieve maximum efficiency.

Maintenance: Poorly maintained units lose efficacy. Severely neglected units can clog, the fixer tank in the processor can overflow, and the developer can be contaminated or internal components damaged. With regard to electrolytic units, excessive corrosion can cause electrical hazards and these corroded elements must be removed. When obtaining silver from the cathode, clean out the bottom of the unit tank and scrub the anodes. Never allow more than 1 in of silver to accumulate on the cathode because the buildup may cause an electrical short circuit or may jam the rotating mechanism used for agitation. The excessive weight of the silver on the cathode also puts stress on the drive motor of this rotating mechanism and shortens its life span.

Green Film

Green film is film that has not been processed, such as film that has expired or film that was exposed to white light accidentally (which occurs when a film bin is opened in white light). Green film is the most valuable because all the silver is in place (usually about 0.4 troy oz/sheet of 14 × 17-in [35 × 43-cm] film). Because of its greater value, it is recommended that green film be separated from other categories of film to be sold and that a greater price per pound be negotiated.

Scrap Exposed Film

Scrap exposed film is film that has been exposed and processed, such as rejects, old sensitometry films, and even dry laser print films obtained from digital systems. This film contains about 0.11 troy oz of silver/14 × 17-in (35 × 43-cm) sheet and is therefore of least value.

Archival Film

Archival film is film that has been exposed and processed, and has outlived its use as a patient record. Most hospitals and associated medical facilities retain images for a minimum of 5 years (except for mammograms, which must be kept by a facility for either 10 years [if the patient never returns for another exam] or 5 years if the patient returns regularly). In general, archival film is released for sale, except for film containing certain pathologic conditions, or film required for litigation or pending litigation. With more imaging departments going digital, many facilities have either digitized or are in the process of digitizing film images from their old case files so they can be added to their current Picture Archiving and Communication System (PACS). This process creates a large quantity of archival film that must be disposed. Any film dated before 1974 contains 20% more silver (0.13–0.18 troy oz/14 × 17-in sheet) than film manufactured since then. The reason is that the price of silver escalated in 1974, and manufacturers responded by developing emulsions that maintain image quality with less silver. Any film in this category should be separated from newer archival film and scrap exposed film so a greater price per pound can be negotiated.

When a refiner obtains films from a diagnostic imaging department, the silver is reclaimed either by incineration (which burns the film and removes the silver from the ash) or chemical treatments (which use chemicals to remove, or leach, the silver from the film).

SUMMARY

In many diagnostic radiology departments, the quality control technologist is given the responsibility of determining the type of silver reclamation to be used, as well as providing unit maintenance and service during operation. A basic understanding of these systems is essential to fulfilling this responsibility.

Refer to the Evolve website at https://evolve.elsevier.com for Student Experiment 6.1: Silver Recovery.

REVIEW QUESTIONS

1. Which of the following units is used for measurement of precious metals such as silver?
   a. Standard ounce
   b. Avoirdupois ounce
   c. Troy ounce
   d. None of the above

2. Which of the following is the largest worldwide consumer of silver?
   a. Photographic industry
   b. Electronics industry
   c. Sterlingware industry
   d. Space program

3. The Resource Conservation and Recovery Act of 1987 limits liquid waste to a toxic level of no more than _____ ppm.
   a. 2
   b. 5
   c. 10
   d. 100

4. From which of the following components do most silver recovery systems reclaim the silver?
   a. Developer solution
   b. Fixer solution
   c. Wash water
   d. Dryer section

5. Which of the following is the simplest and least expensive method of silver reclamation?
   a. Metallic replacement method
   b. Electrolytic method
   c. Chemical precipitation
   d. Resin method

6. Which of the following problems are associated with steel wool metallic replacement cartridges: (1) channeling, (2) rusting, or (3) drain stoppage?
   a. 1 and 2 only
   b. 2 and 3 only
   c. 1 and 3 only
   d. 1, 2, and 3

7. When electrolytic silver recovery units are used, the silver is deposited on which of the following?
   a. Anode
   b. Cathode
   c. Both the cathode and the anode
   d. Neither the cathode nor the anode

CHAPTER 6 Silver Recovery

8. The oldest form of silver recovery is the _____ method.
   a. metallic replacement
   b. electrolytic
   c. chemical precipitation
   d. resin

9. Which of the following are factors that affect the efficiency of silver reclamation systems: (1) dwell time, (2) agitation, or (3) surface area?
   a. 1 and 2 only
   b. 2 and 3 only
   c. 1 and 3 only
   d. 1, 2, and 3

10. What percentage of silver is usually dissolved in the fixer solution during film processing?
    a. 10%
    b. 25%
    c. 50%
    d. 90%

CHAPTER 7

Quality Control of X-ray Generators and Ancillary Radiographic Equipment

KEY TERMS

Actual focal spot
Automatic exposure control
Comparator
Coulomb per kilogram
Detector
Effective focal spot
Focal spot blooming
Grid latitude
Grid uniformity
Half-value layer
High-frequency
Homogenous phantom
Ion chamber
Kilowatt rating
Law of Reciprocity
Linear tomography
Line focus principle
Linearity
Mobile X-ray generator
Objective plane
Photodetector
Pluridirectional tomography
Portable X-ray generator
Reciprocity
Reproducibility
Roentgen
Sensor
Single-phase
Solid-state detector
Three-phase
Voltage ripple

OBJECTIVES

At the completion of this chapter, the reader should be able to do the following:

- Explain the difference between single-phase, three-phase, and high-frequency X-ray generators
- Recognize the voltage waveform characteristics of the three types of X-ray generators
- List the voltage ripple values for the three types of X-ray generators
- Calculate the power output rating for the three types of X-ray generators
- List the three main parts of a quality control program for radiographic equipment
- List and describe the performance tests for radiographic equipment
- List the main components of an automatic exposure control system
- Perform quality control testing of various automatic exposure control parameters
- Describe the quality control parameters for conventional tomographic systems
- Discuss the importance of grid uniformity and alignment on image quality
- Explain the quality control tests performed on mobile equipment

OUTLINE

X-ray Generator
   Single-Phase Generator
      Half-Wave Rectified
      Full-Wave Rectified
   Three-Phase Generator
      Three-Phase, Six-Pulse Generators
      Three-Phase, 12-Pulse Generators
   High-Frequency Generator
      Voltage Ripple
      Power Ratings
   Control or Operating Console
   High-Voltage Generator
   X-ray Tube, Tube Accessories, and Patient Support Assembly
Quality Control Program for Radiographic Units
   Visual Inspection
      Control Console
      Overhead Tube Crane
      Radiographic Table
      Protective Lead Apparel
      Miscellaneous Equipment
   Environmental Inspection
   Performance Testing
      Radiation Measurement

CHAPTER 7 Quality Control of X-ray Generators and Ancillary Radiographic Equipment

OUTLINE—cont'd

Reproducibility of Exposure
Beam Quantity
Filtration Check
Kilovolt (Peak) Accuracy
Voltage Waveform
Timer Accuracy
Milliampere and Exposure Time Linearity and Reciprocity
Focal Spot Size
Beam Restriction System
X-ray Beam–Alignment
Source-to-Image Distance and Tube Angulation Indicators
Overload Protection
X-ray Tube Heat Sensors
Ancillary Equipment
Automatic Exposure Control Systems
  Detectors
    Photodetectors
    Ion Chambers
    Solid-State Detectors
  Comparator
  Automatic Exposure Control Testing
    Backup, or Maximum Exposure, Time
    Minimum Exposure Time
  Quality Control for Automatic Exposure Control
    Reproducibility
    Density Control Function
    Reciprocity Law Failure
Conventional Tomographic Systems
  Quality Control of Tomographic Systems
    Section Uniformity and Beam Path
    Patient Exposure
Grids
  Grid Uniformity
  Grid Alignment
Portable and Mobile X-ray Generators
  Portable X-ray Generator
  Mobile X-ray Generator
  Cordless, or Battery-Powered, Mobile Units
  High Frequency Mobile Units
Summary

Several of the previous chapters have addressed film/screen image receptors (digital image receptors are discussed in a later chapter) and the importance of quality control testing to avoid poor-quality images. However, many other components of diagnostic imaging departments are subject to variability and must have separate quality control protocols established to ensure safe operation and function. One such component is the equipment used as the X-ray source in conventional radiography, including the X-ray generator, the control or operating console, a high-voltage generator, and the X-ray tube, tube accessories, and patient support assembly.

X-RAY GENERATOR

The X-ray generator is the largest component of the radiographic unit. It contains the high-voltage transformers, rectifiers, timing circuitry, and milliampere (mA) and kilovolt (peak) (kVp) selectors. Single-phase, three-phase, and high-frequency X-ray generators are available.

Single-Phase Generator

A single source of alternating current is used to power the generator in a **single-phase generator**. A representation of single-phase alternating current is shown in Fig. 7-1.

The graph in Fig. 7-1 plots the voltage on the y-axis versus time on the x-axis. The peaks in the graph represent the flow of electricity changing direction throughout the circuit. Voltage values range from 0 V to a peak value (hence the term *kilovolts [peak]*) and back to 0 V. The two types of single-phase generators used in

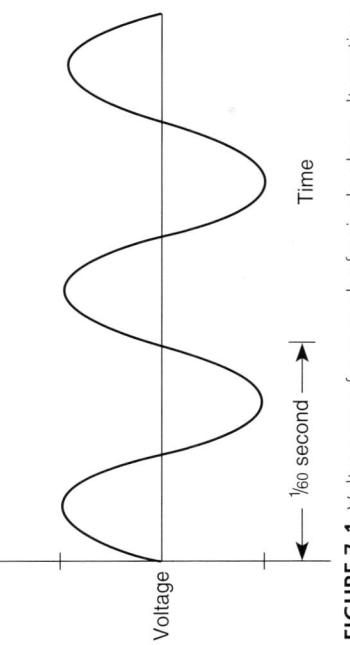

FIGURE 7-1 Voltage waveform graph of a single-phase alternating current.

diagnostic radiography are half-wave rectified and full-wave rectified.

Half-Wave Rectified. In a half-wave rectified generator, one-half the normal alternating current wave is used to power the X-ray tube and the other half is shut off by the addition of one or two rectifiers. This design causes the normal single-phase alternating current waveform graph to appear as shown in Fig. 7-2.

Because the standard frequency of alternating current in the U.S. is 60 Hz, or 60 cycles per second (a cycle represents the current flowing in each direction one time), only 60 pulses of electricity per second can be used to create X-rays. This means the X-rays are emitted in pulses, or spurts, and therefore a longer amount of time is required to obtain a specific quantity of X-rays. For this reason, half-wave rectified units are generally used in dental X-ray units and some small portable X-ray units.

Full-Wave Rectified. Full-wave rectified generators use a combination of four rectifiers to channel all the pulses

92 CHAPTER 7 Quality Control of X-ray Generators and Ancillary Radiographic Equipment

through the X-ray tube during X-ray production. The resulting waveform graph for this type of unit appears in Fig. 7-3.

Because 120 pulses of electricity per second can be used to create X-rays, twice as many X-rays can be created during a given period compared with the half-wave unit. This fact allows full-wave rectified units to be used for many conventional radiographic procedures. However, the X-rays are still emitted in pulses (as demonstrated by the number of times the pulses reach 0 V on the waveform graph) and therefore still require some exposure time to achieve a specific quantity of X-rays. The shortest exposure time available for single-phase X-ray generators is 1/120 second. For this reason, full-wave rectified units are seldom found in larger hospitals but may be found in doctors' offices and small clinics.

Three-Phase Generator

Three-phase X-ray generators are powered by three separate sources of alternating current that are staggered so they are "out of phase" with one another by 120° or one-third of a cycle. The voltage waveform graph for three-phase alternating current appears in Fig. 7-4.

By the time one pulse of current begins to drop toward 0 V, another pulse is heading back up to the maximum value, so the voltage never reaches 0 V and X-rays are produced constantly (eliminating the pulsed effect of single-phase units), which allows exposure time values as low as 1/1000 second (1 ms). The X-rays created with three-phase units also have a greater average energy than those of single-phase units because the voltage is near the peak value for a greater percentage of the time during X-ray production (which can lower patient dose compared with single-phase units). The main disadvantages of three-phase equipment are greater capital cost (at least twice as expensive as a single-phase unit) and the size of the unit (because of the additional electronic components required). In general, the advantages outweigh the disadvantages, and the three-phase X-ray generator has been the most common type of unit in major hospitals and medical centers since the 1970s. The two types of three-phase generators are 6-pulse and 12-pulse generators.

Three-Phase, Six-Pulse Generators.
The six-pulse type of three-phase unit uses six rectifiers and one-half the three-phase alternating current pulses. The resulting voltage waveform appears in Fig. 7-5.

As mentioned previously, one cycle of single-phase alternating current refers to one pulse of electricity traveling each direction one time so that two pulses comprise one cycle. Because 60 cycles occur each second, one cycle requires a time of 1/60 second. In a three-phase, six-pulse X-ray generator, six pulses of electricity exist during the same cycle or 1/60-second time interval (instead of two pulses per 1/60 second in single phase), hence the name *three-phase, six-pulse*. This means that 360 voltage pulses are now available per second.

Three-Phase, 12-Pulse Generators.
The three-phase, 12-pulse type of X-ray generator uses 12 rectifiers (four rectifiers per phase) that direct all the three-phase alternating current pulses through the X-ray tube during X-ray production. This action yields 12 pulses of

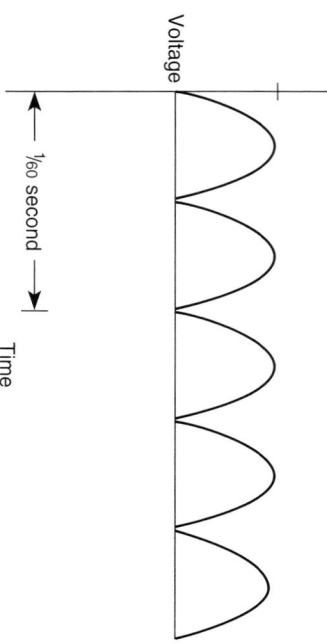

FIGURE 7-2 Voltage waveform graph of a half-wave rectified, single-phase current.

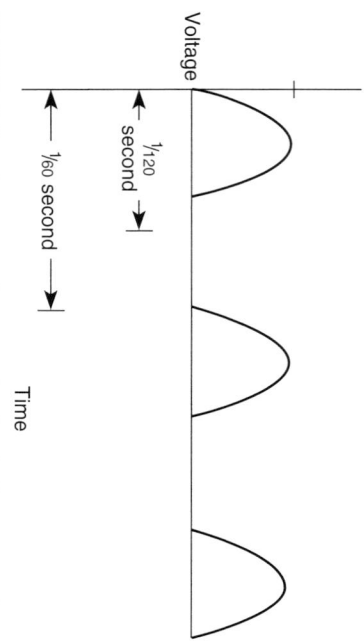

FIGURE 7-3 Voltage waveform graph of a full-wave rectified, single-phase current.

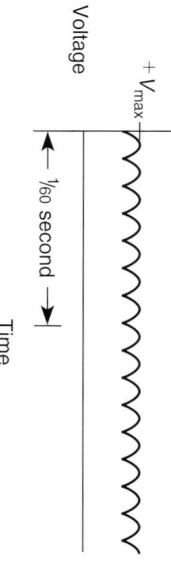

FIGURE 7-4 Voltage waveform graph of a three-phase alternating current.

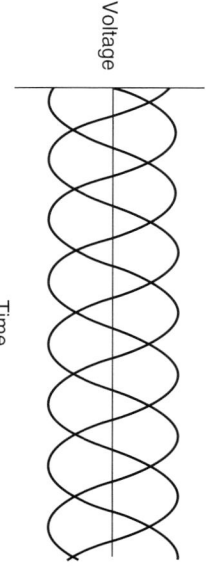

FIGURE 7-5 Voltage waveform graph of a three-phase, six-pulse alternating current.

CHAPTER 7 Quality Control of X-ray Generators and Ancillary Radiographic Equipment

electricity per one-cycle (1/60-second) time interval, for a total of 720 voltage pulses available per second. This unit is more efficient than the three-phase, six-pulse unit but is more expensive in capital cost. The voltage waveform for a three-phase, 12-pulse X-ray generator appears in Fig. 7-6.

High-Frequency Generator

Developed during the late 1970s, **high-frequency** X-ray generators are the newest generators available. They are sometimes referred to as *medium-frequency generators*, depending on the design and manufacturer. These units use either single-phase or three-phase sources of alternating current that are first fed into a microprocessor circuit before entering the high-voltage section. This microprocessor changes the frequency of the alternating current from the standard 60 Hz to as much as 100,000 Hz in some of the more recent models. It is then rectified and smoothed with capacitors before application across the X-ray tube, which causes the pulses to merge together and results in a voltage waveform such as the one that appears in Fig. 7-7.

High-frequency generators and three-phase generators produce similar voltage waveforms. However, the capital cost and power requirements for high-frequency units are far less than those for three-phase units. The transformers in high-frequency units can be smaller because they are much more efficient at higher frequencies (according to Faraday's Law of Electromagnetism), which accounts for the lower capital cost. The transformers also reduce the space requirement for installation. Because these units yield most of the advantages of a three-phase unit but at a fraction of the cost, they have become very common in hospitals, medical centers, clinics, and doctors' offices.

Voltage Ripple. Voltage ripple is a term used often to distinguish the voltage waveforms of each type of X-ray generator. A voltage ripple is the amount of variation from the peak voltage that occurs during X-ray production. For single-phase units, the voltage ripple is considered to be 100% because the voltage drops from its peak all the way to 0 V before increasing again, so 100% of all possible voltages are obtained. For three-phase equipment, the voltage does not decrease all the way to 0 V. One pulse increases as soon as the previous one falls, which yields a voltage ripple of 13% for a three-phase, six-pulse generator and ripple of 3.5% for a three-phase, 12-pulse unit. High-frequency generators can create voltage ripple values between 1% and 15%, which are comparable with those of three-phase units.

Power Ratings The power output of an X-ray generator is used to measure the capacity of X-ray production from the individual unit. This value is measured in kilowatts (kW) and is called the **kilowatt rating**. It is usually calculated by determining the maximum combinations of kilovolts (peak) and milliamperes that can be achieved by a particular generator at an exposure time of 100 milliseconds. These two values are then placed into the following equations:

$$\text{Three-phase and high-frequency kW} = \frac{kVp \times mA}{1000}$$

$$\text{Single-phase kW} = \frac{kVp \times mA \times 0.707}{1000}$$

The rippling effect of the single-phase alternating current requires that the 0.707 multiplier be added to the equation.

CONTROL OR OPERATING CONSOLE

The control or operating console contains all the various controls to operate the X-ray machine (e.g., kilovolt (peak) selector, milliampere selector) and various meters to monitor the production of X-rays. Guidelines by the U.S. Food and Drug Administration (FDA) mandate that diagnostic X-ray machine operating consoles must indicate the conditions of exposure (kilovolt [peak], milliampere-second [mAs]) and when the X-ray tube is energized. The conditions of exposure usually are indicated by the milliampere and kilovolts (peak) selection mechanism (i.e., the milliampere or kilovolt [peak] buttons or computer touch pad keys that are pushed). There is also either an analog or a digital milliamp-second meter to indicate the quantity of X-rays produced by the X-ray unit. These meters also are used to indicate energized X-ray tubes and to detect lights or audible signals. Characteristics for the control booth area, which houses the operating console of a radiographic X-ray unit, include the following:

1. The floor of the control booth must be 7.5 square foot or larger.
2. The exposure switch should be fixed within the booth at a position at least 30 inches from any open edge of the booth wall and should be closest to the examining table.

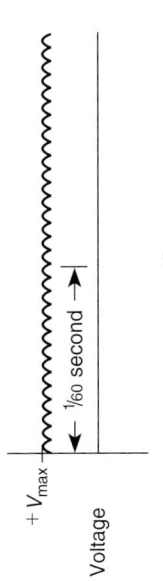

FIGURE 7-6 Voltage waveform graph of a three-phase, 12-pulse current.

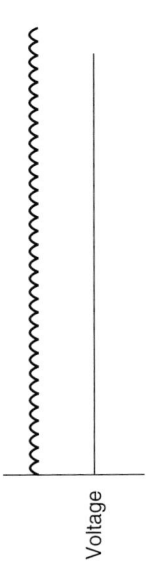

FIGURE 7-7 Voltage waveform graph showing the resulting current through the X-ray tube in a high frequency X-ray generator.

3. X-ray photons must scatter at least twice before they can enter any opening in the control booth. Each time an X-ray photon scatters, its intensity from the scattering object is 1/1000 of the original intensity, at a distance of 1 meter.
4. The control booth window must have the same shielding requirements as the walls (usually a 1.5-mm lead equivalent), be at least 1 square foot in size, and be mounted at least 5 feet above the floor. There should be no obstructions blocking the view of the patient table.
5. The wall of the control booth, facing the radiographic examination table, must be at least 7 feet high and fixed to the floor.
6. Any door on the control booth that is an entrance to the examination room must be interlocked with the control panel so that an exposure cannot be made unless the door is closed.

HIGH-VOLTAGE GENERATOR

The high-voltage generator of the radiographic unit is responsible for converting the relatively low-voltage values supplied by the power companies (usually 220-440 V) to the kilovolt levels necessary for the production of diagnostic radiographs. Included in this generator is a high-tension transformer, which is a shell-type step-up transformer that increases the voltage level selected using an autotransformer to the kilovolts selected on the control console. Also included in the high-voltage generator is a filament (step-down) transformer that feeds a stepped-down voltage level to the filament of the X-ray tube. This area also may contain rectifiers that convert the alternating current of the incoming power supply to a pulsating direct current that is fed to the X-ray tube for X-ray production. The number of rectifiers ranges 4 to 12, depending on the type of X-ray generator, and are usually solid state in nature. The high-voltage generator is normally housed in a metal box that may be found in the X-ray room or in a nearby area, such as the control booth. High-voltage cables (one going to the cathode of the X-ray tube and another to the anode) connect the high-voltage generator to the X-ray tube.

X-RAY TUBE, TUBE ACCESSORIES, AND PATIENT SUPPORT ASSEMBLY

The third main part of any radiographic X-ray unit is a combination of the X-ray tube, X-ray tube support mechanism, patient support assembly (i.e., X-ray examination table), and X-ray tube accessories such as the collimator and added filtration. Most radiographic X-ray tubes are rotating anode X-ray tubes that can withstand greater kilovolt (peak) and milliampere-second combinations than the stationary anode X-ray tubes used in dental offices and in small portable X-ray machines. The X-ray tube must be equipped with a metal housing to prevent leakage of radiation. This housing must confine the leakage amount to less than 100 milliroentgens (mR) per hour when measured at a distance of 1 meter away from the housing. The X-ray tube must also be equipped with a variable-aperture collimator to control the size of the X-ray field (discussed in detail later in this chapter). The X-ray tube support mechanism that holds the X-ray tube in position over the Bucky device must have the following characteristics (the Bucky device contains the image receptor and is taught to x-ray students on the first day of the program):

1. The support mechanism must be strong because the X-ray tube, insulating coil, collimator, and metal housing are heavy.
2. The support mechanism should be counterbalanced to help offset the weight of the X-ray tube and accessory devices. This design makes the assembly more stable and allows it to be moved more easily during patient positioning.
3. Immobilization locks must be incorporated into the support mechanism to hold the X-ray tube in position.
4. The X-ray tube position, in relation to the image receptor, must be indicated clearly (source-to-image distance [SID] indicator) and must be accurate to within 2% of the SID.

In addition, if a radiographic examination table is present (as opposed to an upright Bucky or chest unit), the maximum tabletop thickness over the Bucky assembly is 1 millimeter of aluminum equivalent to prevent the tabletop material from absorbing excessive amounts of radiation before reaching the image receptor (which would, therefore, increase the patient dose).

QUALITY CONTROL PROGRAM FOR RADIOGRAPHIC UNITS

When the X-ray equipment has been installed successfully and has passed all acceptance tests, it needs to be monitored periodically to ensure it continues to perform according to the manufacturer's specifications. This periodic testing is the quality control testing of the equipment. The three parts of a quality control program for radiographic equipment are visual inspection, environmental inspection, and performance testing.

Visual Inspection

Visual inspection includes checking the main components of the equipment for proper function, mechanical condition, and safety. This inspection should be performed at least annually (monthly for American College of Radiology [ACR] accreditation) with a checklist for documentation. An example of this checklist is provided on the Evolve website. The inspection should include the control console, overhead tube crane, radiographic table, protective lead apparel, and miscellaneous equipment.

CHAPTER 7 Quality Control of X-ray Generators and Ancillary Radiographic Equipment

Control Console. The control console contains all the selectors for controlling X-ray production (milliampere, kilovolts [peak], and exposure time) and the various meters that monitor the operation of the generator. Control console inspection includes verifying the proper function of X-ray tube heat sensors and the overload protection indicator (discussed later in this chapter). The proper functioning of all panel lights, meters, and switches must be verified as well. The inspection should ensure a proper view of the exposure room through the window (an unobstructed view of the examination table) and the presence of an up-to-date technique chart.

Overhead Tube Crane. The overhead tube crane is the mounting bracket that holds the X-ray tube over the X-ray table. Items to evaluate in this section include the condition of the high-voltage cables and other wires (are they discolored or frayed?); the condition of the cable brackets, clamps, or tie-downs (are they intact and functioning normally?); the stability of the system; proper movement; SID and angulation indicator function (discussed later in this chapter); detent operation; lock function; the Bucky center light; collimator light brightness (discussed later in this chapter); and interlock function.

Radiographic Table. A patient is usually in contact with the X-ray table throughout the diagnostic procedure, so it must be kept clean and safe. Items to inspect include surface condition and cleanliness of the tabletop, power top and angulation switches, Bucky tray and cassette locks, stability, table angulation indicator (use a protractor to verify the indicator is accurate to within ±2°), and the condition of any footboard or shoulder braces. The tabletop material over the Bucky area should not absorb more than 1.0 millimeters of aluminum equivalent.

Protective Lead Apparel. Lead aprons and gloves should be present in the radiographic room and should have a minimum 0.5 millimeters of lead-equivalent thickness. Standards set forth by accrediting agencies dictate that health care organizations must perform routine inspections on protective lead apparel. They should be radiographed or viewed fluoroscopically (with remote fluoroscopy if possible) on acceptance and then every 6 months thereafter to determine whether any cracks or holes are present (Fig. 7-8). Keep a log of when these inspections are performed, as well as the results and any corrective action. Software programs are available for maintaining inspection reports. When not in use, protective lead apparel should be properly hung to prevent cracks. Lead vinyl sheets and gonadal shields also should be evaluated in the same manner. If a piece of lead protective apparel is no longer usable, it must be disposed of in an appropriate manner. According to the Health Physics Society, lead and other heavy metals meet the criteria for a hazardous material under the Resource Conservation and Recovery Act. The best option for disposal is to recycle the protective apparel so the lead can be reused.

Miscellaneous Equipment. A measuring caliper should be present in radiographic rooms in which the manual technique is used along with a technique chart to establish the correct exposure factors. Ensure that positioning sponges and other patient position aids are clean and free of contrast media. Check the manual integrity of any step stools or intravenous fluid stands as well.

Environmental Inspection

Environmental inspection should be performed at least annually (it may need to be performed more frequently with older equipment), and it involves checking for mechanical and electrical safety. Often, it can be performed along with the visual inspection. One item included in the environmental inspection is evaluation of the condition of the X-ray tube high-tension cables, which is accomplished by checking the covering on the outside of the cables (or any other wires that are visible on the outside of the unit). Any discoloration of the outside insulation, especially where the wire or cable bends, could be an indicator of internal heat and a potential short circuit. Consult a biomedical engineer, medical physicist, or vendor service technician if discoloration is present.

The mechanical condition of the X-ray tube counterweights and tracks (especially in overhead tube stands) must also be included in the environmental inspection. Lubricate the moving parts.

Electrical safety is critical for both the patient and the equipment operator. All radiographic equipment should be grounded and all obvious electrical connections should be intact.

Should the possibility of a short circuit exist, never touch an electrical device with one hand while the other hand is touching any type of conductor; doing so directs the flow of electricity through the heart. If someone is experiencing an electric shock, do not grasp the person directly. Instead, either open the main switch (turn off the power) or use some type of insulator (dry wooden board) to separate the person from

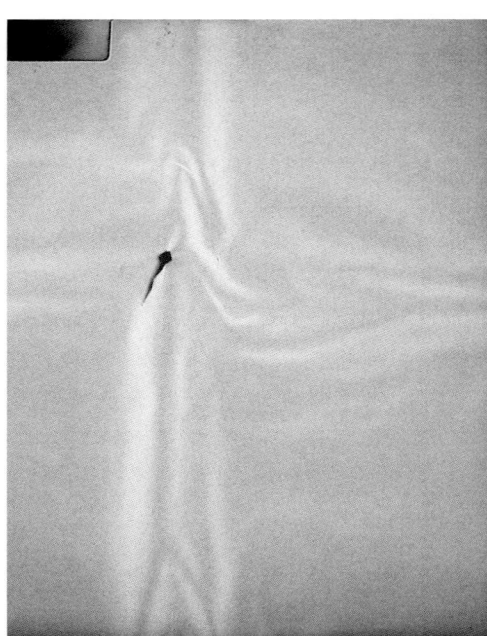

FIGURE 7-8 Image of lead apron with a large hole in the center.

the source of the electricity. A good rule of thumb to remember when dealing with electric current is that the combination of high voltage and low amperage tends to throw a person, whereas a combination of low voltage and high amperage tends to hold a person and is potentially more dangerous. For older equipment or equipment that has a history of problems with electrical safety, a biomedical engineer, medical physicist, or vendor service technician should be consulted for environmental inspections (you may also wish to have them accompany you during these inspections). Many states require that an electrical inspection record be posted on the equipment.

Performance Testing

Performance testing evaluates the performance of the X-ray generator and X-ray tube with specialized test instrumentation, which can range from simple phantoms and test tools to sophisticated computerized systems such as the Noninvasive Evaluation of Radiation Output, or NERO, system (Fig. 7-9), or similar devices available from various manufacturers. These computerized systems make the data gathering for performance evaluations quick and easy, but they cost thousands of dollars. It is more common for facilities to use several smaller devices to gather the necessary data. The results of these tests must be documented for governmental and accreditation agencies. Many states and the ACR require these performance tests be performed by a medical physicist. However, radiographers should know how the tests are performed and how to interpret the results. Sample forms for many of these tests are provided on the accompanying Evolve website.

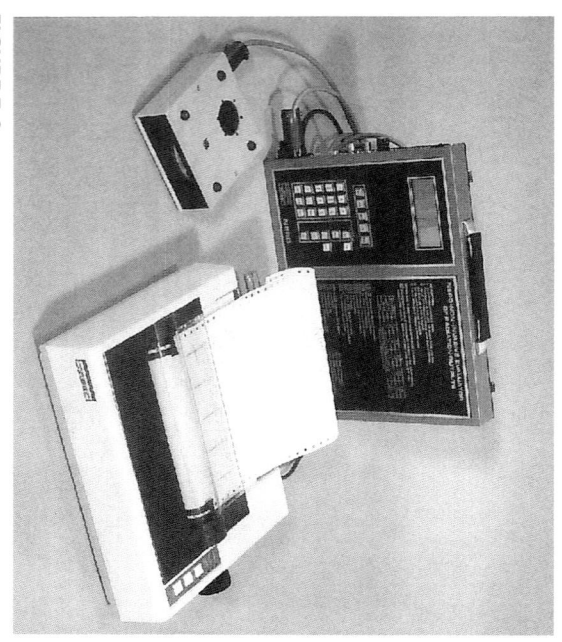

FIGURE 7-9 The noninvasive evaluation of radiation output system is a microprocessor that can be programmed to acquire and analyze exposure data, providing quality control test results for numerous parameters. (From Ballinger PW: Merrill's atlas of radiographic positions and radiologic procedures, ed 9, St Louis, 1999, Mosby.)

Radiation Measurement.
Much of the data obtained during performance testing includes radiation measurement; therefore, some type of radiation detector is a standard piece of equipment for many of these tests. The more common type of detector used in performance testing is the gas-filled chamber. As radiation enters this chamber, it ionizes the gas along its path (Fig. 7-10), which produces a trail of ions that allows the flow of current through the chamber for a split second. This current is converted to a voltage pulse that is amplified and counted. The size of the voltage pulse is proportional to the energy expended in the chamber by the incident radiation. A quenching material may be added to the chamber to speed the return of ions to a stable state. There are three types of gas-filled chamber detectors, which vary according to the chamber voltage (Fig. 7-11): the ion chamber, the proportional counter, and the Geiger-Müller counter.

Ion Chamber.
With 100 to 300 V placed on it, the ion chamber is the least sensitive of the three chambers. The ion chamber is useful for measuring X-rays because a high sensitivity is not required for their detection; ion chambers are often used in performance testing. They usually are available as pocket ionization chambers (also called *pocket dosimeters*) and analog or digital dosimeters (Fig. 7-12). They also can be used as the sensor in automatic exposure control systems and as the detectors in computed tomographic scanners.

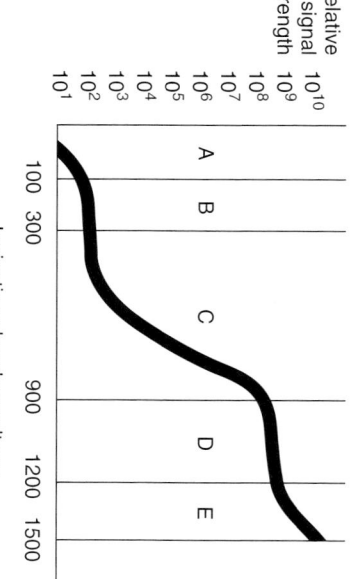

FIGURE 7-10 Schematic diagram of an ion chamber.

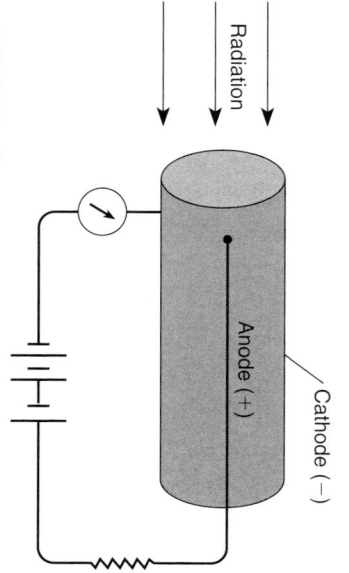

FIGURE 7-11 Graph showing how the intensity of the signal from a gas-filled detector increases as the voltage across the chamber increases. **A**, region of recombination; **B**, ionization region; **C**, proportional region; **D**, Geiger-Müller region; **E**, region of continuous discharge.

CHAPTER 7 Quality Control of X-ray Generators and Ancillary Radiographic Equipment

Proportional Counter. A voltage of 300 to 900 V placed on the chamber increases the sensitivity. Proportional counters are often used in stationary laboratory counters to measure small quantities of radioactive material.

Geiger-Müller Counter. A voltage of 900 to 1200 V placed on the chamber yields the greatest sensitivity. Geiger-Müller counters often are used for contamination control in nuclear medicine departments.

Some newer types of radiation-monitoring devices use a solid-state or semiconducting detector instead of an ionization chamber. These models incorporate a crystal of either silicon or germanium with selected impurities (such as lithium) added to detect the incident radiation. When the crystal is attached to an electric current, little or no current can flow through the crystal because no free electrons are available.

If the crystal is exposed to radiation, electrons are dislodged within its matrix and electric current can flow through it. The increase in current is proportional to the amount of radiation incident on the crystal and is registered with an analog or digital meter. This type of detector is relatively small and accurate but usually costs more than ionization chambers. It is also more sensitive than a gas-filled chamber. In most gases, an average energy of 30 to 40 electron volts (eV) is expended per ion pair produced. In a silicon semiconductor, an ion pair is produced for each 3.5 eV deposited by the incident radiation. For germanium detectors, only 2.9 eV are required to produce an ion pair, which means many more ion pairs are produced in semiconductor detectors (compared with ion chambers) for a given amount of energy absorbed.

The value obtained from the radiation detector is most often the radiation intensity, which can be measured in a special unit called the **roentgen (R)** or in an International System of units called **coulomb per kilogram (C/kg)**.

Because both units measure a relatively large amount of radiation, smaller increments of milliroentgens or microcoulombs per kilogram are most often obtained during performance testing. Some detectors are designed so that the exposure rate (intensity of radiation per unit of time) can be displayed in addition to the radiation intensity, and they are known as *rate meters*. Detectors also can be calibrated to measure absorbed dosage in rads or grays (Gy). One rad is equivalent to 0.01 Gy or 1 cGy. Rads or grays are also used to measure a value known as *air kerma*, which is discussed in Chapter 9.

Reproducibility of Exposure. An X-ray generator should always produce the same intensity of radiation each time the same set of technical factors is used to make an exposure. For example, if 80 kVp, 500 mA, and 0.02 second yields 100 mR radiation when measured with a dosimeter, then at any future time when the same technical factors are entered into the same X-ray generator, the yield, when tested, should be 100 mR. This concept is known as reproducibility. ❶ *The maximum variability allowed in reproducibility is ±5% according to (1020.31(b)), 21 Code of Federal Regulations Subchapter J.* Evaluation of reproducibility variance requires a dosimeter, unless a computerized noninvasive system is used. Reproducibility testing should be performed after equipment installation, after a major system repair, and then annually.

PROCEDURE

1. Place a lead apron on top of a radiographic tabletop with the center of the lead apron in the approximate center of the tabletop. Place a dosimeter on top of the lead apron. The lead apron absorbs backscatter from the tabletop material, which reduces the accuracy of any readings obtained. If a lead apron is unavailable, substitute a sheet of lead vinyl. Center the central ray of the X-ray beam on the dosimeter using a SID of 40 in. Collimate the beam so that the X-ray field is just slightly larger than the dosimeter or remote probe.
2. Make a series of three to five separate exposures of the dosimeter at 80 kVp, 100 mA, and 100 ms. Clear the dosimeter (reset to zero) after each exposure. Record each reading on some type of documentation form, such as the Radiographic Survey Form found on the Evolve website.
3. With the readings obtained, use the following equation to determine reproducibility variance:

$$\text{Reproducibility variance} = \frac{(mR_{max} - mR_{min})}{(mR_{max} + mR_{min})}$$

where mR_{max} is the maximum amount of milliroentgens and mR_{min} is the minimum amount of milliroentgens.

The calculated variance should be less than 0.05 (5%) for a properly functioning X-ray generator. This test should be performed after installation of new equipment and then annually or when service is performed on the X-ray generator or X-ray tube. Variations in X-ray generator performance (e.g., kilovolt (peak) selector, milliamp selector, rectifier failure) or X-ray tube operation (e.g., filament evaporation, arcing) can cause the reproducibility variance to exceed accepted limits, which produces radiographs of inconsistent quality and necessitates repeat patient exposure to radiation.

$1 R = 2.58 \times 10^{-4} C/kg$

$1 C/kg = 3.88 \times 10^{3} R$

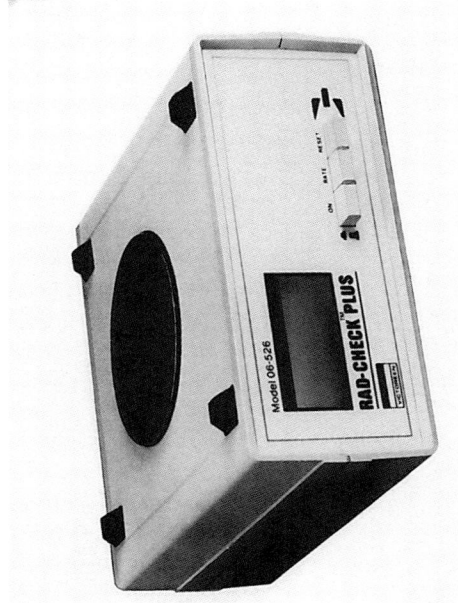

FIGURE 7-12 Digital dosimeter. *(Courtesy Gammex/RMI, Middleton, WI.)*

Beam Quantity. X-ray generators should emit a specific amount of radiation (measured in milliroentgens or microcoulombs per kilogram) per unit of X-ray tube current and time (milliampere-seconds). In addition, similar types of X-ray generators and tubes in a department should emit the same values of milliroentgens per milliampere-seconds (microcoulombs per kilogram per milliampere-seconds) so that technique charts can be valid in all rooms and the number of repeat examinations can be reduced. The original value of milliroentgens per milliampere-seconds (microcoulombs per kilogram per milliampere-seconds) is determined after installation of the unit or at the start of the quality control program. This original value is usually obtained at 80 kVp, 100 cm SID, and 2.5 mm aluminum total filtration. The beam quantity (also known as radiation output) is then measured annually and compared with this original value. The original installation value and future values should be within ±10% of each other in a properly functioning X-ray generator. In addition, values obtained in different radiographic rooms with similar X-ray generators and tubes also should be compared and should fall within ±10% of each other to establish room-to-room consistency. If these rooms exceed the 10% variation limit, they should have separate technique charts provided for each room. The beam quantity for single-phase generators should be approximately 4.0 ± 0.8 mR/mAs at 80 kVp, 100 cm SID, and 2.5 mm aluminum total filtration whereas three-phase and high-frequency units should be approximately 2.5 mm 6.0 ± 1 mR/mAs at 80 kVp, 100 cm SID, and 2.5 mm aluminum filtration.

Many states and TJC require the posting of this value to guarantee the X-ray generator does not emit excessive amounts of radiation exposure for a given combination of kilovolts (peak) per milliamperes-seconds.

The ACR specifies a maximum entrance exposure for chest and abdominal views obtained with an ACR phantom. Chest views should not exceed a maximum exposure of 50 mR (measured with a dosimeter); abdominal views should not exceed 1100 mR.

Filtration Check. Proper filtration is necessary to remove low-energy photons from the X-ray beam (1020.30(m), 21 CFR Subchapter J). A patient's skin dose can increase by as much as 90% if the photons are not removed. This test should be performed after installation and then annually or whenever service is performed on the X-ray tube or collimator. The best method to determine whether adequate filtration exists is to measure the **half-value layer** (HVL), which is the amount of filtration that reduces the exposure rate to one-half its initial value, because it is not usually possible to measure inherent filtration. The reason the measurement is not easily acquired is a result of filament evaporation that takes place continually, which adds a layer of tungsten to the inside of the X-ray tube window. By measuring the HVL (which measures beam quality) instead of the total amount of filtration, it does not matter how much material is in the path of the beam, as long as sufficient beam quality is measured and obtained. Using HVL for determining sufficient filtration is also relatively easy and is noninvasive. The HVL should not vary from its original value (which is established after installation) or its value at the beginning of the quality control program. It is dependent on the kilovolts (peak) used, the total beam filtration, and the type of X-ray generator (Fig. 7-13, Table 7-1).

A quick test to determine whether adequate filtration is present can be performed in cases in which HVL value measurements cannot be made. However, this quick test indicates the presence of adequate filtration only and not the actual amount of filtration; therefore, it should not take the place of HVL measurements during formal quality control testing. Using this method, a dosimeter and a 2.3-mm-thick aluminum plate are used.

Kilovolt (Peak) Accuracy. The X-ray tube voltage (measured in kilovolts [peak]) has a significant effect on image contrast, optical density, and patient dose. Therefore the kilovolts (peak) stated on the control panel should produce an X-ray beam with a comparable and consistent amount of energy. ❶ *Variations between the stated kilovolts (peak) and the X-ray*

PROCEDURE

1. Place a dosimeter on the radiographic tabletop on top of a lead apron or sheet of lead vinyl, with an SID of 40 in or 100 cm (just as in step 1 of the procedure to determine reproducibility).

2. Make an exposure at 80 kVp, 100 mA (large focal spot), and 100 ms (10 mAs). Some physicists recommend that the dosimeter be placed under a homogenous phantom of aluminum or acrylic plates or in the Bucky for this measurement, any of which are satisfactory, but the test must always be performed the same way so the values can be compared for variation.

3. Divide the radiation measurement recorded from the dosimeter by 10 mAs to obtain the value of milliroentgens per milliampere-seconds, or microcoulombs per kilogram per milliampere-seconds. Record this value and repeat the test at least annually (with the same procedure and exposure factors). Compare the current and previous readings, then determine the percent deviation with the following equation:

$$\text{Percent mR/mAs variation} = \frac{(\text{mR/mAs}_{min} - \text{mR/mAs}_{min})}{\text{mR/mAs}_{max}} \times 100$$

❶ *The original installation value and future values should be within ±10% of each other in a properly functioning X-ray generator.* In addition, values obtained in different radiographic rooms with similar X-ray generators and tubes also should be compared and should fall within ±10% of one another to establish room-to-room consistency. If these rooms exceed the 10% variation limit, they should have separate technique charts provided for each room. Variation in milliroentgens per milliampere-seconds (microcoulombs per kilogram per milliampere-seconds) for a single room can occur over time as a result of problems in X-ray generator calibration, timer circuit inaccuracy, and filament evaporation from the cathode of the X-ray tube (some of the tungsten from the filament is deposited on the inside of the window of the X-ray tube, which causes additional filtration of the beam).

CHAPTER 7 Quality Control of X-ray Generators and Ancillary Radiographic Equipment

PROCEDURE

1. Place a dosimeter on the radiographic tabletop on top of a lead apron or lead vinyl (to prevent backscatter).
2. Adjust the tube-to-dosimeter distance to between 60 and 80 cm, and collimate the X-ray beam to an area slightly larger than the dosimeter.
3. Make an exposure at 80 kVp and 50 mAs and record the amount of radiation from the dosimeter on a documentation form such as the HVL Evaluation Form found on the Evolve website.
4. Clear the dosimeter and add a 1-mm-thick aluminum plate between the bottom of the collimator and the dosimeter and expose it. Record the reading and clear the dosimeter. Repeat this procedure, adding aluminum plates in 1-mm increments until a total of 6 to 8 mm are in place.
5. Use semilog graph paper and plot a graph of X-ray intensity (dosimeter readings) on the y-axis versus absorber thickness on the x-axis (see Fig. 7-13). Draw in a curve by connecting the dots in the graph. The HVL is determined by taking one-half the maximum dosimeter reading and then drawing a line from this point on the y-axis to the curve, then drawing another line from this point on the curve down to the x-axis. This value on the x-axis represents the HVL, and it should be greater than 2.3 mm or more because this is the minimum HVL at 80 kVp, according to the FDA. HVL amounts at various kilovolt (peak) values are given in Table 7-1.

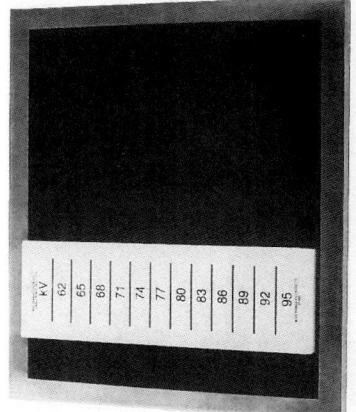

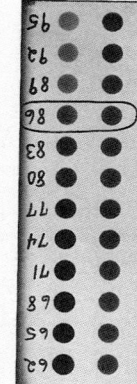

FIGURE 7-14 Wisconsin Test Cassette. (*Courtesy Gammex/RMI, Middleton, WI.*)

beam quality must be within ±5%. For example, if 80 kVp is selected on the control panel, the maximum X-ray beam energy should fall within ±4 kVp of this value. The kilovolt (peak) accuracy can be determined using a specialized test cassette, such as the Wisconsin Test Cassette (Fig. 7-14), Ardan and Crook's cassette, or a digital kilovolt (peak) meter (Fig. 7-15), according to the respective manufacturers' instructions. The

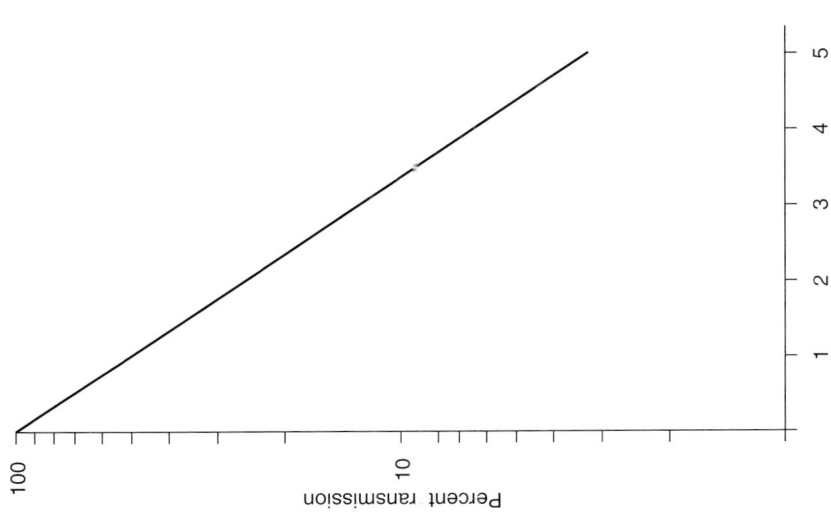

FIGURE 7-13 Semilog plot of radiation intensity versus attenuator thickness for determination of the half-value layer (HVL). HVL, half-value layer.

TABLE 7-1	Minimum HVL Values for Diagnostic X-ray Units		
X-ray Tube Voltage (kilovolt [peak])		Minimum HVL (mm aluminum)	
Designed Operation Range	Measured Operating Potential	Specified Dental Systems	Other X-ray Systems
<50	30	1.5	0.3
	40	1.5	0.4
	49	1.5	0.5
50-70	50	1.5	1.2
	60	1.5	1.3
	70	1.5	1.5
>70	71	2.1	2.1
	80	2.3	2.3
	90	2.5	2.3
	100	2.7	2.7
	110	3.0	3.0
	120	3.2	3.2
	130	3.5	3.5
	140	3.8	3.8
	150	4.1	4.1

HVL, half-value layer.

digital meters are usually more accurate and easier to use (because when they are exposed, the measured kilovolts [peak] appears automatically with a light-emitting diode [LED] readout) but are more expensive than the test cassettes. The test cassettes require that a film be placed inside and exposed to a specific set of technical factors. The resulting image is then analyzed visually or with a densitometer to obtain the measured kilovolts (peak). Whichever device is used for this test, it should estimate the peak voltage at various kilovolt (peak) stations available for the particular X-ray generator being evaluated. This process should be done in 10- to 20-kVp increments, usually beginning with 50 kVp. This test should be performed after installation and then annually or when service is performed on the X-ray generator or tube. Variations in kilovolt (peak) output may be caused by variations in the line voltage supplying the X-ray generator, by faulty high-voltage cables, or by problems with the autotransformer/kilovolts (peak) selection circuitry.

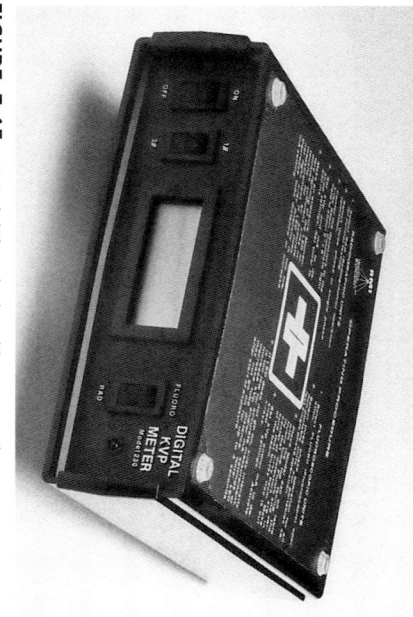

FIGURE 7-15 Digital kilovolt (peak) meter. (Courtesy Gammex/RMI, Middleton, WI.)

PROCEDURE

1. Place the dosimeter on the radiographic table on top of a lead apron.
2. Make an exposure at an SID of 40 in at 80 kVp and 50 mAs and record the reading.
3. Clear the dosimeter and make a second exposure using the same technical factors but with the aluminum plate between the detector and the X-ray source.
4. Place the readings obtained into the following equation:

$$\frac{\text{Exposure with aluminum plate}}{\text{Exposure without aluminum plate}}$$

If adequate filtration is present, the number obtained from the equation should range from 0.5 to 0.75. If the number is less than 0.5, beam filtration is inadequate. If the number is greater than 0.75, excessive filtration exists, which is legally acceptable but can be an indicator of pending X-ray tube failure because of excessive tungsten deposits on the X-ray tube window resulting from filament evaporation.

Voltage Waveform. As discussed previously, each type of X-ray generator creates a distinctive voltage waveform. If the waveform could be displayed on an oscilloscope screen during X-ray production, considerable information could be obtained concerning kilovolt (peak) accuracy, timer accuracy, rectifier malfunctions, loading characteristics, contact or switching problems, and high-voltage cable or connector arcing (Fig. 7-16) because these variables affect the size or shape of the waveform. An oscilloscope is hooked up electronically (only by personnel with an extensive electronics background such as physicists, biomedical engineers, or service engineers) to specific areas of the X-ray generator, or it can be attached to a commercially available X-ray output detector (Fig. 7-17). This detector is placed in the X-ray beam, and the output cable is connected to the oscilloscope input. Newer versions of the output detector can be attached to a laptop computer, iPad, or similar

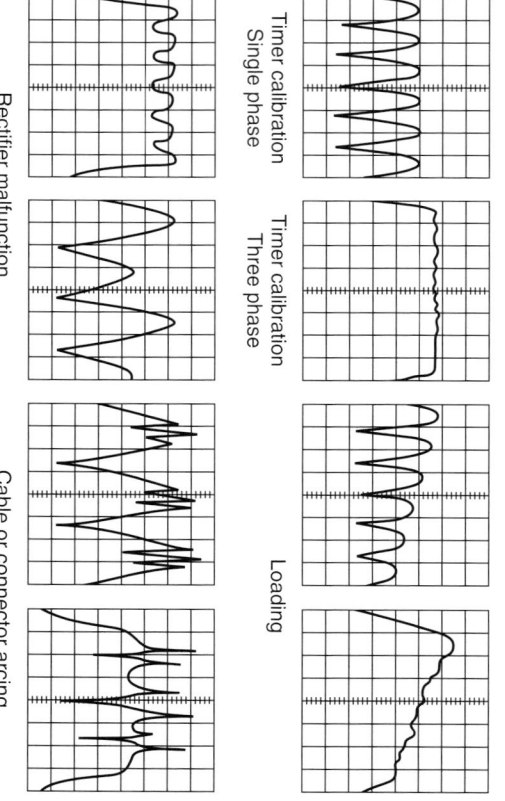

Timer calibration Single phase · Timer calibration Three phase

Rectifier malfunction · Loading · Cable or connector arcing

FIGURE 7-16 Voltage waveforms indicating various conditions within the X-ray generator.

CHAPTER 7 Quality Control of X-ray Generators and Ancillary Radiographic Equipment

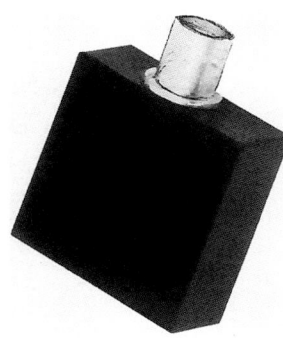

FIGURE 7-17 Output detector for obtaining voltage waveforms. (*Courtesy Nuclear Associates, Inc., Carle Place, NY.*)

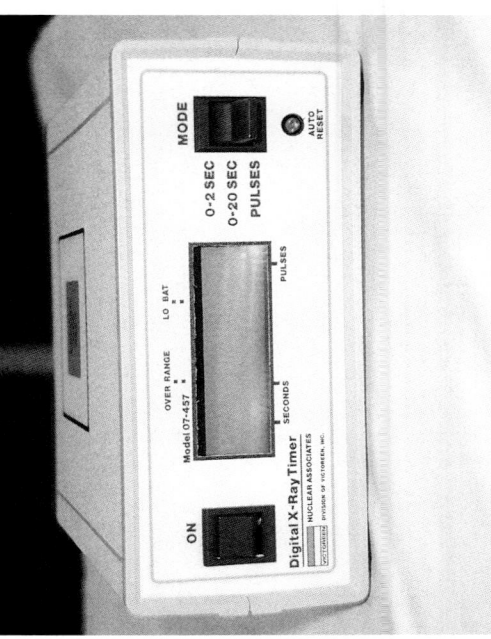

FIGURE 7-18 Digital timer for radiographic units. (*Courtesy Nuclear Associates, Inc., Carle Place, NY.*)

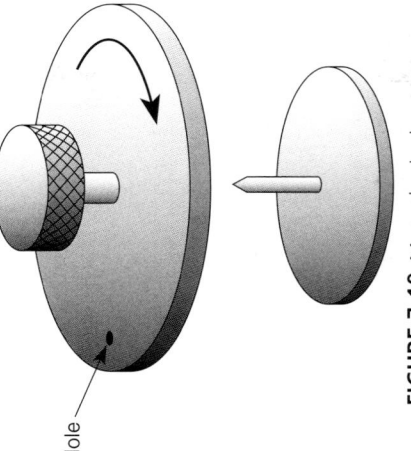

FIGURE 7-19 Manual spinning top.

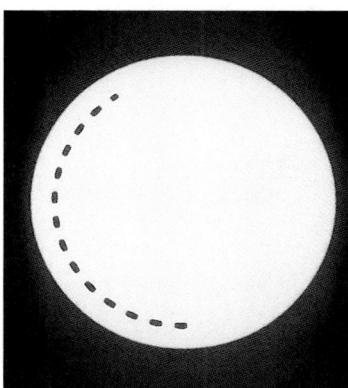

FIGURE 7-20 Image from manual spinning top on a single-phase X-ray generator.

device to view the output waveform. The display is then analyzed for potential problems and is documented for future reference. These waveforms should appear to be stable to within ±5% from initiation to at least 100 milliseconds and should show no spikes or dropouts during any exposure. The rise time (when voltage increases from 0 V to the peak voltage) should represent less than 1% of the total exposure time whereas the fall time (when the voltage decreases from the peak back to 0 V at the end of the exposure) should represent less than 10% of the total exposure time. This test should be performed on installation and then annually or after X-ray generator service and should be documented with a form such as the Radiographic Survey Form on the Evolve website.

Timer Accuracy. Exposure time affects directly the total quantity of radiation emitted from an X-ray tube; therefore, an accurate exposure timer is critical for acquiring properly exposed radiographs and reasonable patient radiation exposure. *The variability allowed for timer accuracy is ±5% for exposure times longer than 10 milliseconds and ±20% for exposure times less than 10 milliseconds.* Timer accuracy should be determined on installation and then annually, or when service is performed on the X-ray generator or if technique problems arise suddenly. The easiest method to validate timer accuracy is the use of a digital X-ray timer available from various manufacturers (Fig. 7-18). These timers usually incorporate a solid-state detector that measures the total time of X-ray production and then displays the time by means of a digital LED readout. These devices cost several hundred dollars, so other lower cost methods can be used. One of the oldest methods is the spinning top test, which includes a spinning top consisting of a metal disk with a hole or slit cut into the outside edge. If a single-phase X-ray unit is being evaluated, a manual spinning top can be used (Fig. 7-19). Single-phase generators emit X-rays in pulses, and therefore, each pulse creates a dot on the radiograph made of the spinning top (Fig. 7-20). The number of dots appearing on this radiograph is then compared with the number that should, theoretically, appear at the particular time station selected on the control panel for each exposure. The shortest exposure time available on most single-phase X-ray units is 1/120 second (8.3 ms). The number of dots that should, theoretically, appear is determined by the following equations:

Half-wave rectified:

Correct number of dots = Exposure time (second) × 60

Full-wave rectified:

Correct number of dots = Exposure time (second) × 120

Exposures should be made at 1/10, 1/20, 1/30, and 1/40 of a second for single-phase equipment.

For three-phase and high-frequency generators, X-ray production is constant, so a solid line or arc appears instead of a series of dots. For this reason, a manual spinning top cannot be used; a synchronous or motor-driven spinning top is used instead (Fig. 7-21). The synchronous spinning top is also used to evaluate single-phase equipment. The electric motor in the synchronous spinning top rotates at a constant speed of 1 revolution per second (rps) so that at the end of 1 second, a 360° circle is made. When placed on an image receptor and exposed with a three-phase or high-frequency X-ray generator, this device creates an arc on the processed image that is some fraction of 360° at exposure times less than 1 second. These X-ray units are capable of creating exposure times as short as 1/1000 second (1 ms). The arc size on the image is measured with a protractor (Fig. 7-22) and then inserted into the following equation to determine the actual exposure time (as a fraction) that occurred:

$$\text{Actual exposure time} = \frac{\text{Arc size}}{360}$$

For example, if the image yields an arc size of 72°, 72/360 equals a 1/5-second exposure time (0.2 second or 200 ms). At least four different time stations should be tested for three-phase equipment.

Many of the newer high-frequency units come equipped with milliampere-second timers instead of separate milliampere and time stations. Because the exposure time is regulated by the internal microprocessor circuitry, the actual time is unknown. A digital milliampere-second meter must be used instead of the digital timer or spinning top test. These devices have electrical probes that must be attached to the circuitry of the unit to obtain a reading. Only a person with adequate training on the use of these devices should attempt to access the circuitry.

Another option to determine timer accuracy is to use an oscilloscope to display the voltage waveform, which was discussed in the previous section.

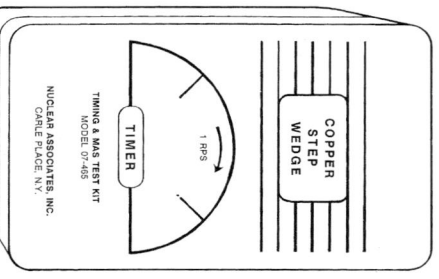

FIGURE 7-21 Synchronous spinning top. (*Courtesy Nuclear Associates, Inc., Carle Place, NY.*)

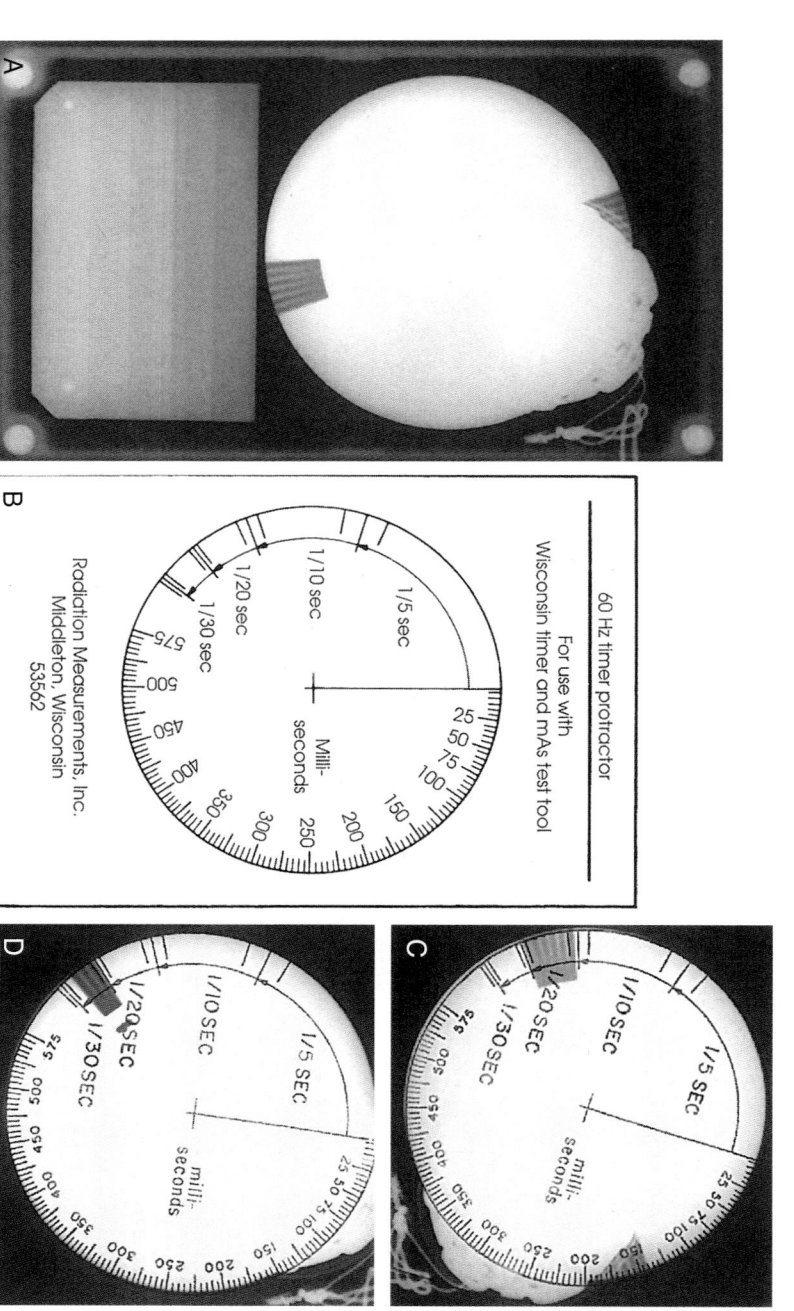

FIGURE 7-22 **A,** Radiograph produced at 200 mA and a 1/20-second exposure. **B,** RMI protractor template. **C,** Radiograph A with template showing acceptable results for a 1/20-second exposure. **D,** Radiograph produced at 200 mA and 1/30 of a second showing unacceptable results. mAs, milliampere-second. (*From Ballinger PW: Merrill's atlas of radiographic positions and radiologic procedures, ed 9, St Louis, 1999, Mosby.*)

CHAPTER 7 Quality Control of X-ray Generators and Ancillary Radiographic Equipment

Milliampere and Exposure Time Linearity and Reciprocity.

The milliampere selector in an X-ray generator is used to regulate the X-ray tube filament temperature, which, along with the exposure time, ultimately determines the quantity of X-rays in the X-ray beam. Therefore, the accuracy of the milliampere selected is equally important to the accuracy of the exposure timer. One method of testing milliampere accuracy is to make a 1-second exposure while watching the milliampere-second meter on the control panel. A better method is to determine the milliampere **reciprocity** and **linearity**.

Reciprocity refers to the same milliampere-second being selected but with different combinations of milliamperes and exposure time. The radiation output should be the same as long as the kilovolt (peak) is kept constant. For example, an exposure of 70 kVp, 50 mA at 1 second should produce the same amount of radiation as an exposure of 70 kVp, 100 mA at 1/2 second because both yield 50 mAs. **Any variation in reciprocity must be ±10%.**

PROCEDURE

1. Place a dosimeter, 40 in from the focal spot, on the radiographic tabletop on top of a lead apron or lead vinyl.
2. Make three to five exposures at 80 kVp and 20 mAs. Each exposure should be at a different milliamperes and time combinations. Be sure to reset the dosimeter after each exposure.
3. Record the dosimeter readings from each exposure and then divide each by 20 mAs to yield the milliroentgens per milliampere-second, or microcoulombs per kilogram per milliampere-second, value.
4. The minimum, maximum, and average of three to five of these values are then used to determine the reciprocity variance with the following equation:

$$\text{Reciprocity variance} = \frac{(mR/mAs_{max} - mR/mAs_{min})}{mR/mAs_{average}} \div 2$$

Adequate reciprocity exists when the variance is less than 0.1 (10%). If a dosimeter is unavailable, images of an aluminum step wedge or homogenous phantom made of aluminum or acrylic can be created with the use of a similar procedure to the one described earlier. Using a 10 × 12-inch image receptor, make three to five exposures at 80 kVp and 5 mAs (be sure to use lead vinyl strips so you can fit all three to five images on a single image receptor). After the image is processed, take optical density readings of the same area from each of the three to five images with a densitometer and then compare them. The readings should be within an optical density value of ±0.1.

Linearity means that sequential increases in milliampere-seconds should produce the same sequential increase in the exposure measured. In other words, if factors of 70 kVp and 10 mAs produced 50 mR of exposure on a dosimeter, then 70 kVp and 20 mAs on the same X-ray generator should produce an exposure of 100 mR if the milliampere station and timer are accurate. **Any variation must be within ±10% according to (1020.31(c)), 21 CFR Subchapter J** and can be evaluated in a manner similar to reciprocity.

PROCEDURE

1. Place the dosimeter on the radiographic table on a lead apron or strip of lead vinyl, just like in the reciprocity procedure.
2. For mA or mAs linearity, make four exposures using 70 kVp, 0.1 second (100 ms), at milliampere stations of 50, 100, 200, and 400. These yield milliampere-second values of 5, 10, 20, and 40 (each exposure twice the previous one). These factors can be modified if the X-ray generator does not have these milliampere-second stations. If only mAs selection is available on the control console, you can make the four exposures at the mAs values listed above.
3. To determine timer linearity (for units with separate mA and exposure time selection only), repeat step two using the same mA and exposure times that are double the previous exposure.
4. Record each reading and determine the milliroentgen/milliampere-second value for each exposure, along with the maximum, minimum, and average milliroentgen/milliampere-second values, then determine mA and timer linearity (on units that have separate mA and time stations) or mAs linearity (for units with only mAs selection available) using the following equation:

$$\text{Linearity variance} = \frac{(mR/mAs_{max} - mR/mAs_{min})}{mR/mAs_{average}} \div 2$$

Adequate linearity exists when the variance is less than 0.1 (10%). This variance also can be determined without a dosimeter, with a step wedge or homogenous phantom and image receptor. Make an exposure of the phantom or step wedge onto an image receptor using the previously mentioned technical factors. After the image is processed, compare the optical density readings of the same area to determine whether they are within ±0.1 of each other. Problems with the X-ray generator, such as the milliampere selector, timer circuitry, or rectifier failure, can cause the linearity variance to exceed accepted limits.

Focal Spot Size.

The area of the anode bombarded by projectile electrons is called the *focal spot*. Because these projectile electrons lose their kinetic energy at this point, this spot is also the source of X-ray photons in the X-ray tube. This area can be viewed from two perspectives: the actual rectangular surface on the target where electrons strike, called the **actual focal spot**, and the actual focal spot viewed from the perspective of the image receptor, called the **effective** (apparent or projected) **focal spot**. The effective focal spot always appears smaller than the actual focal spot because of the angle of the **line focus principle** (Fig. 7-23). This effect is the result of the angle of the anode surface (the smaller the anode angle, the smaller the effective focal spot size). The effective focal spot size has a significant impact on the amount of recorded detail and spatial resolution in a radiographic image because an increase in the effective focal spot size decreases the amount of recorded detail and spatial resolution. Therefore, focal spot size should remain relatively constant throughout the life of the X-ray tube. However, focal spot size can increase with age and use and with increases in the milliampere station selected. This phenomenon is known as **focal spot blooming**. Several performance tests are used to evaluate the degree of focal spot blooming.

Pinhole Camera. As shown in Fig. 7-24, a pinhole camera is made up of a plate of gold platinum alloy with

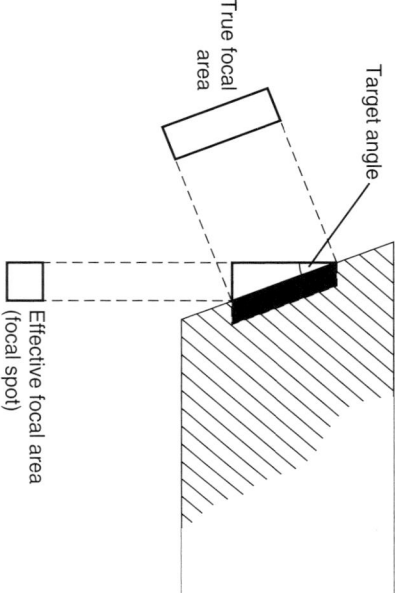

Relationship between true and effective focal areas

$$\text{Sine of target angle} = \frac{\text{Opposite}}{\text{Hypotenuse}}$$

FIGURE 7-23 Line focus principle.

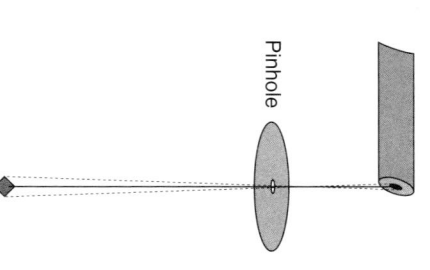

FIGURE 7-24 Concept of the pinhole camera.

a tiny hole of a specified shape and size cut into its center. A 0.03-mm hole is used for measuring focal spots smaller than 1 mm. A 0.075-mm hole is used for measuring focal spot sizes from 1 to 2.5 mm, and a 0.1-mm hole is used for measuring focal spot sizes greater than 2.5 mm. When placed on a stand over an image receptor (preferably a fine-grain film placed in a nonscreen holder or an extremity cassette) and then exposed, an image of the focal spot is projected on the film and can be measured with a ruler or micrometer after processing. The image is then compared with the stated, or nominal, focal spot size supplied by the X-ray tube manufacturer.

Focal Spot Test Tool. As shown in Fig. 7-25, an image of this test tool is obtained, and the resulting image is compared with a chart supplied by the manufacturer (Table 7-2).

Resolution Chart. Resolution charts are tools that project a chart pattern of various shapes or lines onto a film when radiographed. These charts can be used to estimate focal spot size. The two basic types are star charts (Fig. 7-26) and slit charts. Slit charts usually yield the amount of spatial resolution in line pairs per millimeter, which then correspond to a certain focal spot size used to

PROCEDURE

1. Place the pinhole camera stand on the radiographic tabletop and align it with the central ray and image receptor. If computed radiology (CR) is used, set preprocessing image data recognition to fixed mode (the CR image receptor acts like a film/screen cassette).
2. Adjust the pinhole-to-image receptor distance and SID to obtain the proper enlargement factor. For focal spots less than 2.5 mm, an enlargement factor of two should be selected. This means the pinhole-to-image receptor distance should be 60 cm and the X-ray source-to-pinhole distance should be 30 cm. For focal spots larger than 2.5 mm, the enlargement factor should be one, which is obtained with a source-to-pinhole distance of 40 cm and a pinhole-to-image receptor distance of 40 cm.
3. Expose the image receptor to 75 kVp and 50 mAs (100 mAs if a nonscreen image receptor is used). These factors should yield an optical density between 0.8 and 1.2 on the resulting image.
4. Measure the pinhole area on the processed image with a ruler or calipers along both the x-axis and the y-axis (with the long axis of the X-ray table and transverse to the long axis of the X-ray table). If CR is used, use the measuring software or print a hard copy of the image using a dry laser printer.
5. Divide the measurements by the enlargement factor obtained in step 2 to obtain the dimensions of the focal spot.

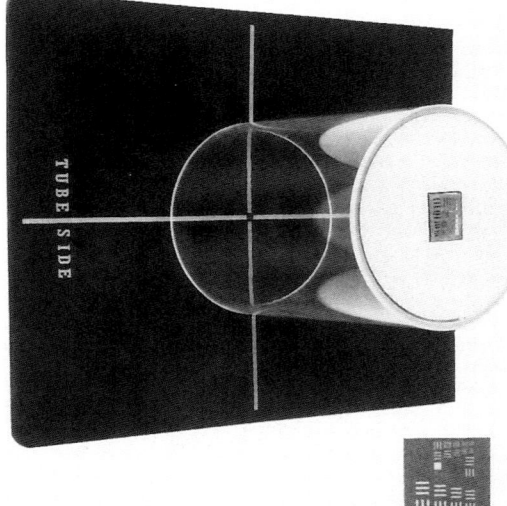

FIGURE 7-25 Image from the focal spot test tool. (Courtesy Nuclear Associates, Inc., Carle Place, NY.)

create the image (discussed in detail in Chapter 3 because this also determines the spatial resolution of imaging systems). When a star pattern resolution chart is used, the pattern is imaged on a fine-grain film (preferably in a nonscreen holder) and the image diameter (D_i) is measured from the resulting film. When this is compared with the actual diameter of the star pattern (D_o), the magnification factor (M) can be calculated with the following equation:

$$M = \frac{D_i}{D_o}$$

The diameter of the blur zone, or zero contrast band, in millimeters is measured from the image with a ruler (the diameter measured in both the x and y dimensions can

CHAPTER 7 Quality Control of X-ray Generators and Ancillary Radiographic Equipment

PROCEDURE

Washer or Coin Method

If a beam alignment tool is unavailable, the following procedure also can be used to determine X-ray beam–Bucky tray alignment.

1. Bring a metal coin, a steel washer, or a lead number zero, along with an 8 × 10-inch image receptor, into a radiographic room. If CR is used, set preprocessing image data recognition to fixed mode (the CR image receptor acts like a film/screen cassette).
2. Place the image receptor in the Bucky tray (with the long axis of the image receptor in the same direction as the long axis of the radiographic table) and center the X-ray field to the image receptor. Set the SID for 40 in (100 cm).
3. Turn on the positioning light and place the coin, lead zero, or steel washer in the center of the crosshairs. Place another coin or some other lead number in the light field, near the edge closest to where you are standing. This allows you to determine in which direction the alignment may be off when analyzing the resulting image.
4. Make an exposure using 50 kVp and 1 mAs (you may have to increase this amount, depending on the image receptor speed). Process the image.
5. Using a ruler, measure the distance from the middle of the outside of the long axis of the image to the washer, coin, or lead zero (with CR systems, use the electronic measuring software). If proper beam alignment exists, the distances are exactly the same. If they are not the same, the image of the washer, coin, or lead zero should be within 0.4 in of the center of the image or a service person should be notified to repair the system.

user should call a service technician to repair the system. No one should engage the expose button because serious X-ray tube damage can result if the overload protection system is malfunctioning. The overload protection mechanism should be evaluated at installation and then annually or when service is performed on the X-ray generator.

X-ray Tube Heat Sensors. As just mentioned, most X-ray generators are equipped with overload protection circuits to prevent excessive tube heat in a single exposure. In general, they do not protect against cumulative heat buildup that can occur when several exposures are made within a relatively short period. To guard against this accumulated heat, radiographers can rely on anode cooling charts or housing cooling charts supplied by the tube manufacturer. Use of these charts is especially critical during fluoroscopy and angiography, during which considerable heat can be produced quickly. Many newer units are equipped with X-ray tube heat sensors that provide an LED readout of the percentage of heat capacity remaining inside the X-ray tube housing. *Heat sensors should provide a warning when anode heat reaches 75% of the maximum.* These devices should be checked at installation and then every 6 months. Checking involves taking several exposures at a known heat unit value and then comparing the total with the known maximum heat capacity of the X-ray tube provided by the manufacturer.

PROCEDURE

1. Place a radiopaque object (e.g., a metal plate about 2 in long) at a distance from the focal spot mark on the X-ray tube housing. Measure and record the exact distance from the focal spot to the object. This value is known as d_1 (Fig. 7-32). Also measure and record the exact size of the object.
2. Using a 40-in SID, make an image of the object using an image receptor. If CR is used, set preprocessing image data recognition to fixed mode (the CR image receptor acts like a film/screen cassette). Make sure the object is positioned in the beam so that it is covered completely by the beam and the image receptor is large enough to contain the image produced.
3. Process the image and measure the size of the radiopaque object recorded in the image. The SID ($d_1 + d_2$) can then be calculated using the similar triangles equation and inserting the measured values of d_1, object size, and image size:

$$\frac{d_1}{\text{Object dimension}} = \frac{d_1 + d_2 \text{ (SID)}}{\text{Image dimension}}$$

ANCILLARY EQUIPMENT

The creation of diagnostic radiographs in a modern radiology department requires more than just an X-ray generator, X-ray tube, and X-ray table. Several types of ancillary equipment are also involved in the imaging chain to help create or enhance the radiographic image, regulate X-ray production, and protect the patient and radiographer, including automatic exposure control systems, conventional tomographic systems, grids, and portable and mobile X-ray generators. Because variation in this equipment can occur during use, quality control protocols must be in place to minimize repeat examinations.

Automatic Exposure Control Systems

The automatic exposure control (AEC) system has been used in radiography since the 1960s. It functions as a regulator for the exposure time and provides constant exposure to the image receptor regardless of the kilovolt (peak) or milliampere selected, or thickness of the part being imaged. This type of system involves some type of

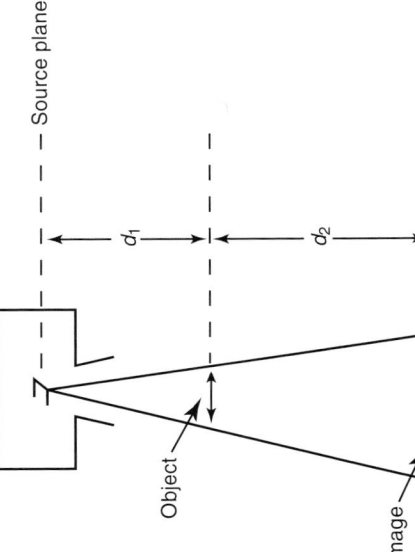

FIGURE 7-32 Similar triangle configuration for determination of source-to-image distance.

CHAPTER 7 Quality Control of X-ray Generators and Ancillary Radiographic Equipment

radiation detection device that measures the quantity of X-rays received by the patient or image receptor. When this exposure reaches a level corresponding to a predetermined value, the system causes the X-ray generator to terminate the exposure. This value is set by a service engineer on the basis of the image receptor system used in the department. A postreading milliampere-second indicator should be present on the control console and should display accurately the total milliampere-seconds delivered during the exposure. An AEC system has two main parts, the detector and the comparator.

Detectors. The **detector**, also known as the **sensor**, is a radiation detector that monitors the radiation exposure at or near the patient and produces a corresponding electric current proportional to the quantity of X-rays detected. Detectors are sometimes referred to as *cells* or *chambers*. Normally, three detectors are available for use by the radiographer, one in the midline and one on either side of the midline (Fig. 7-33). Units also are available with one or as many as five detectors. The X-ray machine control console should have indicators present that reflect which detectors are active. Three different types of radiation detectors have been used in AEC systems: photodetectors, ion chambers, and solid-state detectors.

Photodetectors. The **photodetector**, or **photocell**, uses a scintillation crystal (usually sodium iodide) coupled with a photomultiplier tube (Fig. 7-34). When radiation interacts with the crystal, light is created and it enters the photomultiplier tube. This light then releases electrons through the process of photoemission. The electrons multiply in number and form an electric current proportional to the original amount of radiation that struck the photocell. The photodetector was the original detector used as a sensor and was marketed under the name *phototimer*. This name is still used commonly to describe AEC systems, although the photodetector is seldom used in modern systems. These sensors are placed behind the image receptor to measure the exposure because they are not radiolucent. Care must be taken with these systems so that the lead in the back of the cassettes (normally present to control backscatter) is not excessive.

Ion Chambers. The **ion chamber** (discussed earlier in this chapter) consists of a gas-filled chamber. It is smaller than a photocell and can be made of a radiolucent material, which allows it to be placed between the grid and the front of the image receptor so that any type of cassette design can be used. An ion chamber is the most common type of sensor found in current AEC systems and is often marketed under the name *ionomat*.

Solid-State Detectors. The **solid-state detector** uses a small silicon or germanium crystal, which is more sensitive but also more expensive than photocells or ion chambers. The crystals are radiolucent and can be placed between the grid and image receptor. The solid-state detector is often marketed under the name *autotimer*.

Comparator. The **comparator** is an electronic circuit that receives the current signal sent by the sensor. An internal capacitor stores a voltage as long as this current is flowing. When the voltage in the capacitor becomes the same as a preset reference voltage, a switch is opened and it terminates the exposure. Changing the density selector switch changes this reference voltage and, therefore, the quantity of radiographs produced by the generator. Each step on the density selector should change the radiation exposure by 25% to 30%. Typical selector settings are shown in Fig. 7-35. The radiographer also must select

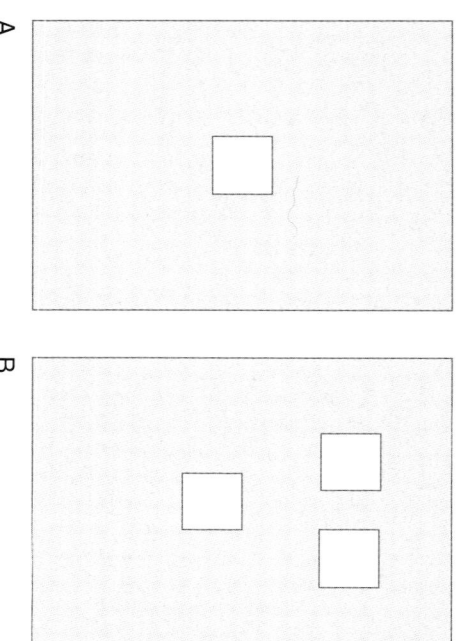

A

B

FIGURE 7-33 Sensor cell location for automatic exposure control systems. **A**, Single-cell option. **B**, Three-sensor option.

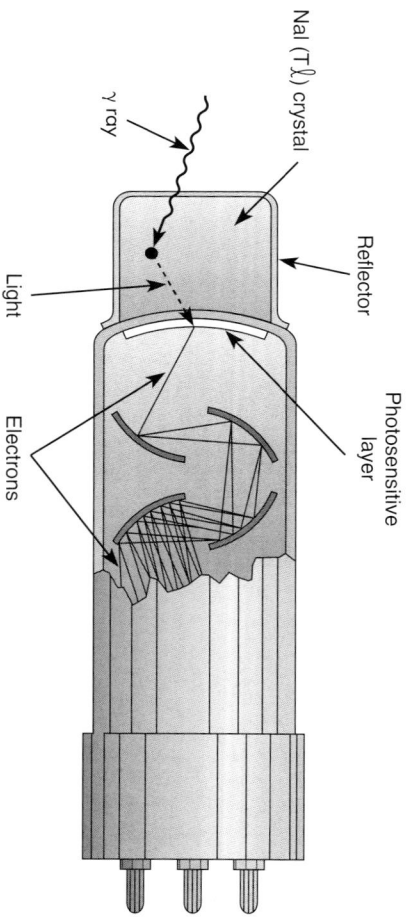

FIGURE 7-34 Schematic for photomultiplier tube and scintillation crystal.

CHAPTER 7 Quality Control of X-ray Generators and Ancillary Radiographic Equipment

the proper chamber, kilovolts (peak), and milliamperes; verify the properly positioned patient and X-ray tube; and verify backup time in case of system failure.

Automatic Exposure Control Testing. It is becoming more common for radiographic examinations to be performed with AEC systems. It is estimated that more than 60% of all hospital radiology departments have radiographic equipment that uses an AEC system or anatomically programmed units (which contain a microprocessor circuit with preprogrammed technical factors). The advantage of AEC is that it delivers consistent optical density on film screen (or image brightness on digital) radiographs over a wide range of patient thickness and kilovolt (peak) settings. Proper system performance should therefore be monitored through quality control procedures at installation and then semiannually or whenever work is performed on the system. Items that should be monitored include backup, or maximum exposure, time and minimum exposure time. Results should be recorded as pass or fail on a documentation form. A sample form for AEC system evaluation is available on the Evolve website.

Backup, or Maximum Exposure, Time. Because the exposure is controlled by the sensor and comparator combination instead of a conventional timer, care must be taken to avoid excessive patient exposure and heat in the X-ray tube in the case of system failure or during the examination of an extremely large patient. This is accomplished by setting a backup timer on the control unit. ⓖ *The backup timer should terminate the exposure within 6 seconds or 600 mAs, whichever comes first*, and can be checked with the following procedure.

PROCEDURE

1. Place a lead apron over the AEC detector cells and make an exposure at 70 kVp and 100 mA.
2. Watch the milliampere-second meter on the control panel, in addition to using a stopwatch, to determine whether the backup system terminates the exposure within the 6-second or 600-mAs limit. If not, release the expose button so the X-ray tube is not damaged.

Minimum Exposure Time. The detector and comparator combination requires a certain period to detect the radiation, compare it with the preset value, and then terminate the exposure (usually around 10 ms). If a particular X-ray examination requires an exposure less than this amount, the AEC system cannot respond in time and the resulting image is overexposed. For this reason, distal extremity radiographs are, in general, not performed with AEC. Certain lung diseases such as emphysema can also require less than the minimum exposure time, so it is important to lower the milliamperes before making the exposure. The manufacturer's literature should be checked regarding the minimum exposure time available, and then the technologist should be instructed regarding which radiographic examinations and kilovolt (peak) and milliampere combinations can and cannot be used with AEC.

Quality Control for Automatic Exposure Control

Consistency of Exposure with Varying Milliamperes. The AEC system should be able to adjust the exposure time and maintain optical density with any changes in milliamperes on the control panel. ⓖ *Any variation cannot exceed ±10%.* To evaluate this parameter, use the following procedure (Fig. 7-36).

PROCEDURE

1. Obtain a **homogenous phantom**, which is uniform in thickness, made of acrylic plastic (Plexiglas or Lucite) that is at least 10 cm in thickness (see Fig. 7-36).
2. Make a series of four radiographs of the phantom on a 10 × 12-inch (25 × 30-cm) image receptor using 70 kVp, 40-in SID Bucky, and a normal density setting, with each at a different milliampere station. If CR is used, set preprocessing image data recognition to fixed mode (the CR image receptor acts like a film/screen cassette).
3. Process each radiograph and use a densitometer to measure the optical density of the center of each image. For CR images, print a hard copy of the image using a dry laser printer or measure the pixel brightness at the center of the image. ⓖ *The optical density values should measure the same or be within an optical density of ±0.2 or no more than a 30% difference in pixel brightness.* If not, inconsistent optical density or image brightness in the resulting radiographs can occur, leading to repeat exposures. This is usually the result of a malfunctioning comparator.

Consistency of Exposure with Varying Kilovolts (Peak). The AEC system should be able to adjust the exposure time and maintain optical density with any changes in kilovolts (peak) on the control panel. Consistency can be evaluated with the same homogenous phantom mentioned previously.

Consistency of Exposure with Varying Part Thickness. The AEC system should be able to adjust the exposure time and maintain optical density with any changes in part thickness. System evaluation again uses a homogenous phantom.

	Density setting
Weak, very young Very old, debilitated	−2
Thin Easy to penetrate	−1
Average Normal build	0/Neutral
Muscular	+1/+2

FIGURE 7-35 Automatic exposure control density selector settings.

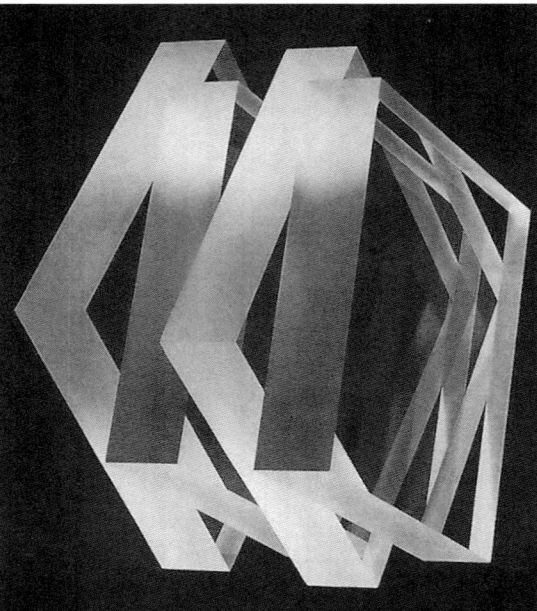

FIGURE 7-36 Automatic exposure control test tool consisting of acrylic sheets of varying thickness. (Courtesy Nuclear Associates, Inc., Carle Place, NY.)

PROCEDURE

1. Make four exposures of the phantom on a 10 × 12-in image receptor using 100 mA, a normal density setting, 40-in SID Bucky, and values of 60, 70, 80, and 90 kVp. If CR is used, set preprocessing image data recognition to fixed mode (the CR image receptor acts like a film/screen cassette).
2. Process the four radiographs and take optical density readings of the center of each image, using a densitometer. For CR images, print a hard copy of the image using a dry laser printer or measure the pixel brightness at the center of the image. ⊕ *The optical density values should measure the same or be within an optical density of ±0.3 or no more than a 50% difference in pixel values.*

PROCEDURE

1. Make three exposures on separate 10 × 12-in image receptors at 70 kVp, 100 mA, a normal density setting, and 40-in SID Bucky. Make each exposure with a phantom thickness of 10, 20, and 30 cm. If CR is used, set preprocessing image data recognition to fixed mode (the CR image receptor acts like a film/screen cassette).
2. Process each image and take density readings of the center. For CR images, print a hard copy of the image using a dry laser printer or measure the pixel brightness at the center of the image. ⊕ *The optical density values should measure the same or be within an optical density of ±0.2 or no more than a 30% difference in pixel values.*

Consistency of Exposure with Varying Field Sizes. The AEC system should be able to compensate for changes in the area of field, provided the detector remains in the area of field. Radiographs of the homogenous phantom can also be used to evaluate this parameter.

Consistency of AEC Detectors. Most AEC systems use a configuration of three detectors. Each detector should provide the same exposure or exposure time as the other two. For evaluation, use the following procedure.

PROCEDURE

1. Make a series of three exposures of the phantom using 70 kVp, 100 mA, a normal density setting, and 40-in SID. If CR is used, set preprocessing image data recognition to fixed mode (the CR image receptor acts like a film/screen cassette).
2. Make each exposure with a different field size of 6 × 6, 10 × 10, and 14 × 14 in, with an appropriate image receptor size. Be sure the X-ray beam is centered on the detector chamber.
3. Process the images and record the optical density from the center of each. For CR images, print a hard copy of the image using a dry laser printer. ⊕ *The optical density values should measure the same or be within an optical density of ±0.1 or no more than a 20% difference in pixel values.*

PROCEDURE

1. Make a series of three radiographs of the homogenous phantom using a different detector selection for each. Be sure the phantom is placed over the appropriate detector. Use exposure factors of 70 kVp, 100 mA, a normal density setting, and 40-in SID Bucky. If CR is used, set pre-processing image data recognition to fixed mode (the CR image receptor acts like a film/screen cassette).
2. Process the radiographs and compare the optical density readings from the center of each image. For CR images, print a hard copy of the image using a dry laser printer or measure the pixel brightness at the center of the image. ⊕ *The optical density values should measure the same or be within an optical density of ±0.2 or no more than a 30% difference in pixel values.*

Reproducibility. Exposures made at the same kilovolt (peak) and milliampere stations of the same phantom thickness should produce the same optical density on the resulting image. This is referred to as reproducibility.

PROCEDURE

1. Make three exposures of the homogenous phantom using 80 kVp, 200 mA, a normal density setting, a 10 × 12-in image receptor size, and 40-in SID Bucky. If CR is used, set preprocessing image data recognition to fixed mode (the CR image receptor acts like a film/screen cassette).
2. Process each radiograph and compare the optical density readings taken from the center of each image. For CR images, print a hard copy of the image using a dry laser printer or measure the pixel brightness at the center of the image. ⊕ *The readings should be within an optical density of ±0.10 of each other or no more than a 20% difference in pixel values.*

An alternative method of evaluating reproducibility is to make the same three exposures but not to use an image receptor to record an image. Instead, place a radiation detector and homogenous phantom over the appropriate sensor chamber and record the readings obtained in each exposure. For valid results, the radiation detector should be radiolucent. The reproducibility variance can then be calculated with the equation used earlier in this chapter. ⊕ *The reproducibility variance must be within 0.05 (5%).*

CHAPTER 7 Quality Control of X-ray Generators and Ancillary Radiographic Equipment

Density Control Function. The density selector switch should allow for changes in radiation exposure of 25% to 30% for each increment. Accuracy can be evaluated by the following procedure.

PROCEDURE

1. Make a series of five radiographs of the homogenous phantom using 70 kVp, 100 mA, and 40-in SID Bucky, and using the density selector settings of normal (0/neutral), +1, +2, −1, and −2 (these settings vary according to manufacturer). Be sure to mark each image with a lead number or some other identifier. If CR is used, set preprocessing image data recognition to fixed mode (the CR image receptor acts like a film/screen cassette).
2. Take optical density readings from the center of each of the processed images and compare. For CR images, print a hard copy of the image using a dry laser printer or measure the pixel brightness at the center of the image. Each should increase in optical density by a value of 0.2 to 0.25 (30% difference in pixel values), from the lowest to the highest density setting (−2 to +2).

Reciprocity Law Failure. The Law of Reciprocity states that the same amount of radiation should be created at any milliampere-second value regardless of the milliampere/time combination used; therefore, the optical density of any resulting image also should be the same. Film/screen image receptor systems can experience reciprocity failure at very short exposure time values (<10 ms) and very long exposure time values (>1 second).

- Phantom images of either a homogenous phantom or an anthropomorphic (lifelike) phantom should be made at 70 kVp, a normal density setting, 40-in SID Bucky, and the lowest milliampere station possible on the control panel (so that a long exposure time is used). Another image should be made with the highest milliampere station available (to yield a short exposure time).
- Optical density readings should be obtained from the center of each image and compared. If reciprocity failure exists, the optical density of the images varies by more than a value of ±0.2.

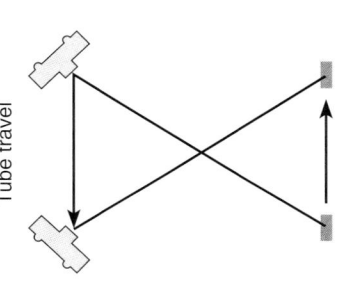

FIGURE 7-37 Principle of linear tomography.

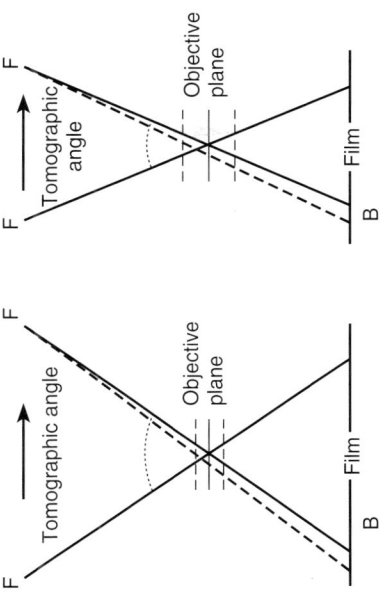

FIGURE 7-38 Effect of tomographic angle on section thickness. (F, focal spot; B, Bucky)

Conventional Tomographic Systems

Many radiographic units are equipped with a conventional tomographic system that is used to image certain "slices" of the body, whereas all other slices are blurred. This system helps remove superimposition and improves radiographic contrast in the area of interest. There are two basic types of conventional tomography: linear tomography and pluridirectional tomography.

In **linear** (sometimes called *rectilinear*) **tomography** the X-ray tube and image receptor move longitudinally in opposite directions during the exposure (Fig. 7-37). The plane through the fulcrum or pivot point remains in focus, whereas structures that are above and below this plane are blurred by the motion of the tube and film. This plane is called the **objective plane**, or tomographic section. The fulcrum level determines the level of the objective plane and is measured from the radiographic tabletop upward. For example, a 5-cm tomographic section means the objective plane is 5 cm above the tabletop. The thickness of the tomographic section is determined by the tomographic angle, which is the angle between the central ray at the beginning of the exposure and at the end of the exposure. The greater the tomographic angle, the thinner the tomographic section because of the greater motion of the tube and film (Fig. 7-38).

In **pluridirectional tomography**, the X-ray tube and film move in a variety of patterns such as circular, elliptical, hypocycloidal, and trispiral (Fig. 7-39). These units produce sharper images than rectilinear units because of the increased motion of the tube and film. Because of this complexity of motion, pluridirectional units are dedicated usually only to tomographic imaging, which has limited their use on a widespread basis because most radiology departments cannot afford to have a room dedicated solely to this type of unit, with a relatively small number of patients who might benefit.

Quality Control of Tomographic Systems. Because tomography involves motion of the X-ray tube and image receptor, considerable variation can occur in the performance of these systems with age and use. In addition,

CHAPTER 7 Quality Control of X-ray Generators and Ancillary Radiographic Equipment

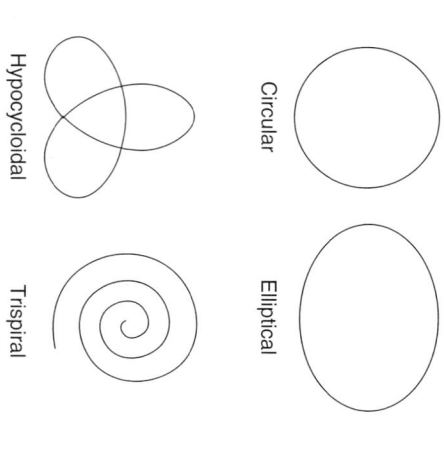

FIGURE 7-39 Pluridirectional tomographic patterns.

Circular
Elliptical
Hypocycloidal
Trispiral

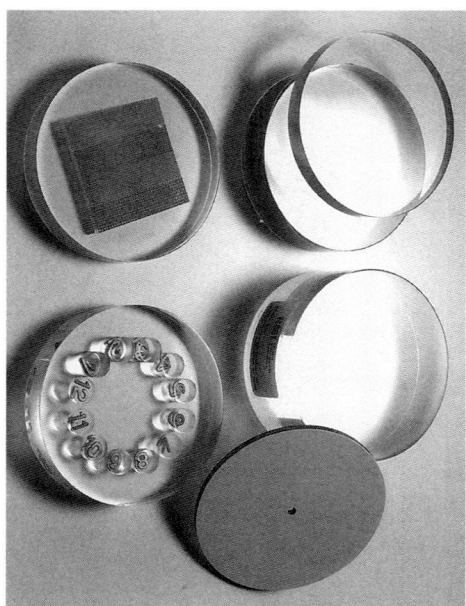

FIGURE 7-40 Tomographic test tool. (Courtesy Gammex/RMI, Middleton, WI.)

most X-ray generators for tomographic systems may not be calibrated for extremely low milliampere/long exposure time combinations used during these procedures. Mechanical instabilities can manifest in the tube system as a result of the large mass of the X-ray tube and housing. This manifestation can cause inconsistencies in the exposure and asymmetry in tube motion, and can lead to poor image quality; therefore, specific quality control tests should be performed at installation and then annually. Specialized test tools and phantoms should be used for these evaluations (Fig. 7-40). Factors to evaluate include section level, section thickness, level incrementation, exposure angle, spatial resolution, section uniformity and beam path, and patient exposure.

Section Level. ◉ *The level of the tomographic section (fulcrum level) indicated on the equipment and the actual level of the tomographic section imaged above the tabletop should be the same or within ±5 mm (some manufacturers suggest ±1 mm for pluridirectional units).* Evaluation is made with a test tool that has a series of lead numbers at various depths that are imaged on the image receptor (Fig. 7-41). A tomographic exposure is made of the test tools at various fulcrum levels. The

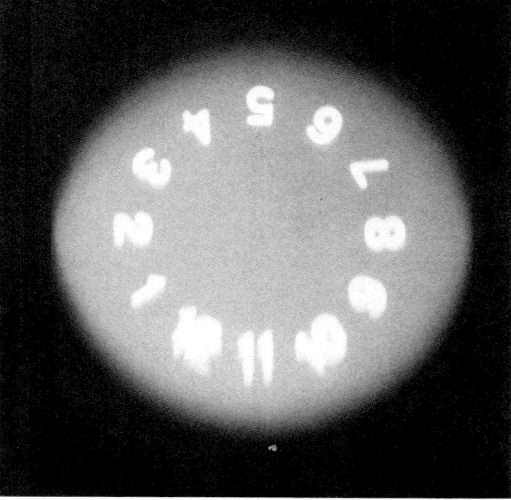

FIGURE 7-41 Image from a tomographic test tool indicating the level of tomographic section.

TABLE 7-4	Section Thickness at Various Tomographic Angles
Tomographic Angle (degrees)	Section Thickness (mm)
50	1.1
40	1.4
30	2
10	6
5	11
0	—

resulting image is then analyzed for the number that appears the sharpest. For example, if the fulcrum for the exposure is set for 5 cm, the number 5 should be the sharpest number visible.

Section Thickness. The thickness of the tomographic section depends on the tomographic angle. Table 7-4 lists the section thickness at various tomographic angles. Evaluation is made with a special test tool according to the manufacturer's instructions (Fig. 7-42).

Exposure Angle. The exposure angle determines the thickness of the tomographic section so it can be used as an alternative to measuring section thickness. ◉ *It is important that the value indicated on the equipment and the actual angle be the same or within ±5° for units operating at angles greater than 30°. For exposure angles less than 30°, the maximum variation allowed is ±2°.* Accurate measurement of this variable is difficult and is best accomplished by evaluating the section thickness with the appropriate phantom. Variations in section thickness are usually the result of improper exposure angles.

Level Incrementation. All tomographic units have some type of ruler or other device to indicate the level of the tomographic section. ◉ *A ruler should be constructed so that changing from one tomographic section to the next is accurate to within ±2 mm.* Evaluation can be

CHAPTER 7 Quality Control of X-ray Generators and Ancillary Radiographic Equipment

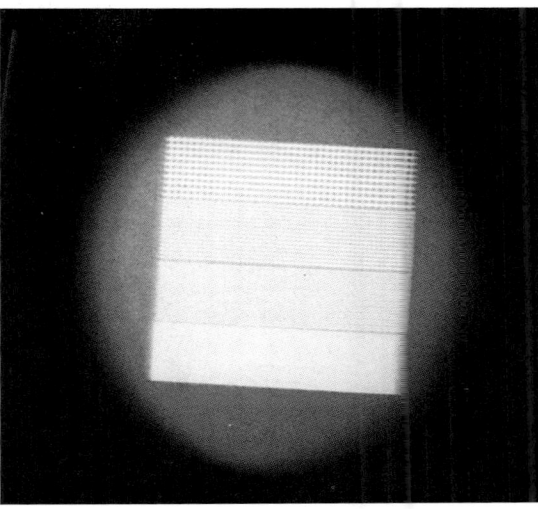

FIGURE 7-42 Multipurpose tomographic test tool with section thickness ruler.

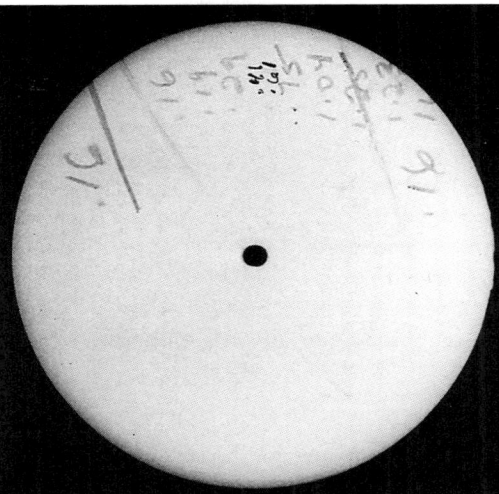

FIGURE 7-43 Image from a tomographic test tool indicating the resolution pattern.

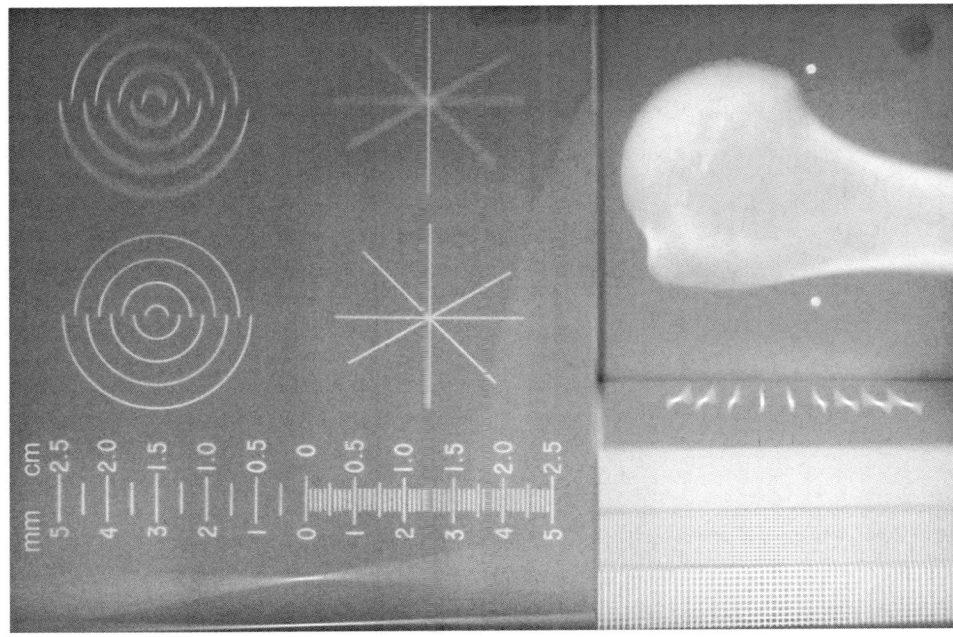

FIGURE 7-44 Lead aperture of a tomographic test tool.

accomplished with the same test phantom and procedure used in section-level determination.

Spatial Resolution. Spatial resolution in tomographic imaging is the ability of the tomographic system to resolve objects within the tomographic section. The structures within the tomographic section must be demonstrated with sufficient spatial resolution to make an accurate diagnosis possible. Fig. 7-43 shows an image of a tomographic resolution test tool with brass or copper wire mesh patterns of 20 holes per inch (0.8 holes/mm), 30 holes per inch (1.2 holes/mm), 40 holes per inch (1.6 holes/mm), and 50 holes per inch (2 holes/mm). Most tomographic units should be able to resolve a mesh screen pattern of at least 40 holes per inch. Variations in resolution are usually the result of asymmetry in tube motion.

Section Uniformity and Beam Path

The amount of radiation emitted should be consistent throughout the tomographic exposure so the optical density of the image is uniform. Consistency can be evaluated with a test tool consisting of a lead aperture (Fig. 7-44). When an exposure is made on a linear tomographic unit, a thin line should appear on the resulting image (Fig. 7-45). Optical density readings should be taken throughout the line and compared. *Any variation should be within an optical density value of ±0.3.* This same device can also be used for evaluation of beam path. Any asymmetry in motion or inconsistencies in the exposure alters the normal shape of the beam path. Linear units should demonstrate a straight line, as shown in Fig. 7-45. Pluridirectional units should create images that are appropriate to the pattern selected. Fig. 7-46 shows an image created with an elliptical pattern. *Path closure in pluridirectional units should be within ±10% of the path length.*

Patient Exposure. As the X-ray tube and film move in opposite directions during tomography, different patient thicknesses exist at various points within the exposure; therefore, the number of milliampere-seconds is greater during conventional tomography than with conventional radiography of the same view. The tomographic exposure should not exceed two times the nontomographic exposure for the same part. For example, if 50 mAs is required for an anteroposterior (AP) projection of the kidneys, an AP tomographic cut of the same kidneys should be obtained at 100 mAs or less. For departments equipped with more than one tomographic unit, patient exposure should not vary by more than 20% if the units have comparable X-ray tubes and generators. Evaluation can be made by exposing an abdomen or skull phantom to create both tomographic and nontomographic images.

PROCEDURE

1. Using either an abdomen or skull phantom, make a nontomographic exposure with an appropriate-size image receptor and the kilovolts (peak) and milliampere-seconds specified for your particular unit. If CR is used, set preprocessing image data recognition to fixed mode (the CR image receptor acts like a film/screen cassette).
2. Using the same phantom, make a tomographic image at the same kilovolts (peak) and appropriate milliampere-seconds specified for your particular unit.
3. Process the images and use a densitometer to obtain density readings of the same anatomic structure from each image (e.g., middle of the L4 vertebra and middle of the sella turcica). For CR images, print a hard copy of the image using a dry laser printer or measure the pixel brightness at the center of each image. The readings should be the same or within an optical density value of ±0.1 or no more than a 20% difference in pixel values.
4. If the optical density readings are similar, compare the milliampere-second values used for each exposure. The tomographic exposure should not be more than double the milliampere-seconds required for the nontomographic exposure.

Grids

The grid is the most common device for controlling scattered radiation (assuming collimation to the appropriate field size has been performed). Improper use of a grid can cause grid cutoff (resulting in an underexposed radiograph)

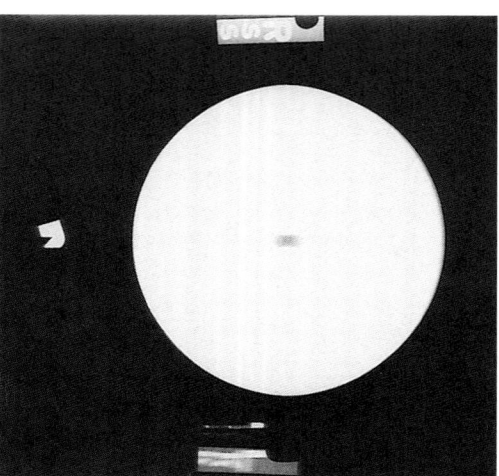

FIGURE 7-45 Image of a lead aperture with linear tomography.

or grid artifacts (e.g., grid lines and moiré patterns). These artifacts are discussed in detail in Chapter 10. Grid artifacts also occur because of imperfections during the manufacturing process or mishandling during clinical use (dropping the grid). Barium or other contrast media also creates artifacts and must be removed. The grid variables to be evaluated are grid uniformity and grid alignment, which should occur at installation and then annually.

Grid Uniformity

All the lead strips in the grid must be spaced uniformly or a mottling effect may appear in the image, which can mimic a pathologic condition. Nonuniformity occurs from manufacturing defects or by dropping a grid on its edges. For evaluation of **grid uniformity**, the following procedure may be used.

PROCEDURE

1. Place an image receptor under a grid and make an image of a homogenous phantom (made of either aluminum Lucite or a pan of water), using a kilovolt (peak) comparable for use with the grid ratio and enough milliampere-seconds to create an optical density of 1.5.
2. After processing, take optical density readings of the center and the four quadrants (and any suspicious areas) of the image and compare. ⓖ *All density readings should be within an optical density value of ±0.10 for proper uniformity.* For CR or DR systems, measure pixel brightness in each of the previously mentioned areas. There should not be more than a 20% difference in pixel brightness. Stationary grids on grid cassettes may require more frequent evaluation.

Grid Alignment

Grids that are misaligned attenuate more of the primary X-ray beam, and this attenuation results in a loss of

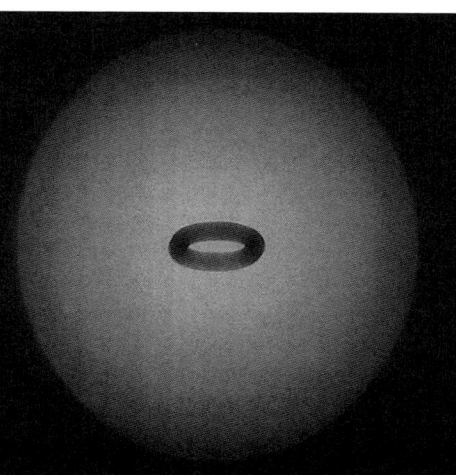

FIGURE 7-46 Image of a lead aperture with elliptical motion. *(Courtesy Central DuPage Hospital, Winfield, IL.)*

CHAPTER 7 Quality Control of X-ray Generators and Ancillary Radiographic Equipment

image quality and greater patient dosing. Proper alignment refers to centering the X-ray field with the focused grid and maintaining the proper grid focusing distance. Grid focusing distance is the proper distance from the X-ray source that a focused grid can be used, because the angle of the lead strips in the grid and the angle of divergence of the X-ray photons being emitted match at a specific range of distance values only. Alignment is more critical with greater grid ratios such as 10:1, 12:1, and 16:1, because grid latitude is less. **Grid latitude** is the margin of error in centering the X-ray beam on the center of the grid before significant grid cutoff appears in the resulting image. The alignment must be within the grid latitude specified by the manufacturer (usually within 1 in). The grid latitude value is found either on the grid front or in the literature supplied by the manufacturer. A commercial grid alignment tool is available (Fig. 7-47) and should be used according to the manufacturer's specifications.

Portable and Mobile X-ray Generators

Many radiographic examinations must be performed with mobile X-ray generators in hospitals and medical centers because patients' conditions may prevent them from being transported to the main X-ray department. Most of the variables mentioned earlier in this chapter, such as reproducibility, linearity, and focal spot size, can be tested with the same test tools and procedures used for standard radiographic equipment. Testing should occur at installation and then annually (some states require semiannual inspection) or when service is performed. Electrical safety and grounding are critical for safe operation of mobile equipment. A policy also must be in place regarding the storage of the keys that are required to operate this equipment. Federal and state regulations prohibit leaving keys in mobile equipment when this equipment is not in use and stored in a public area. This is a safety indicator of TJC. Some type of lockbox with a combination lock, a key storage area within the radiology department, and a key allotment policy for radiographers are just some of the possible ways to address this concern. A distinction should be made between portable and mobile X-ray generators.

Portable X-ray Generator. A portable X-ray generator is small enough to be carried from place to place by one person. It consists of an oil-filled metal tank or casing that contains a stationary anode X-ray tube and transformers. A smaller control unit, containing the exposure switch and timer circuitry, attaches to the casing by means of a 6-ft (1.8-m) cord. A metal stand or tripod holds the casing in place. The maximum output for portable units is 75 kVp and 15 mA, so use is confined generally to chest and extremity examinations in nursing homes, to battlefield use by the military, and to field veterinary use.

Mobile X-ray Generator. A mobile X-ray generator is a smaller version of a radiographic unit that is mounted on wheels and pushed from one location to the next. Mobile units are most often found in hospitals for the examination of patients who are too ill or injured to be taken to the main radiology department. Often, mobile units are mistakenly called "portables." There are several types of mobile X-ray generators (Table 7-5).

Direct-Power Units. Direct-power units are usually equipped with stationary anode X-ray tubes and have a plug that is placed into a standard 110/120-V outlet. The maximum output for most of these units is 100 kVp and 15 mA. These units are subject to power fluctuations in line voltage.

Capacitor Discharge Units. Capacitor discharge units are equipped with a high-tension capacitor that

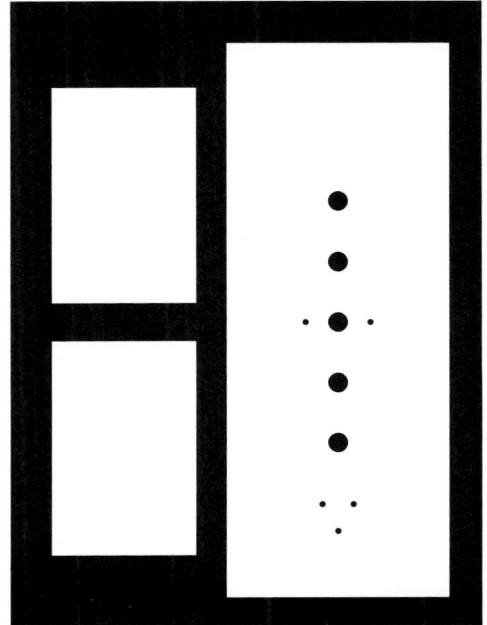

FIGURE 7-47 Grid alignment tool. (*Courtesy Nuclear Associates, Inc., Carle Place, NY.*)

TABLE 7-5	Comparison of Mobile Radiographic Units			
Direct Power	**Capacitor/Discharge**	**Battery Powered**	**High Frequency**
Single-phase output	Constant potential (X-ray production constant)	Constant potential (X-ray production constant)	Constant potential (X-ray production constant)
Limit of 15 mA	Limited to short exposure time	Unit is relatively large and heavy	Unit is small and lightweight
Subject to power fluctuations	No power fluctuation	No power fluctuation while battery is being charged	High kilovolts (peak) and milliampere-seconds available
Requires standard outlet in immediate area of operation	Requires standard outlet in immediate area of operation	No need for outlet in immediate area of operation	Requires standard outlet in immediate area of operation

must be precharged before each exposure. For the unit to operate properly, it must be plugged in to the main power supply, and the appropriate kilovolts (peak) and milliampere-seconds are selected. A charge button is then activated on the control panel that allows the capacitor to charge up to the selected value, which usually takes about 10 seconds. A green light indicates a full charge. The X-ray exposure should be made immediately after the indicator light appears because the charge on the capacitor begins to leak. If the kilovolts (peak) drops below 2 kVp of the selected value, the green light deactivates and no exposure can be made until the unit is recharged. Because the voltage drops during the exposure (at about 1 kV/mAs), the exposure time should be kept short to keep the kilovolts (peak) at the desired level. This effect also makes testing for kilovolt (peak) variation difficult for these units; therefore, an average kilovolt (peak)/milliampere-second value should be established on installation and then maintained throughout the life of the unit. Any variation of the kilovolt (peak)/milliampere-second value must be within ±5%. X-ray output is constant, much like that of a three-phase or high-frequency X-ray generator.

Cordless, or Battery-Powered, Mobile Units. Cordless, or battery-powered, mobile units use a series of lead or nickel-cadmium wet-cell batteries (usually three) that must be kept charged when the unit is not in use (with a built-in charger that is plugged into the main power supply). The batteries are used to power a drive motor that propels the unit and a polyphase electric generator that produces the electric current that energizes the X-ray tube. These units can usually attain a maximum output of 100 kVp and 25 mA, with a constant X-ray output. The batteries should be removed from the unit, cleaned, discharged completely, and then recharged every 6 months to maintain a continued optimum charge.

High-Frequency Mobile Units. Like their larger counterparts, high-frequency mobile units are equipped with a microprocessor circuit that increases the frequency of the alternating current to create a nearly constant potential. Some systems are plugged in to a standard outlet, whereas others have batteries that must be kept charged. These systems usually achieve as much as 133 kVp and 200 mAs, with a minimum exposure time of 3 milliseconds. For battery-powered systems, the milliroentgen/milliampere-second output should be determined when the unit is fully charged and again after it has been used for a length of time comparable with what occurs during clinical use. Radiation output should decrease by no more than 20% between the two values.

SUMMARY

Through visual inspections, environmental inspections, and performance testing, variation in the functioning of radiographic equipment can be kept to a minimum, which should increase department efficiency, lower the repeat rate, and reduce the number of unnecessary exposures. In addition, ancillary equipment used in conjunction with radiographic units must function within specific parameters to obtain consistent and acceptable quality images. Therefore, quality control testing is also required to monitor this level of performance.

Refer to the Evolve website at https://evolve.elsevier.com for Student Experiments 7.1: Radiographic Unit Visual Check; 7.2: Half-Value Layer Measurement and Filtration; 7.3: Milliampere and Exposure Time Linearity; 7.4: Reproducibility, Milliampere-Second Reciprocity, and Milliroentgen per Milliampere-Second; 7.5: Collimation, Beam Alignment, and Perpendicularity; 7.6: Automatic Exposure Control Reproducibility; 7.7: Automatic Exposure Control and Patient Positioning; and 7.8: Grid Alignment.

REVIEW QUESTIONS

1. The indicated level of the tomographic section and the actual level of the section must correspond to within _____ mm.
   a. 2
   b. 5
   c. 10
   d. 15

2. A three-phase X-ray generator can operate at a maximum of 100 kVp and 500 mA at 100 ms. What is the kilowatt rating of this generator?
   a. 5 kW
   b. 35 kW
   c. 50 kW
   d. 500 kW

3. The backup timer for an automatic exposure control system should terminate the exposure at _____ second(s) or _____ mAs, whichever comes first.
   a. 1; 100
   b. 3; 300
   c. 6; 600
   d. 9; 900

4. How large of an arc appears during a spinning top test of a three-phase X-ray generator at 50 ms?
   a. 18°
   b. 20°
   c. 36°
   d. 90°

5. Which of the following should a quality control program for radiographic equipment include: (1) visual inspection, (2) environmental inspection, or (3) performance testing?
   a. 1 and 2 only
   b. 2 and 3 only
   c. 1 and 3 only
   d. 1, 2, and 3

CHAPTER 7 Quality Control of X-ray Generators and Ancillary Radiographic Equipment

6. The minimum half-value layer for X-ray units operating at 80 kVp is _____ mm of aluminum.
   a. 1.3
   b. 1.5
   c. 2.3
   d. 2.5

7. The maximum variability allowed for the reproducibility of exposure is ± _____ %.
   a. 2
   b. 5
   c. 10
   d. 20

8. Any variations between the stated kilovolt (peak) on the control panel and the measured kilovolt (peak) must be ± _____ %.
   a. 2
   b. 5
   c. 10
   d. 20

9. The variability allowed for timer accuracy in exposures less than 10 ms is ± _____ %.
   a. 2
   b. 5
   c. 10
   d. 20

10. The variability allowed for milliampere and time linearity is ± _____ %.
    a. 2
    b. 5
    c. 10
    d. 20

CHAPTER 8

Quality Control of Fluoroscopic Equipment

KEY TERMS

Air kerma
Automatic brightness control
Automatic brightness stabilization
Automatic gain control
Brightness gain
Charge-coupled device
Cinefluorography
Flat-panel sensor (detector)
Flux gain
High-contrast resolution
Image intensifiers
Image lag
Image-orthicon
Low-contrast resolution
Minification gain
Multifield image intensifier
Orthicon
Photoemission
Photofluorospot
Pincushion distortion
Plumbicon
Relative conversion factor
S distortion
Veiling glare
Vidicon
Vignetting

OBJECTIVES

At the completion of this chapter, the reader should be able to do the following:

- List the main components of a modern fluoroscopic system
- Discuss how the brightness of fluoroscopic images is maintained
- Describe the various methods of monitoring fluoroscopic images
- Perform visual and environmental inspections of a fluoroscopic system
- List and describe the performance tests for fluoroscopic equipment

OUTLINE

Introduction to Fluoroscopic Equipment
Image Intensifiers
  Components
  Image Brightness
  Multifield Image Intensifiers
  Image Intensifier Artifacts
Image Monitoring Systems
  Closed-Circuit Television
  Mirror Optics
  Cinefluorography
  Photofluorospot, or Spot Film,
    Camera
  Film/Screen Spot Film
    Devices
  Digital Image Recorders
Quality Control of Fluoroscopic Equipment
  Visual Inspection
  Environmental Inspection
  Performance Testing
    Reproducibility of Exposure
    Focal Spot Size
    Filtration Check
    Kilovolt (Peak) Accuracy
    Voltage Waveform
    Milliampere Linearity
    X-ray Tube Heat Sensors
    Grid Uniformity and
      Alignment
    Automatic Brightness
      Stabilization Systems
    Automatic Gain Control
    Maximum Entrance Exposure
      Rate
    Standard Entrance Exposure
      Rates
    High-Contrast Resolution
    Low-Contrast Resolution
    Source–Skin Distance
    Distortion
    Image Lag
    Image Noise
    Relative Conversion Factor
    Veiling Glare, or Flare
    Fluoroscopic Systems for
      Cardiac Catheterization and
      Interventional Procedures
    Video Monitor Performance
Summary

CHAPTER 8 Quality Control of Fluoroscopic Equipment

Fluoroscopic imaging is used widely in radiology to visualize the dynamics of internal structures and fluids. The image produced is a dynamic, or real-time, image compared with conventional radiography, which creates a static image. Because of the real-time image created, fluoroscopy is used widely for gastrointestinal (GI) studies, vascular and cardiac studies, and interventional procedures. Many of these studies and procedures involve a considerable length of X-ray exposure time for the patient. For this reason, fluoroscopy is considered the principle source of medical radiation to the population of the United States. In particular, upper GI tract fluoroscopy is the most commonly conducted fluoroscopic procedure in the United States and contributes the greatest effective radiation dose to the U.S. population.

Strict quality control guidelines and protocols should be in place to minimize variation in equipment performance so patient dose is as low as possible. Federal guidelines for fluoroscopic equipment are found in Title 21 of the Code of Federal Regulations Part 1020 (21 CFR 1020) Subchapter J, which uses input from the American College of Radiology (ACR), the American Association of Physicists in Medicine (AAPM), and various other groups. Many states have or will be adopting fluoroscopic protocols developed by the Nationwide Evaluation of X-ray Trends committee of the Conference of Radiation Control Program Directors (CRCPD). This chapter contains many of the mentioned guidelines and protocols, but regulations in the state of practice also must be checked.

INTRODUCTION TO FLUOROSCOPIC EQUIPMENT

The three main parts of a typical fluoroscopic unit are the X-ray tube and generator, the image intensifier, and the video monitoring system. The X-ray generators in modern fluoroscopic units are either three-phase or high-frequency units, for maximum efficiency. Fluoroscopic units equipped with cinefluorography require fast exposure times, on the order of 5 to 6 ms for a framing rate of 48 frames/s; therefore, the X-ray generators must offer a high output—that is, a 130- to 200-kW power rating. The X-ray tubes are usually higher capacity tubes (at least 500,000 heat units) compared with general radiographic tubes (about 300,000 heat units). In general, the X-ray tube and generator generally must perform according to the same standards as radiographic units and are evaluated in a similar way. Factors such as filtration (half-value layer [HVL]), focal spot size, X-ray tube heat sensors, overload protection, kilovolt (peak) (kVp) accuracy, reproducibility, linearity, output wave forms, automatic exposure control (AEC) (for spot film devices), and grid uniformity and alignment all should be tested at least every 6 months with the methods and test tools discussed in previous chapters.

Image Intensifiers

Components. Fluoroscopic systems must use an image intensifier, which brightens electronically the image obtained during fluoroscopy. The most common type of image intensifier in fluoroscopic systems is the tube-type image intensifier, which works by converting a low-intensity, full-size image to a high-intensity minified image. This type of device was first developed in 1948 by Coltman, who used technology similar to an electron microscope (Fig. 8-1). A newer alternative to the tube-type image intensifier is the **flat-panel detector** made up of an active matrix array very similar to digital radiographic systems, which are discussed in detail in Chapter 9. The essential parts of the tube-type image intensifier are the glass envelope, input phosphor, photocathode, electrostatic focusing lenses, anode, and output phosphor.

Glass Envelope. A tube-type **image intensifier** is a vacuum tube that allows the free flow of electrons

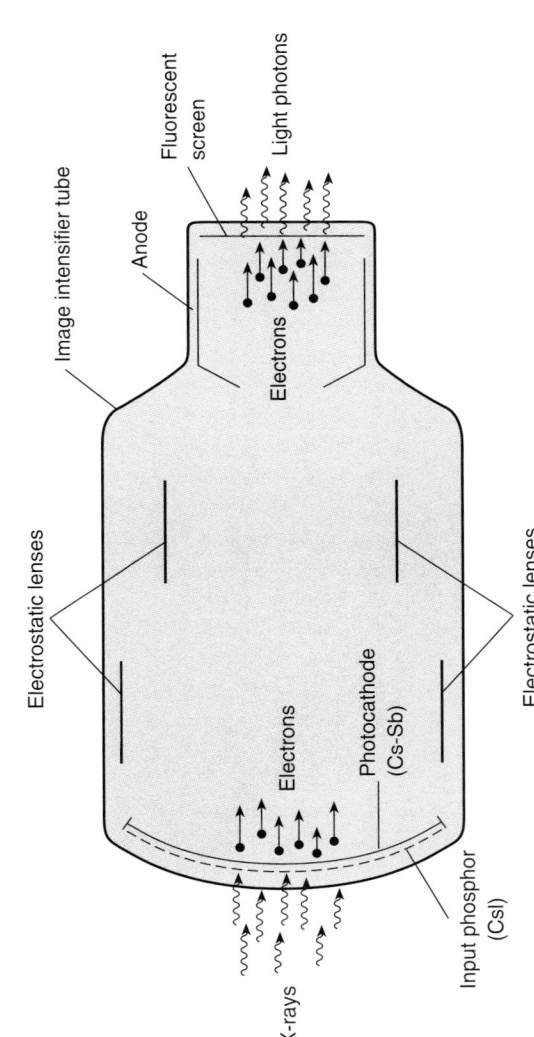

FIGURE 8-1 Schematic of an image intensifier tube. CsI, cesium iodide; Cs-Sb, cesium antimony.

from one side of the device (photocathode) to the other (anode). The glass envelope is necessary to contain this powerful vacuum, which can experience as much as 1 ton of force from the outside air pressure pushing against it. Breakdown of vacuum integrity is the usual cause of the limited life of the image intensifier.

Input Phosphor. On entry into the image intensifier, the X-rays strike the input phosphor, which absorbs them and converts their energy into visible light. The image intensifier ranges in diameter from 6 to 16 inches (15-40 cm) and is curved to maintain an equal distance between all points on the input and output phosphors. An input phosphor consists of either a glass or thin aluminum base (used in most newer input phosphors) with a coating of sodium-activated cesium iodide crystals placed in a layer 0.1-0.2 mm thick. The crystals form long, needlelike shapes that act as light pipes to emit light with minimal divergence (Fig. 8-2). The light emitted has a wavelength of about 4200 Å (420 nm), which places it in the blue portion of the color spectrum.

Photocathode. Light photons from the input phosphor strike the photocathode immediately, which is a thin layer of antimony and cesium compounds. The light photons release electrons from the photocathode through the process of photoemission.

Anode. The anode is a positively charged electrode that attracts the electrons toward the output phosphor. The potential difference between the anode and photocathode is 25 to 35 kV.

Electrostatic Focusing Lenses. Electrostatic focusing lenses are positively charged metal plates that focus and accelerate the electrons as they travel toward the output phosphor.

Output Phosphor. Output phosphor is usually a piece of glass or aluminum about 1 inch (2.54 cm) in diameter and is coated with a thin layer (4-8 μm) of zinc cadmium sulfide (also known as P20). When electrons from the photocathode strike these crystals, light is emitted with wavelengths between 5000 and 6500 Å (500-650 nm), which places it in the yellow-green portion of the color spectrum. Because the light is placed in the approximate center of the visible light spectrum, video cameras (and the human eye) can detect this light easily. **Image Brightness.** The image intensifier increases the brightness of the image by the following two processes:

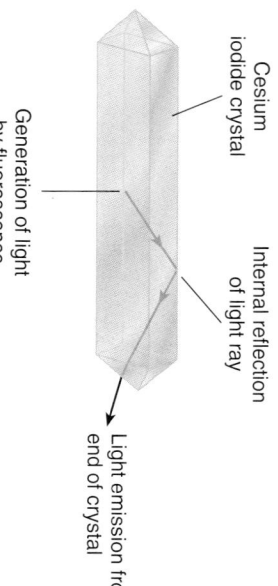

Cesium iodide crystal

Internal reflection of light ray

Generation of light by fluorescence

Light emission from end of crystal

FIGURE 8-2 Cesium iodide light pipe.

1. The image from the larger input phosphor is condensed onto the smaller output phosphor. Because the image is emitted from a smaller area, it appears to be brighter. This increase in brightness is known as **minification gain** and is calculated with the following equation:

$$\text{Minification gain} = \frac{\text{Input diameter}^2}{\text{Output diameter}^2}$$

2. High voltage accelerates the electrons from the photocathode and their kinetic energy is increased, releasing many times more light photons from the output phosphor surface. This increase in brightness is known as the **flux gain**. At 25 kV, one electron incident on the output phosphor releases 50 light photons. The flux gain is then considered to be 50 times.

The total **brightness gain** is determined by multiplying the minification gain by the flux gain. Brightness gain may be referred to as the amount of brightness of an image-intensified image versus a nonimage-intensified fluoroscopic image. The brightness level of a fluoroscopic image is affected by milliamperes (mA), kilovolts (peak), **automatic brightness control** (ABC), variable tube current, and variable pulse width, as shown in Box 8-1.

Multifield Image Intensifiers. The **multifield image intensifier** allows the fluoroscopic image to be magnified electronically by changing the voltage on the electrostatic focusing lenses, which decreases the amount of the input phosphor image sent to the output phosphor. The resulting image is then magnified (Fig. 8-3). Because the minification gain is decreased, the milliamperes must be increased to maintain image brightness, which results in significantly increased entrance skin exposure. Another disadvantage is that the field of view is decreased. This type of image intensifier is used in digital fluoroscopic units and interventional, vascular, and cardiac studies.

The two basic types of multifield image intensifiers are dual focus and trifocus.

Dual Focus. The dual-focus multifield image intensifier allows for a choice of two different fields of view to be used. The most common dual-focus option is called the 9/6, which means the input phosphor can vary from a 9-inch diameter for a normal field of view to a 6-inch diameter for a magnified field of view (also called 23/15 for centimeter diameter measurement).

Trifocus. The trifocus option provides the user a choice of three input phosphor diameters, the most common of which is the 10/7/5 (in inches) or the 25/18/12 (in centimeters).

Image Intensifier Artifacts. The use of image intensifiers in fluoroscopic systems may lead to five basic types of artifacts: veiling glare, or flare; pincushion distortion; barrel distortion; vignetting; and S distortion.

Veiling Glare, or Flare. Veiling glare, or flare, is caused by light being reflected from the window of the output phosphor, which reduces image contrast. This

CHAPTER 8 Quality Control of Fluoroscopic Equipment

BOX 8-1 Factors Affecting the Brightness of Fluoroscopic Images

Milliamperes
An increase in the fluoroscopic X-ray tube milliamperes multiplies the number of X-ray photons incident on the image intensifier, and therefore image brightness increases.

Kilovolts (Peak)
An increase in the fluoroscopic X-ray tube potential difference (i.e., kVp) multiplies the number of X-ray photons reaching the image intensifier. Causing an increase in image brightness.

Patient Thickness and Tissue Density
An increase in patient thickness and tissue density reduces the number of X-ray photons reaching the image intensifier, thereby decreasing the image brightness.

Automatic Brightness Control or Automatic Brightness Stabilization
Automatic brightness control, or **automatic brightness stabilization**, allows the fluoroscopic unit to maintain the brightness level of the image automatically for variations in patient thickness and attenuation. This maintenance is accomplished by one of the following three methods, depending on the manufacturer:

- *Variable kilovolts (peak)*. Variable kilovolt (peak) systems use a motor-driven autotransformer that varies the kilovolts (peak) in response to image brightness-sensing electrodes. These electrodes monitor the output phosphor directly or use a signal generated by a video camera. This method covers a wide range of patient thicknesses. However, it is slow, and the images may demonstrate quantum noise and low image contrast at high kilovolt (peak) values.
- *Variable tube current*. A variable tube current system varies the milliamperes or tube current in response to image brightness-sensing electrodes, which requires a large-capacity X-ray generator.
- *Variable pulse width*. Using the variable pulse width method, the X-ray output is pulsed with a grid-controlled X-ray tube at a sequence rapid enough to avoid image flicker. A faster pulsing sequence is selected by the equipment to increase fluoroscopic image brightness and vice versa.

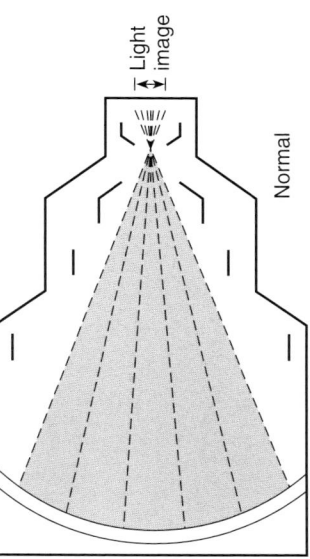
Normal

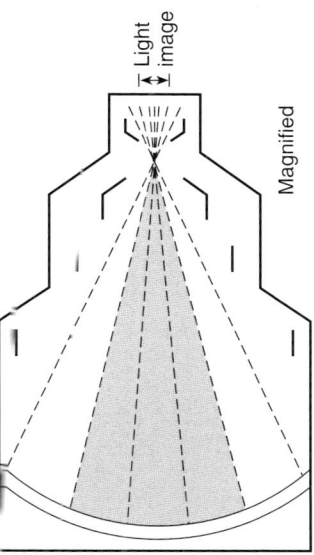
Magnified

FIGURE 8-3 Multifield image intensifier showing normal and magnification modes.

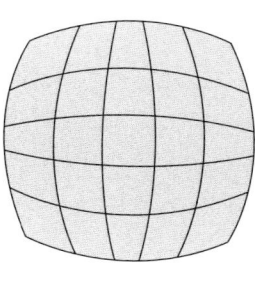
Image displaying "S" distortion

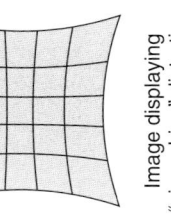
Image displaying "pincushion" distortion

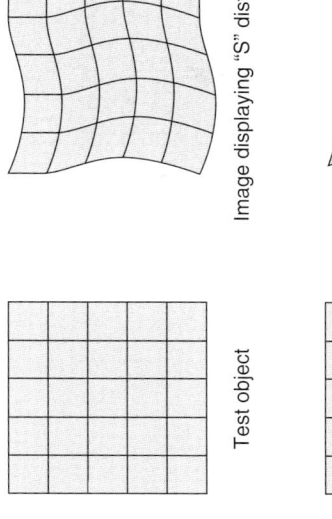
Image displaying "barrel" distortion

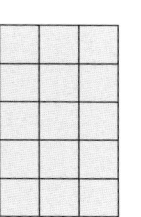
Test object

Test object

Test object

FIGURE 8-4 S, pincushion, and barrel distortion.

artifact occurs most often when moving from one portion of a patient's anatomy to another (such as when imaging the chest and moving down to the abdominal area), causing a sudden increase in image brightness. Most manufacturers incorporate designs to reduce veiling glare to minimize this effect.

Pincushion Distortion. Pincushion distortion is caused by projecting an image from a curved surface (input phosphor) onto a flat surface (output phosphor). This effect is similar to that of a carnival mirror that distorts appearance and is greater toward the lateral portions of the image. With pincushion distortion, magnification increases toward the periphery (Fig. 8-4).

Barrel Distortion. Barrel distortion is similar to pincushion distortion and is caused, again, by projecting from a curved surface to a flat one (or vice versa), but magnification is reduced toward the periphery (also seen in Fig. 8-4).

Vignetting. Vignetting is a decrease in image brightness at the lateral portions of the image and is caused by a combination of pincushion distortion and the coupling of the television camera to the output phosphor.

S Distortion. An S distortion artifact is a warping of the image along an S-shaped axis and is the result of strong magnetic fields changing the trajectory of the electrons moving across the image intensifier tube.

Image Monitoring Systems

Because the output phosphor is only 1 inch (2.54 cm) in diameter, the image projected is relatively small and, therefore, must be magnified and monitored by an additional system. The main methods used include mirror optics, closed-circuit television (CCTV) monitoring, cinefluorography, photofluorospot, film/screen spot devices, and digital image recorders.

Mirror Optics. Mirror optics is the oldest method of monitoring the image from an image intensifier. It uses a system of mirrors and lenses. The final image is projected onto a 6-in-diameter mirror mounted on the side of the image intensifier tower. The field of view is small, so only one person can view the image at a time. Image resolution of this system is 3 to 4 line pairs per millimeter (lp/mm). This method is rarely used today.

Closed-Circuit Television Monitoring. CCTV is the most common method for monitoring the fluoroscopic image. A television camera is focused onto the output phosphor and then displayed on a monitor. The components necessary for television monitoring are a television camera, linkage from the camera to the output phosphor, and a television monitor.

Television Camera. The television camera converts visible light images into electronic signals. Four basic types of television cameras have been in use throughout the years: the **orthicon**, **plumbicon**, **vidicon**, and **charge-coupled device**.

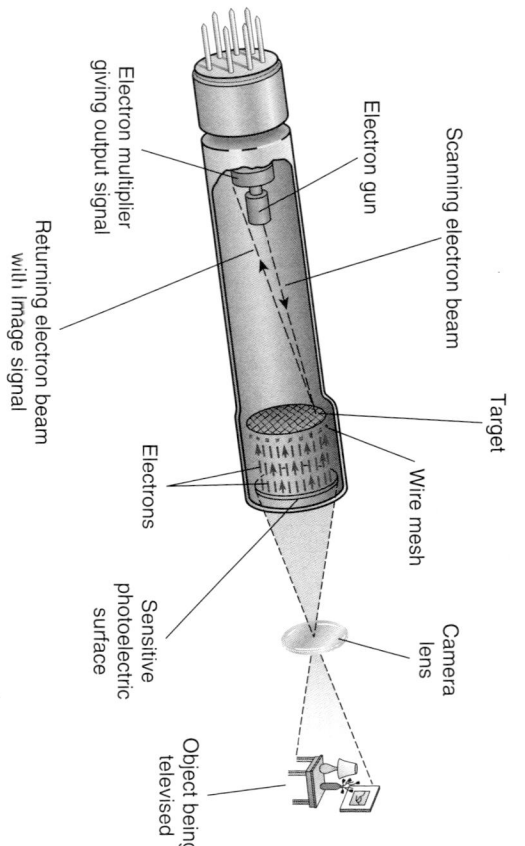

FIGURE 8-5 Orthicon television camera tube.

Orthicon. The **image-orthicon** is the largest and most sensitive type of television camera, and it functions as both an image intensifier and a television pickup tube. Image quality is excellent and completely free of lag; however, it is expensive, extremely sensitive to temperature changes, and requires a long warm-up time (Fig. 8-5).

Plumbicon. The **plumbicon** camera uses lead oxide as the target phosphor and is often used in digital fluoroscopy because of its short lag time.

Vidicon. The **vidicon** camera is currently the most common type of video camera in fluoroscopic systems. Target material in the camera is antimony trisulfide, which has a relatively long lag time (helpful in GI studies) to help reduce image noise.

Charge-Coupled Device. The **charge-coupled device** (CCD) does not use a photoconductive target inside of a glass tube to convert light images to electronic signals (as in the first three types of cameras). Instead, an array of 100 to 1000 tiny (5–20-μm) photodiodes on a solid-state computer chip form pixels to create the signal (Fig. 8-6). When light strikes these photodiodes, electrons are released in direct proportion to the amount of incident light. These electrons build up charges that form electronic pulses. These pulses then form the electronic video signal containing the image information. Most home video cameras use CCD technology, as do digital photographic cameras. More fluoroscopic units are being equipped with CCD cameras, a trend that should increase as the number of pixels increases (which increases resolution). The CCD cameras exhibit virtually no lag and very low electronic noise. They are also more sensitive than video tubes (meaning, they can detect lower amounts of light) and have a much longer life than video camera tubes (because they do not have a heated cathode). The CCD cameras also consume less electrical power during operation than tube cameras (operating costs are lowered) and are not as fragile (because there is no glass envelope).

CHAPTER 8   Quality Control of Fluoroscopic Equipment

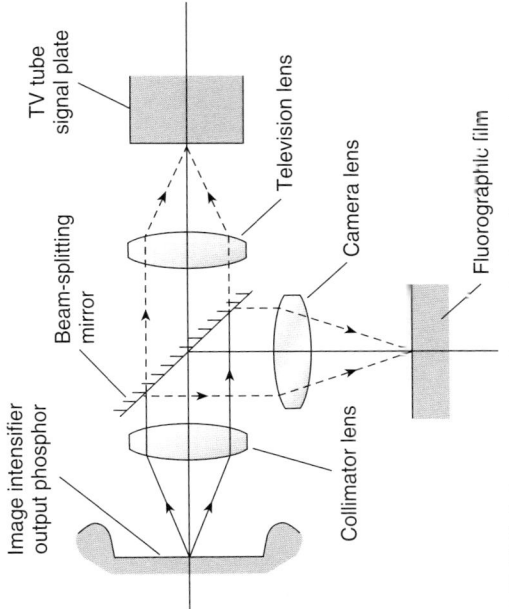

FIGURE 8-6 Representation of a photodetector/pixel arrangement in a charge-coupled device.

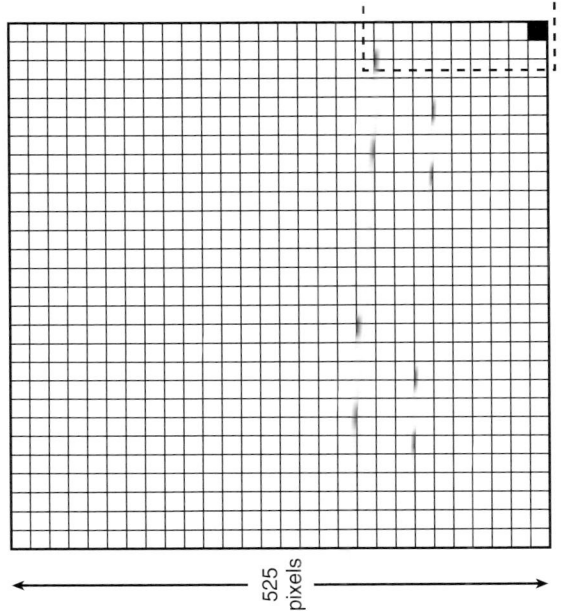

FIGURE 8-7 Principle of fiber optics.

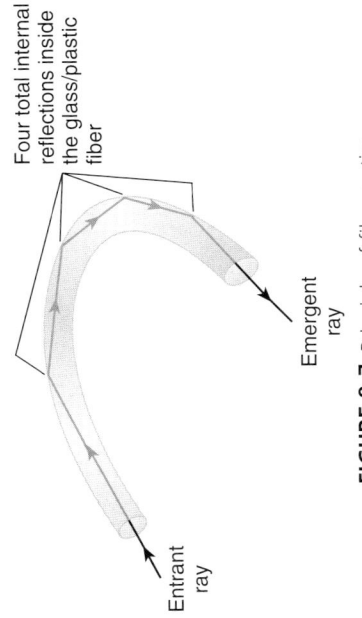

FIGURE 8-8 Split mirror for monitoring fluoroscopic images.

Linkage from the Television Camera to Output Phosphor.
The television camera must be coupled, or linked, to the output phosphor so that image quality is maintained. To maintain image quality, one of two methods is used: fiber optics and lens coupling.

Fiber Optics. Fiber optics linkage uses flexible glass or plastic fibers in which total internal reflection occurs (Fig. 8-7). This device is small, rugged, and relatively inexpensive but cannot accommodate auxiliary units such as cine or spot film cameras.

Lens Coupling. The lens coupling method uses a system of lenses and mirrors to split the image so auxiliary devices can view the image simultaneously with the television camera (Fig. 8-8).

Television Monitor. The television monitor found on an older system uses a cathode ray tube (CRT) to display the fluoroscopic image. The CRT monitor uses the Electronics Industries Association's RS-170 standard for closed-circuit black-and-white television, which uses 525 lines per frame, with 30 separate frames appearing each second and an aspect ratio of 4:3. Standard monitors use a method called *interlaced horizontal scanning* to avoid flicker, which involves scanning the odd-numbered lines in the first half of the frame and the even-numbered lines during the second half, rather than all 525 at once. This type of monitor can resolve between 2 and 2.5 lp/mm. Noninterlaced, or progressive, scan monitors (which scan all lines in order and have a frame rate of 60 frames/s) also are available and are used in most personal computer displays. These monitors are preferred in angiographic and interventional procedures because of their reduced flickering. High-resolution monitors with up to 1023 lines per frame are available and demonstrate 2.5 to 5 lp/mm. Newer fluoroscopic systems are now incorporating high-resolution flat-panel monitors in which a liquid crystal display is used instead of a CRT monitor. The next chapter contains a more complete discussion of viewing monitors. As high-definition television systems have become more cost effective, and have rapidly replaced CRT monitors.

Cinefluorography. With the *cinefluorography* method, a motion picture camera is used to monitor the image from the output phosphor. This high-speed motion picture camera records the image of fast-moving objects, and it is ideal for cardiac catheterization studies (95% of all cine studies involve cardiac studies). The film used is either 16 mm or, most often, 35 mm (98% of all cine studies) black-and-white motion picture film. The larger size yields better image quality but requires a greater patient dose. The camera is capable of recording framing frequencies of 7.5, 15, 30, 60, and 120 frames/s, depending on the motion of the object. The greater the framing frequency, the greater the ability to minimize motion in the resulting image. However, it also results in an increased patient dose. The X-ray beam is pulsed with a grid-controlled X-ray tube to match the framing frequency. Quality control tests on cine equipment are discussed in Chapter 9.

Photofluorospot, or Spot Film, Camera.

The photofluorospot, or spot film, method uses a spot film camera that takes a static photograph of the fluoroscopic image with a lens-coupling device. The lens has a longer focal length than that of cine cameras to cover a larger film format. These cameras use 70-, 90-, 100-, or 105-mm roll or cut film sizes. The larger the film format, the better the image quality, but the patient receives a greater dose. The patient dose with this method is less than that from film/screen spot filming. In addition, the cost of film and processing is less than that of film/screen spot filming. Quality control tests on these cameras are discussed in Chapter 9.

Film/Screen Spot Film Devices.

Film/screen spot film devices do not monitor the fluoroscopic image from the image intensifier; rather, they use a fluoroscopic X-ray tube to create a radiograph on a standard cassette. This cassette is usually kept in a lead-shielded compartment until the spot film device is activated. It is then placed into the X-ray beam path behind a grid, and a field format is selected (e.g., one on one, two on one) (Fig. 8-9). The fluoroscopic X-ray tube is then changed from approximately 3 mA to as much as 1000 mA, and the exposure is made and then controlled with an AEC system. The images created with this method have a greater contrast and spatial resolution than photofluorospot images. Spot film devices are preferred for most angiographic procedures, air contrast GI examinations, endoscopic retrograde cholangiopancreatography, arthrography, and sialography.

Digital Image Recorders.

Digital image recorders now are being used in many fluoroscopic systems to view fluoroscopic images at a later time. These systems are discussed in Chapter 9.

QUALITY CONTROL OF FLUOROSCOPIC EQUIPMENT

The procedure for evaluating fluoroscopic systems involves much of the same processes as the evaluation of radiographic systems, with the components of visual inspection, environmental inspection, and performance testing.

Visual Inspection

A fluoroscopic system visual inspection should be performed at least every 6 months, using a checklist, by either a quality management technologist or a medical physicist. A sample checklist is included at the Evolve website. The following should be included in the checklist:

- *Fluoroscopic tower and table locks.* Operate all locks manually to verify function.
- *Power assist.* Activate the power assist. The tower should move smoothly over the tabletop.
- *Protective curtain.* Ensure that a protective curtain or drape is in place and moves freely so that it can be placed between the patient and any personnel in the

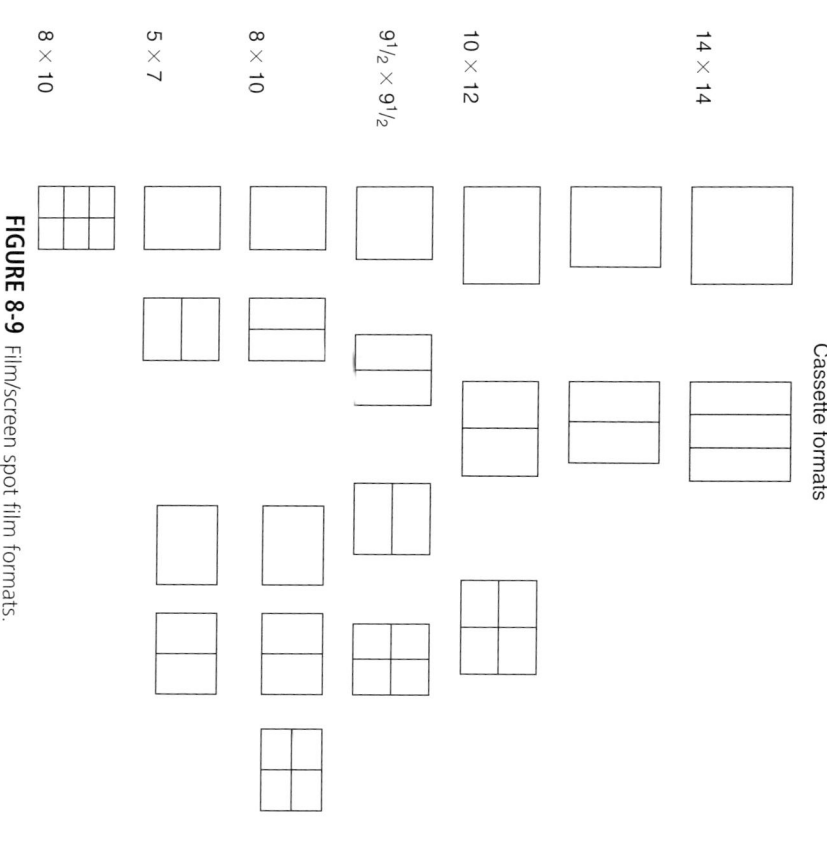

Cassette formats

14 × 14

10 × 12

9½ × 9½

8 × 10

5 × 7

8 × 10

FIGURE 8-9 Film/screen spot film formats.

CHAPTER 9

Digital and Advanced Imaging Equipment

KEY TERMS

Active matrix array
Amorphous
Analog-to-digital converter
Application program interface
Aspect ratio
Capture element
Cinefluorography
Collection element
Computed radiography
Coupling element
Detective quantum efficiency
Digital Imaging and Communications in Medicine group
Digital fluoroscopy
Digital radiography
Digital subtraction angiography
Digital X-ray radiogrammetry
Direct-to-digital radiographic systems
Dose creep
Dual-energy X-ray absorptiometry
F-center
Fill factor
Flat fielding
Frame rate
Image contrast
Image enhancement
Image management and communication system
Image restoration
Interpolation
Liquid crystal display
Nyquist frequency
Photostimulated luminescence
Picture archiving and communication system
Pixel pitch
Preprocessing
Postprocessing
Refresh rate
Saturation
Special procedures laboratory
Specular reflection
Teleradiology
Thin-film transistor
Window level
Window width

OBJECTIVES

At the completion of this chapter, the reader should be able to do the following:

- Describe the basic methods of obtaining digital radiographs
- State the advantages and disadvantages of digital radiography versus conventional film/screen radiography
- Discuss the quality control (QC) procedures for evaluating digital radiographic systems
- Describe the basic methods of obtaining digital fluoroscopic images
- Explain how digital subtraction angiography is performed
- Discuss the QC procedures for evaluating digital fluoroscopy
- Describe the basic principle of image production from multiformat cameras, laser cameras, dry laser printers, cathode-ray tube cameras, videotape and videodisc recorders, and cinefluorographic equipment and discuss the QC procedures for each
- Describe the various types of electronic display devices and discuss the applicable QC procedures
- Explain the basic image archiving and management networks and discuss the applicable QC procedures
- Describe the basic QC process for special procedures equipment
- Explain the various methods for obtaining bone mineral density measurements

OUTLINE

Digital Radiographic Imaging Systems
   Secondary Capture
      Laser Scanning Digitizer
      Charge-Coupled Device Scanner
Computed Radiography (CR)
   Advantages of Computed Radiography versus Conventional Radiography
   Disadvantages of Computed Radiography versus Conventional Radiography
Digital Radiography
   Indirect-conversion or Scintillator Digital Radiography System
   Direct-conversion or Photoconductor Digital Radiography System

CHAPTER 9 Digital and Advanced Imaging Equipment

OUTLINE—cont'd

Comparison of Computed Radiography with Digital Radiography
Quality Control of Digital Radiographic Imaging Systems
Digital Fluoroscopy
  Last Frame-Hold
  Road Mapping
  Digital Temporal Filtering
  Image Enhancement
  Image Restoration
  Image Intensifier Tube Digital Fluoroscopy Systems
  Flat-Panel Digital Fluoroscopy Systems
  Continuous Fluoroscopy Mode
  Pulsed Interlaced Scan Mode
  Pulsed Progressive Scan Mode
  Slow Scan Mode
  Digital Subtraction Angiography
  Temporal Mask Subtraction
  Time-Interval Difference Subtraction
  Dual-Energy Subtraction
  Quality Control of Digital Fluoroscopy Units
Electronic Display Devices
  Cathode-Ray Tube Displays
  Liquid Crystal Displays
  Plasma Displays
  Quality Control of Electronic Display Devices
Multiformat Cameras
  Components
  Brightness
  Contrast
  Exposure Time
  Quality Control of Multiformat Cameras
Laser Cameras
  Components
  Quality Control of Laser Cameras
Dry Laser Printers
Cathode-Ray Tube Cameras
  Components
  Quality Control of Cathode-Ray Tube Cameras
Videotape, Videodisc, and Digital Recorders
  Components
  Quality Control of Analog and Digital Recorders
Cinefluorography and Photofluorography
Image Archiving and Management Networks
Miscellaneous Special Procedures Equipment
  Film Changers
  Pressure Injectors
Bone Densitometry Systems
  Single-Photon Absorptiometry
  Single-Energy X-ray Absorptiometry
  Dual-Photon Absorptiometry
  Dual-Energy X-ray Absorptiometry
  Quantitative Computed Tomography
  Quantitative Ultrasound
  Digital X-ray Radiogrammetry
  Quality Control of Bone Densitometry Equipment
Summary

DIGITAL RADIOGRAPHIC IMAGING SYSTEMS

Virtually all diagnostic imaging systems can be considered to have three key components: image acquisition, image processing, and image display. Since the late 1890s, radiographic images were acquired by exposing a screen/film combination that required chemical processing and was displayed on a viewbox illuminator. In digital imaging, an image acquisition system obtains image data in the form of an electronic signal, which is processed electronically in a computer memory whereby the image exists as electronic values in a computer matrix (rather than as grains of silver on a sheet of polyester plastic), and displayed on an electronic display device (computer monitor). The computer matrix is made up of tiny squares called pixels (a contraction of the term *picture element*). The more pixels in a matrix, the smaller each pixel becomes, thereby increasing spatial resolution (Fig. 9-1). The production of digital radiographic images has virtually replaced this method of film/screen radiography. Creating radiographic images in a digital format has many advantages over the analog format (film/screen images), including:

- reducing repeat images resulting from technique error (Most overexposures and slight underexposure can be corrected with software and not have to be repeated, but gross underexposure cannot.),
- **postprocessing** of the image (Detail and contrast can be enhanced by the computer software.),
- transmitting the electronic images (This allows quick access to images by referring physicians and for consultation over large distances.).

Currently, digital images can be acquired by using one of three methods: secondary capture, **computed radiography** (CR), or digital radiography (DR).

Secondary Capture

This method of creating digital images involves the initial creation of an analog image (on film) and then its conversion into a digital format. One method of accomplishing this conversion would involve taking a photograph of a film radiograph with a digital camera. This method has been used for years by diagnostic imaging educators to obtain

In recent years, diagnostic imaging has undergone an explosion in technology with the advent of computerized imaging, magnetic resonance imaging (MRI), and digital archiving and retrieval systems. All of these technologies are now commonplace in diagnostic imaging departments and can be subject to variations with age and use; therefore, QC protocols should be in place to monitor for these variations so that they can be kept to a minimum.

REPEAT ANALYSIS WORKSHEET

SURVEY PERIOD _____ to _____   LOCATION _____

REPEAT CATEGORY EXAMINATION	POSITION	OVER-EXPOSED	UNDER-EXPOSED	MOTION	ARTI-FACTS	OTHER	TOTAL	%
Chest								
Ribs								
Shoulder								
Humerus								
Elbow								
Forearm								
Wrist								
Hand								
C-Spine								
T-Spine								
L-Spine								
Skull								
Facial								
Sinuses								
Abdomen								
Pelvis								
Hip								
Femur								
Knee								
Lower leg								
Ankle								
Foot								
UGI								
LGI								
IVP								
Other								
Total								
%								

FIGURE 10-1 Repeat analysis worksheet (Film/screen). C-Spine, Cervical spine; IVP, intravenous pyelography; LGI, lower gastrointestinal tract; L-spine, lumbar spine; T-spine, thoracic spine; UGI, upper gastrointestinal tract.

180 CHAPTER 10 Outcomes Assessment of Radiographic Images

CR/DR Repeat Analysis Form

Room # _____ Date: _____ Technologist: _____

Patient ID	Exam	positioning	overexpose	underexpose	motion	wrong exam code	collimation	artifact	No exposure	Double expose	No marker	Marker over part	Wrong exam code	other

FIGURE 10-2 Repeat analysis worksheet (CR/DR). CR, Computed radiography; DR, digital radiography.

the analysis because image viewer differences can affect the outcome of the repeat analysis study. The worksheet should include the radiographic procedures performed in the department, along with the possible causes of rejection such as positioning, overexposure, underexposure, motion, **artifacts**, and miscellaneous causes. Once the data have been recorded for the specified period, the causal repeat rate and the total department rate should be determined. The causal repeat rate is the percentage of repeats from a specific cause such as positioning error or technique error and is calculated with the following equation:

$$\text{Causal repeat rate} = \frac{\text{Number of repeats for a specific cause}}{\text{Total number of repeats}} \times 100$$

For example, if a radiology department has a total of 185 repeat images during a 1-month period and 67 of the 185 are the result of positioning errors, then the percent of repeats caused by positioning error is 36%. Many radiology information systems can calculate the causal repeat rate when department staff enter the number and cause of repeat images into the system.

Total Repeat Rate

The total department repeat rate is determined with the following equation:

$$\text{Total repeat rate} = \frac{\text{Number of repeat images}}{\text{Total number of views taken}} \times 100$$

For example, if a department performs a total of 1160 views during a 1-month period and 132 are rejected and must be repeated, then the total department repeat rate is 11.4%. Some automatic film processors have a counting device that records the total number of images processed that can be used as the "total number of views taken" in the equation (most CR and DR systems have software that can access the total number of images processed during a given period to obtain the same information). Many factors influence this rate, such as the quality of the equipment, the competence of the technical staff, the patient population, data collection method, shift (weekend, evening, or day shift), and the number of images accepted by radiologists to diagnose.

Data from the repeat analysis are used to identify which of these factors is a major contributor to the overall repeat rate. If a particular piece of equipment is often identified as being at fault for repeat images, data from the repeat analysis can be used to justify repair or replacement costs. If certain employees demonstrate an abnormally high number of repeats, additional in-service education or other corrective action can be used to help alleviate the problem. Repeat rates for radiographic *procedures should not exceed 4% to 6% and should be less than 5% for mammographic procedures. Mammographic repeat rates cannot change by more than ±2% each quarter.* However, this may not be practical in all departments when the amount of variation that may be present in imaging equipment, technologist experience level, institutional image quality acceptance standards,

CHAPTER 10 Outcomes Assessment of Radiographic Images

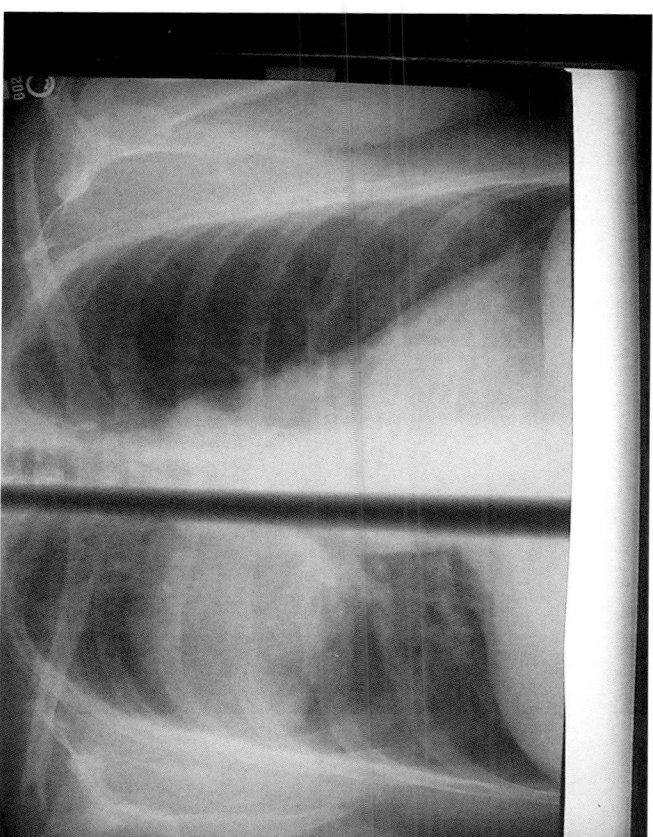

FIGURE 10-24 Shading occuring during hardcopy printing. *(Courtesy of Pamela Verkuilen, Saint Alexius Medical Center, Hoffman Estates, IL.)*

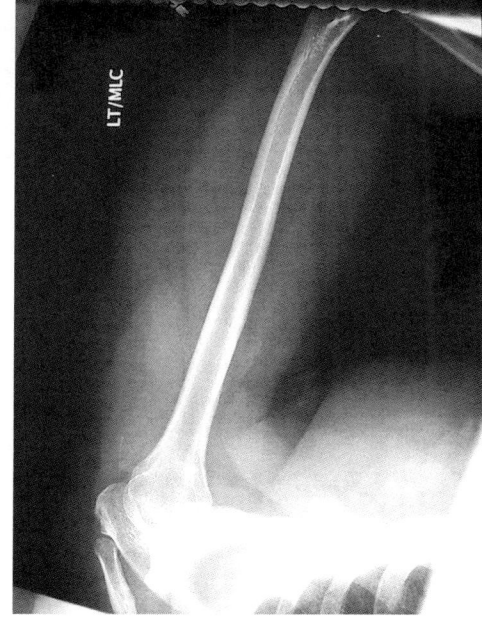

FIGURE 10-25 Corduroy effect. *(Courtesy of Pamela Verkuilen, Saint Alexius Medical Center, Hoffman Estates, IL.)*

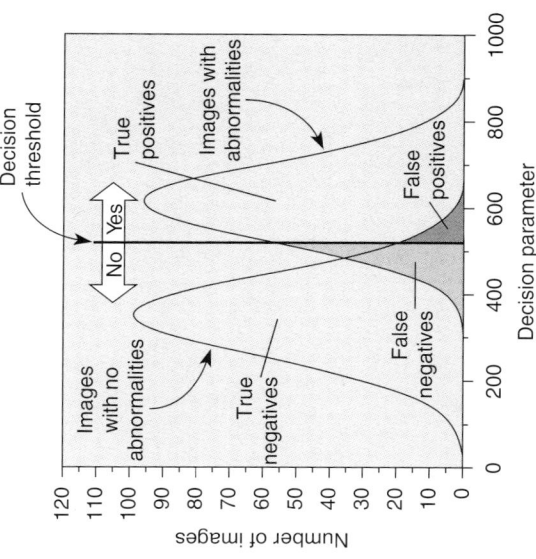

FIGURE 10-26 Graph showing patients with disease versus healthy patients.

affected by factors such as image quality (for which the technical staff is responsible) and the competency of the radiologist to interpret the image (determining whether the anatomy demonstrated in the image is healthy). In images of certain anatomic structures, the distribution of healthy patients follows a bell-shaped normal distribution. The distribution of patients with diseases also follows a normal distribution but with a different mean value (which can be larger or smaller depending on the patient population studied). Fig. 10-26 shows the distribution of these two groups. The two means are relatively far apart, so it should be easy to distinguish between the two.

The region where the two groups overlap indicates less of a distinction between them, and accurate diagnosis is more difficult. A diagnostic cutoff or threshold level is placed to distinguish a healthy diagnosis from a diagnosis of disease. Patients in whom the disease has been diagnosed are considered positive. If a test result (such as a biopsy) reveals that the diagnosis is correct, a designation of *true positive* (TP) is given. Patients are designated as *false positive* (FP) if further study indicates that they do not have the disease despite the positive finding from the image. Healthy patients with no disease present are considered negative. If a diagnosis of negative is determined from an image and supported by follow-up studies, it is designated as *true negative* (TN). If a negative diagnosis is given to a patient who later has the disease, then a designation of *false negative* (FN) is assigned. This information can be obtained from patient medical records and should be determined for high-risk studies such as angiographic procedures. The FDA mandates

light-colored specks similar to those that occur with dirty intensifying screens in film/screen radiography (Fig. 10-23).

Dropped Pixels. Sometimes detector elements in an active matrix array can stop functioning, which means that no data from that area are included in the final image. Because each pixel is relatively small (40 to 100 μm) and there are five or more megapixels in the image, this usually will not be visible. If several detector elements in a specific area all stop at once, white specks can appear in the image that can mimic certain pathologies. Equalization (also known as flat-fielding) software can often correct for dropped pixels, but care should be taken with DR active matrix arrays (especially cassette-based systems) because rough handling can damage them, causing dropped pixels.

Halo Artifacts. Halo artifacts appear as dark bands at the interfaces of structures that differ widely in brightness level such as barium examinations or metal prosthesis.

Printer Errors. Both CR and DR systems rely on dry laser printers to produce hard copies of images. Even though these devices are generally more reliable than wet film processors, they are still subject to problems including incorrect density calibration, light leaks, transport problems, and laser misalignment. These can lead to artifacts such as shading, which results in dark areas in the image (Fig. 10-24) and the "corduroy effect" (Fig. 10-25), where scan lines caused by transport problems also appear in the image. The corduroy artifact can also appear in DR images, where they are caused by a combination of uniformly spaced components within the detector and the sampling rate of the signal. Usually a software update can change the sampling rate and eliminate the artifact.

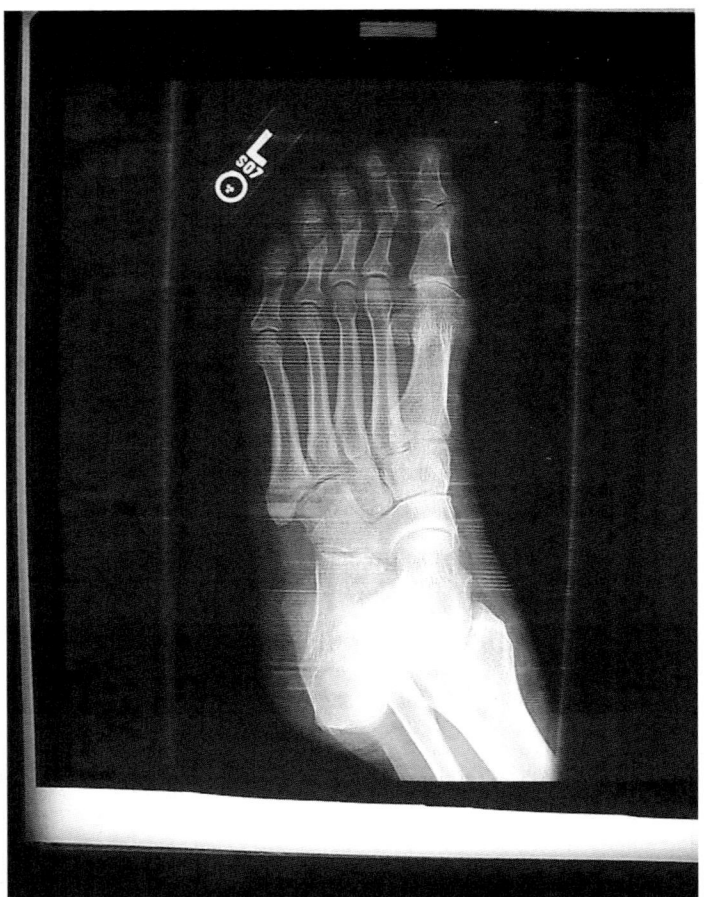

FIGURE 10-22 Scan lines appearing on digital image. (Courtesy of Janet Petersen, Elmhurst Memorial Hospital, Elmhurst, IL.)

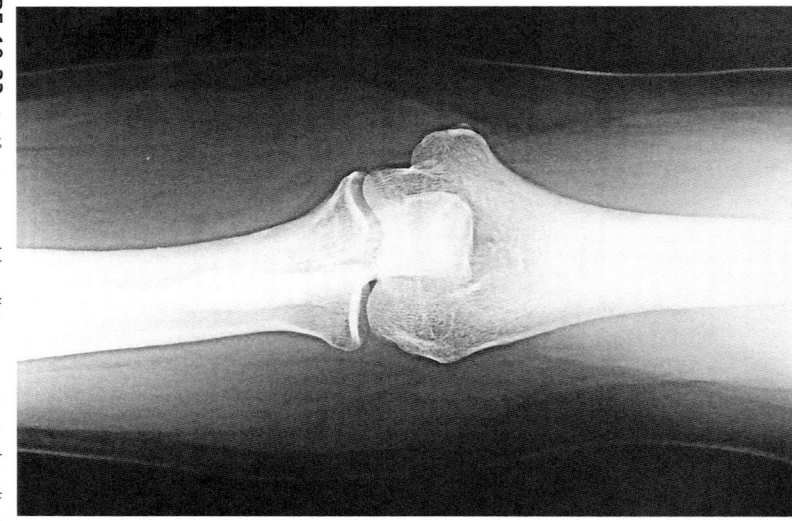

FIGURE 10-23 Artifact caused by dirt on computed radiography (CR) imaging plate.

DIAGNOSTIC PERFORMANCE MEASUREMENT

The main outcome of a diagnostic imaging examination is an accurate diagnosis of a patient's condition so that proper treatment can be administered. This is

CHAPTER 10 Outcomes Assessment of Radiographic Images

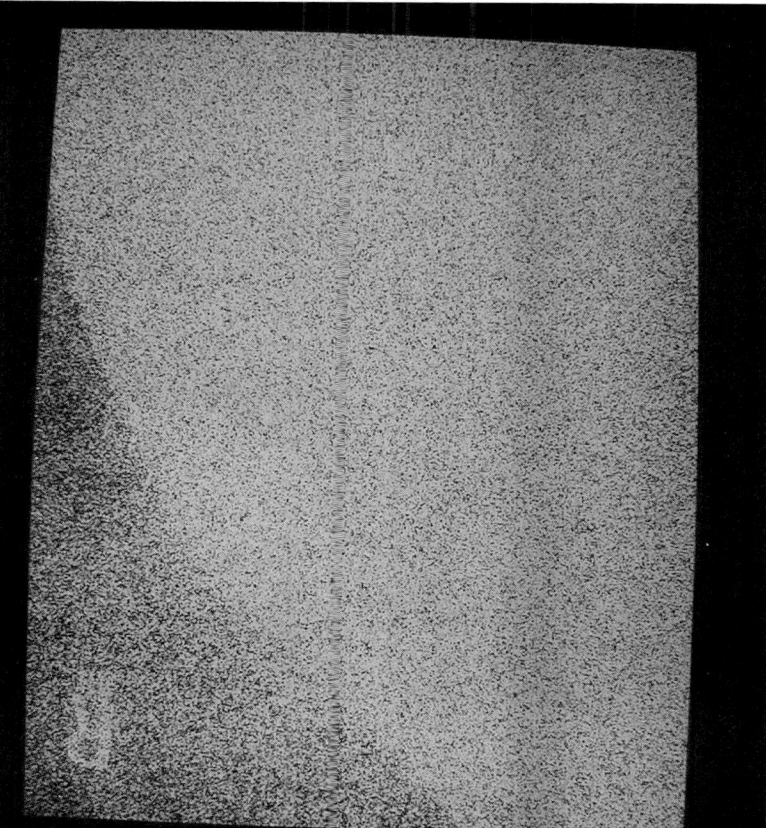

FIGURE 10-20 Phantom image caused by incomplete erasure of computed radiography (CR) imaging plate. *(Courtesy of Janet Petersen, Elmhurst Memorial Hospital, Elmhurst, IL.)*

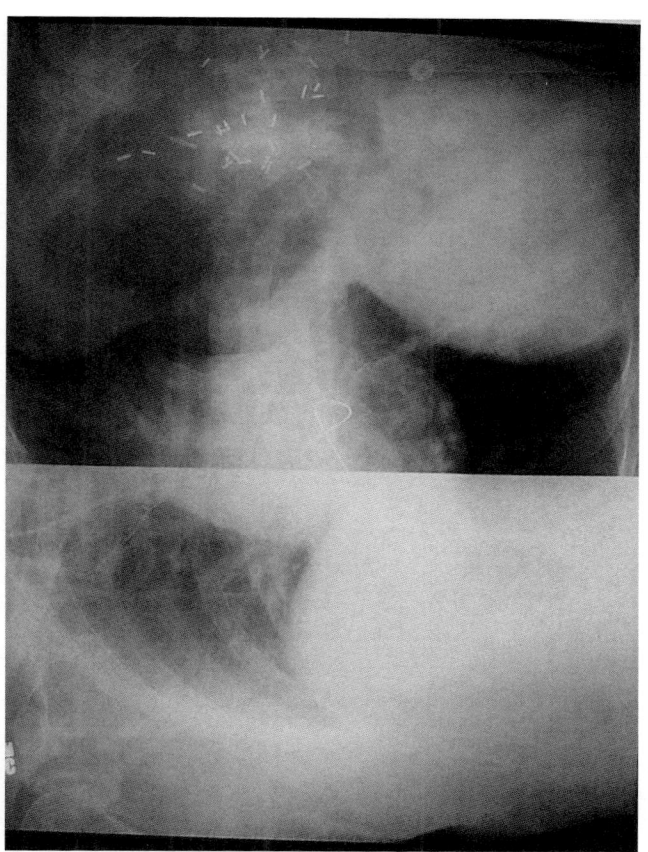

FIGURE 10-21 Double exposure. *(Courtesy of Pamela Verkuilen, Saint Alexius Medical Center, Hoffman Estates, IL.)*

Increased Sensitivity to Scatter. Both CR and DR systems have image receptors that are much more sensitive to scattered radiation due to lower K-edge values. This means that the effects of scatter (and background radiation) can cause a decrease in image contrast that postprocessing software may not be able to correct.

Double Exposure. As with film/screen image receptors, CR imaging plates can be double exposed, leading to both images being lost because data are entered during preprocessing functions (Fig. 10-21).

Computed Radiography Scanner Malfunction. CR scanner malfunction can cause skipped scan lines, missing pixels, and distorted images (Fig. 10-22). These also can be caused by memory problems, digitization problems, or communication errors. Dust and debris also can collect on the rotating polygonal mirror or light collection optics in the IRD. Lasers also have a limited life and must be replaced periodically.

Foreign Objects. Dirt and debris can find their way to CR image plates and DR flat panels, causing

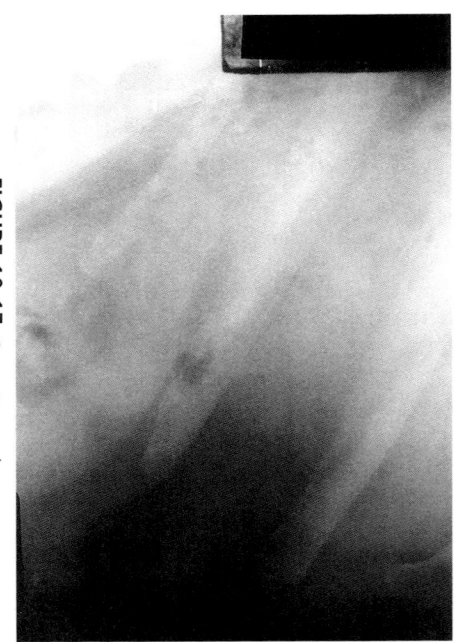

FIGURE 10-17 Cassette marks.

Heat Blur. This is a blurring of the image that can occur when a CR system imaging plate is exposed to intense heat before being processed within the CR reader system.

Improper Image Brightness. When CR systems are used, improper image brightness (optical density when placed onto a hard-copy image) can occur when an incorrect preprocessing histogram is selected (e.g., an adult histogram for the radiography of a pediatric chest). This is known as **histogram error.** Improper optical density with CR systems also can occur because of nonparallel collimation. For the histograms used by CR systems to process the final image, the collimation edges of the radiation field should be parallel to the sides of the imaging plate. This way, the preprogrammed histogram in the CR system, the histogram created by the imaging plate match, and the computer can assign the correct optical density values to the appropriate region of the image. When collimation is not parallel, the histograms do not match correctly and the system then may be unable to determine the appropriate optical density value.

Electronic Noise. Each detector element (DEL) in the active matrix array of a DR system has a certain amount of electronic noise associated with it. This is also known as dark noise and can be present even though no exposure of the image receptor has occurred.

Quantum Mottle. Just as with film/screen systems (or any imaging system that relies on photons to cover an area of interest), quantum mottle can occur with digital imaging systems and create the same "grainy" appearance. Often, it is even more common in digital systems as radiographers may use lower mAs values to decrease patient dose and then use computer software to correct image brightness (Fig. 10-18).

Defects in the Imaging Plate. Scratches, scuff marks, or cracks in a CR image plate can mimic fractures and signs of pneumothorax (Fig. 10-19); therefore, image plates must be inspected periodically, and damaged plates must be removed from service.

Phantom Image Artifact. CR image plates must be properly erased before use, or data from previous images will interfere with current image data (Fig. 10-20). In

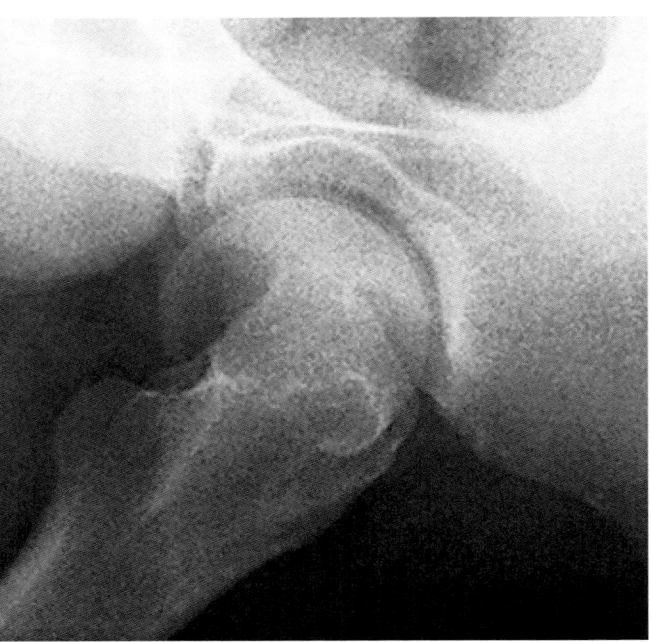

FIGURE 10-18 Quantum mottle occurring in a computed radiography (CR) image.

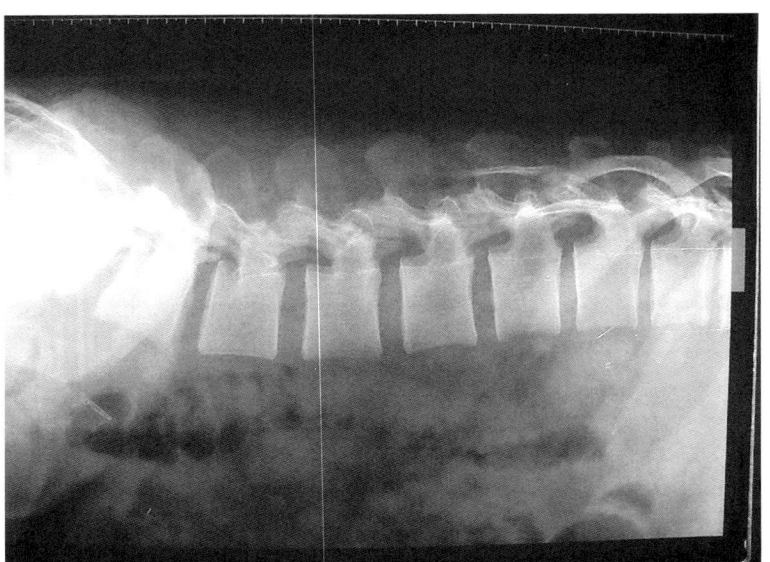

FIGURE 10-19 Artifact caused by scratches on a computed radiography (CR) image plate. (Courtesy of Janet Petersen, Elmhurst Memorial Hospital, Elmhurst, IL.)

DR imaging, this artifact is known as electronic memory artifact or "ghosting" and can be caused by exposures that are taken in too rapid a sequence resulting in not enough time for each previous exposure to transfer the entire signal.

186 CHAPTER 10 Outcomes Assessment of Radiographic Images

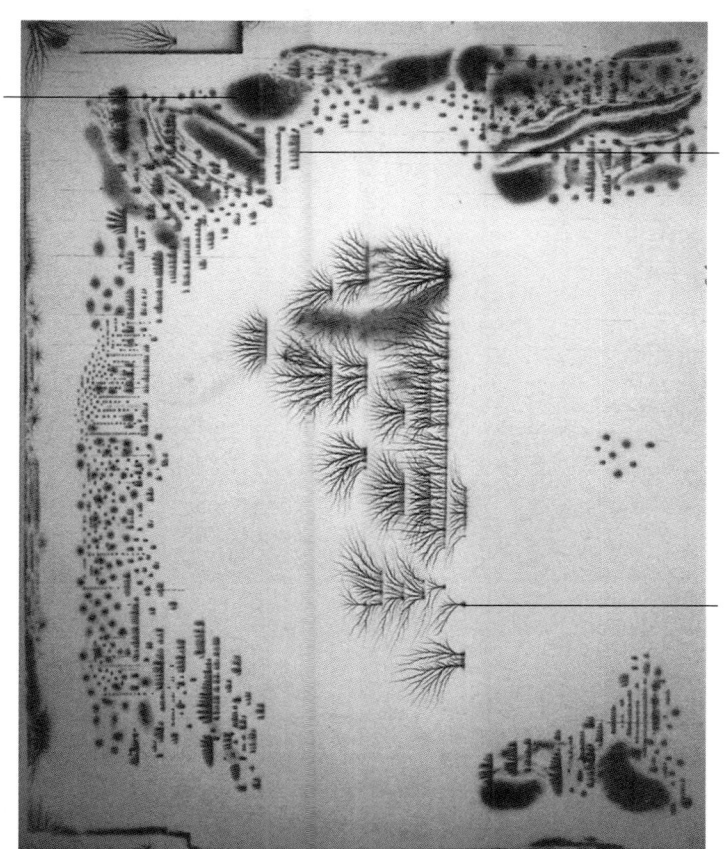

FIGURE 10-15 Image demonstrating static artifacts.

Smudge Static. Smudge static consists of dark areas where excessive amounts of light have exposed the film and is usually caused by rough handling in the film processing area.

Crescent or Crinkle Marks. Crescent or crinkle marks are half-moon-shaped marks of increased optical density caused by bending of the film before processing (Fig. 10-16). The bending of a processed film image can result in crescent marks that are of decreased optical density because some of the silver can be moved from the area where the bending has occurred.

Scratches. Scratches are areas where the emulsion has been removed by sharp objects such as fingernails or sharp points on surfaces.

Cassette Marks. Cassette marks are white specks on the image caused by dirt or debris inside the cassette. This foreign matter blocks the light from the screen from reaching the film. Regular cleaning of the screens with an antistatic cleaner can minimize these artifacts (Fig. 10-17).

Computed Radiography and Digital Radiography Artifacts

Even though liquid processing and film/screen image receptors are not used with CR and DR systems, artifacts can still occur and therefore must have their sources recognized by radiographers in order to minimize their occurrence. This is in addition to the exposure artifacts listed earlier in the section on film/screen artifacts—these

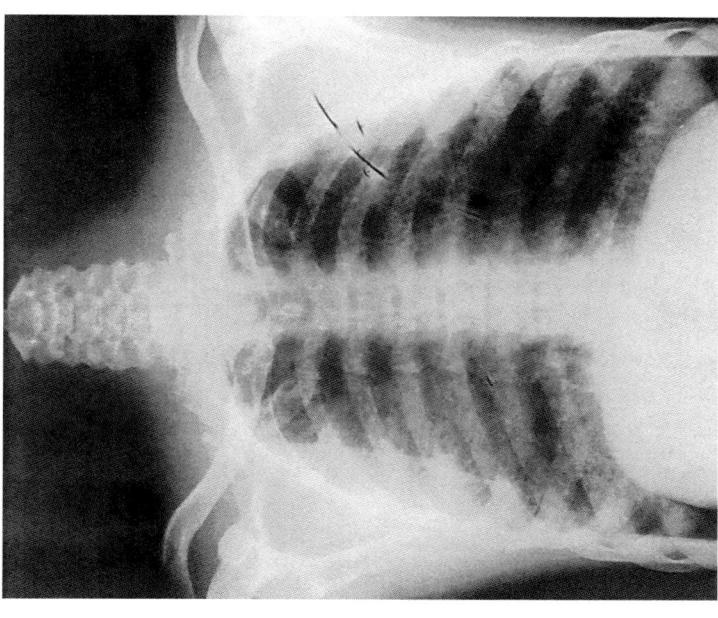

FIGURE 10-16 Crescent marks.

also will occur with CR and DR systems (except for poor film/screen contact). Artifacts occurring during preprocessing functions often cannot be corrected, whereas those occurring during postprocessing tend to be recoverable.

FIGURE 10-12 Grid lines.

FIGURE 10-13 Grid cutoff.

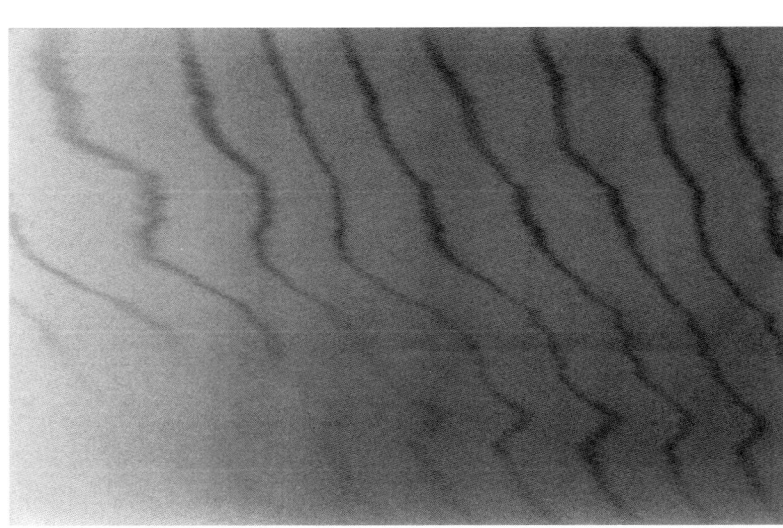

FIGURE 10-14 Moiré effect, or zebra pattern, artifact.

a warm, humid environment. It results in a lower image contrast.

Safelight Fog. Safelight fog is caused by an improper safelight filter, cracks or pinholes in the safelight filter, incorrect wattage of the safelight bulb, incorrect distance between the safelight and work surfaces, or widely open sodium vapor lamp shutters.

Radiation Fog. Radiation fog appears in film that has been exposed to ionizing radiation before development.

Pressure Marks. Excessive pressure, such as a heavy object placed on the film before development, causes pressure marks, which are areas of increased optical density. Pressure marks occur because the pressure splitting the bond between the silver and the halide ion in the film emulsion results in the presence of black metallic silver after processing. Film should be stored vertically to minimize the risk of pressure artifacts.

Static. The sparks from static electricity expose film and produce three types of static artifacts: tree static, crown static, and smudge static (Fig. 10-15).

Tree Static. Tree static resembles trees or bushes without leaves and is usually caused by low humidity conditions in the film processing area.

Crown Static. Crown static marks radiate in one direction so that they resemble a crown. Excessive friction from the pulling of the film (such as in a daylight system, in which the film is "squeezed" too tightly between the intensifying screens) can produce these marks.

Light Fog. The light of any improper color that strikes the film before development fogs the film and therefore lowers the image contrast. Fog is any noninformational optical density present in a film image.

Age Fog. Age fog may occur in film that has been processed beyond the expiration date or has been stored in

image receptor position by the technologist or improper collimation, which can clip the anatomy of interest.

Quantum Mottle. Quantum mottle is a grainy appearance in a radiograph that is caused by statistical variations in the number of X-ray photons covering a specific area. This is usually present when there is an insufficient amount of radiation reaching the image receptor or detection device. This can occur with film/screen radiography, CR, DR, fluoroscopy, computed tomography, and nuclear medicine imaging. This is discussed later in this chapter under Computed Radiology and Digital Radiography Artifacts.

Poor Film-to-Screen Contact. Poor film-to-screen contact results in localized blurring of the radiographic image, which also may demonstrate slightly increased optical density in these regions.

Double Exposure. Double exposure occurs when an image receptor is exposed more than once before the image is processed.

Grid Artifacts. Improper use of a grid causes grid artifacts, which include grid lines, grid cutoff, and moiré effect.

Grid Lines. Grid lines are shadows of the lead strips that appear on the resulting image and are caused by failure of the grid to move during the exposure, improper grid-focusing distance, improper angulation of the central ray with respect to the grid lines, or improper centering (Fig. 10-12).

Grid Cutoff. Grid cutoff is a decrease in optical density caused by primary radiation being absorbed by (or cut off by) the grid (Fig. 10-13). Any improper use of a grid can cause grid cutoff.

Moiré Effect. Moiré effect, or zebra pattern artifact, is a double set of grid lines caused by the placement of a grid cassette in a bucky (Fig. 10-14). This artifact also can occur in CR systems when a stationary grid having a grid frequency in the range of 85 to 100 lines per inch is used, and the grid lines are parallel to the CR reader scan lines. This is due to the scan frequency of the laser in the image reader device (IRD) closely matching the grid frequency. To eliminate this particular cause of Moiré effect, the following steps can be taken:

1. Ensure grids are moving during the exposure.
2. Use a grid with a higher grid frequency.
3. Use a crosshatch grid or a multihole grid.
4. Change the orientation of the grid so that the grid lines are perpendicular to the CR reader scan lines.

Handling and Storage Artifacts

Handling and storage artifacts occur during darkroom handling or during storage before use.

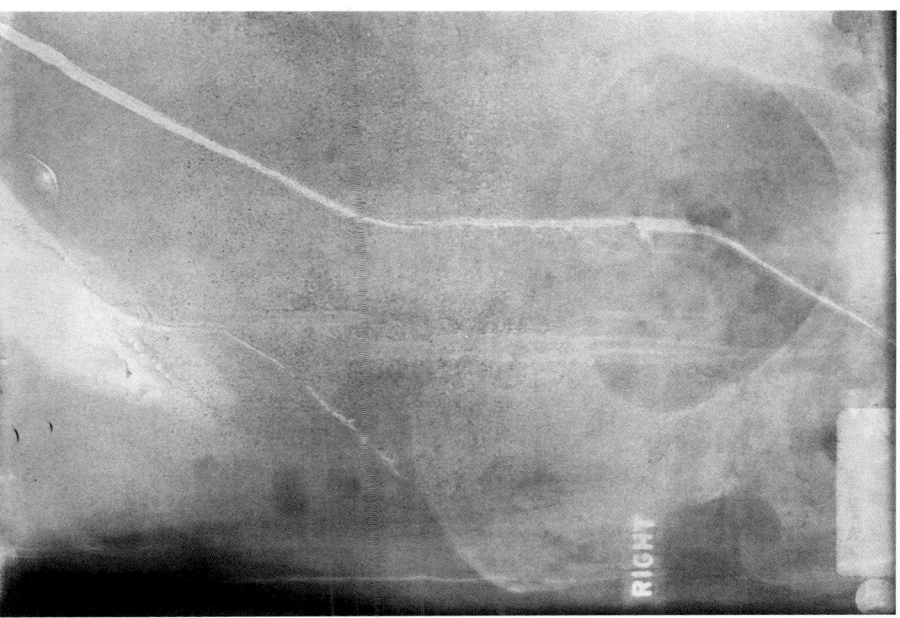

FIGURE 10-10 Wet-pressure sensitization.

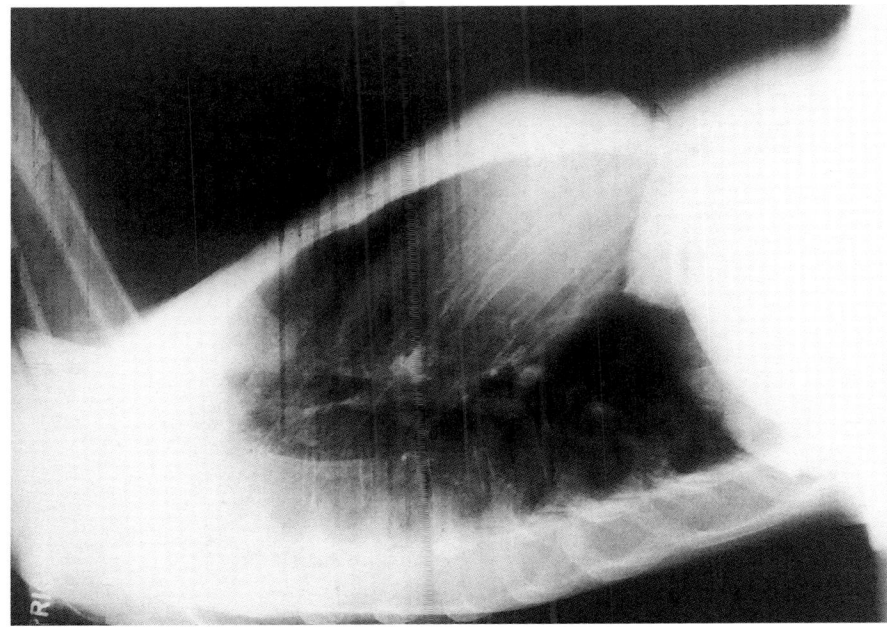

FIGURE 10-11 Hyporetention.

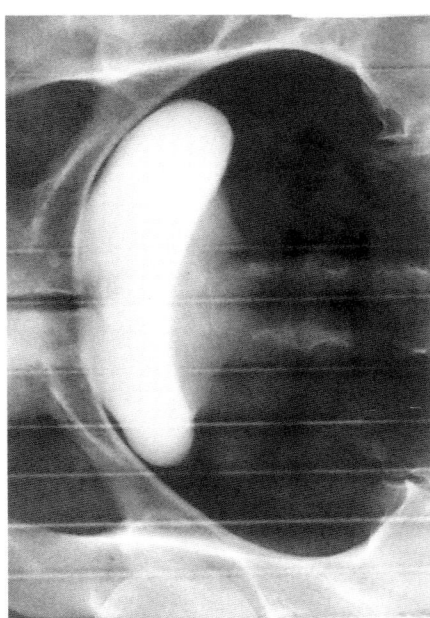

FIGURE 10-8 Hesitation marks.

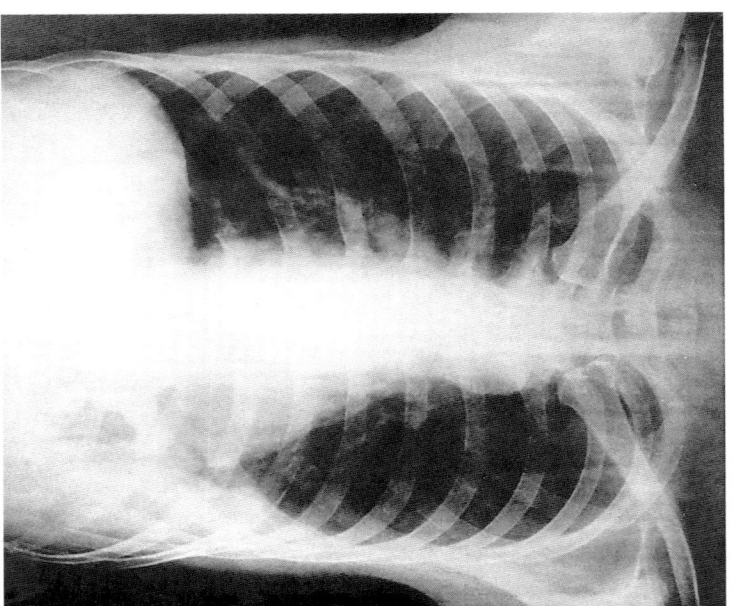

FIGURE 10-7 Streaking.

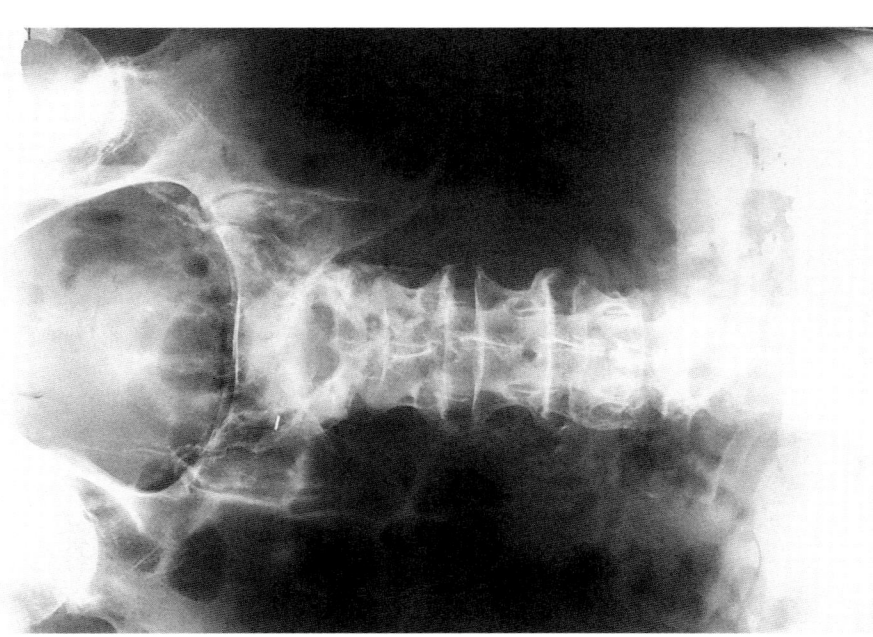

FIGURE 10-9 Water spots.

Hyporetention. Hyporetention is a white, powdery residue that remains on the film surface because of incomplete washing (Fig. 10-11). This residue forms when the fixer chemicals crystallize as the film dries. A lesser degree of hyporetention can result in brown dichroic stains, which were discussed previously.

Insufficient Optical Density. Images that lack sufficient optical density as a result of processing problems can occur because of the following conditions: developer temperature that is below accepted limits, insufficient developer time, underreplenished developer solution, a developer that is contaminated by the fixer, developer pH that is too low, or insufficient developer concentration.

Excessive Optical Density. Images with excessive optical density as a result of processing problems can occur because of the following conditions: the extension of the developer temperature's accepted limits, excessive developer time, overreplenishment, higher accepted limits of the developer pH, or excessive developer concentration.

Exposure Artifacts

Exposure artifacts are caused by the patient, the technologist, or the equipment during a diagnostic procedure.

Motion. A motion artifact is a blurring of the image caused by the motion of the patient, X-ray source, or image receptor. This results in a significant loss of recorded detail. Patient motion can be reduced with short exposure time, immobilization, and proper instructions to the patient.

Patient Artifacts. Patient artifacts are caused by items that can be either on or within the patient when a diagnostic procedure is performed. Examples of patient artifacts include buttons, snaps, necklaces, earrings, hairpins, wet hair, and body piercing jewelry.

Improper Optical Density. Improper selection of technical factors by the technologist or improper cell selection with automatic exposure control results in improper optical density.

Improper Patient Position or Missing Anatomy of Interest. Improper patient position or missing anatomy of interest is the result of improper patient, X-ray, or

182 CHAPTER 10 Outcomes Assessment of Radiographic Images

FIGURE 10-5 Guide shoe marks.

marks caused by crossover assemblies usually occur at the top surface of the film. Guide shoe marks from turnaround assemblies tend to occur at the bottom surface of the film. These scratches run parallel to (in the same direction as) the direction of film travel.

Pi Lines. Pi lines are artifacts that occur relative to the circumference of a roller and therefore occur at regular intervals (Fig. 10-6). These marks run perpendicular to the direction of film travel and are usually caused by dirt or debris on the rollers.

Chatter. Chattering artifacts appear as bands of increased optical density that occur perpendicular to film direction. Chatter is caused by inconsistent motion of the transport system, usually because the drive gears or drive chain slips. Chemical buildup on gears or gears not seated properly can cause chatter marks that are approximately 1/8 inch apart. A rusty or loose drive chain can cause chatter marks that are about 3/8 inch apart.

Dichroic Stain. The term *dichroic* refers to "two colors," brown and greenish yellow. The presence of brown stains on a radiograph could indicate a film processed in oxidized developer or hyporetention that has been present during several years of storage. The greenish yellow type of stain indicates the presence of unexposed and undeveloped silver halide crystals remaining on the film after processing and is caused by incomplete fixation.

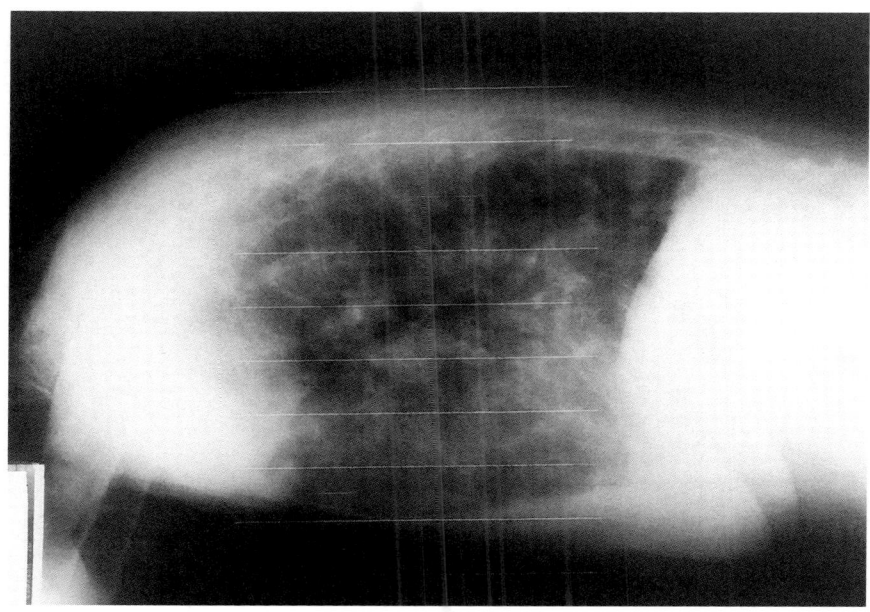

FIGURE 10-6 Pi lines.

Reticulation Marks. When uneven solution temperatures cause excessive expansion and contraction of the film emulsion during processing, the result is a network of fine grooves in the film surface (**reticulation marks**).

Streaking. Streaking is uneven development of the image that can be caused by the failure of agitation in manual processing or the failure of the circulation system in automatic processing (Fig. 10-7).

Hesitation Marks. Hesitation marks (also known as *stub lines*) are stripes of decreased optical density where transport rollers are left in contact with the film and further the development is prevented (Fig. 10-8). These artifacts occur when the processor is turned off or loses power while the film is in the developer section or if the film becomes jammed while in the developer section. They also can occur if the transport system speed decreases significantly.

Water Spots. Should water or other liquid come in contact with an unprocessed image, a pattern of increased optical density appears after processing (Fig. 10-9).

Wet-Pressure Sensitization. The entrance rollers on most processors are made of soft rubber with grooves on the surface to grab the film from the feed tray. Should these rollers or the film become wet before the film is introduced, the combination of the pressure and the water marks forms a series of dark stripes that match the grooves on the rollers (Fig. 10-10). The marks also may occur if the tension on the entrance rollers is too great. These marks run in the same direction as film travel. These artifacts also are known as *entrance roller marks*.

ARTIFACT ANALYSIS

One cause of rejected images listed in the repeat analysis worksheet is the presence of image artifacts. An artifact is anything on a finished radiograph that is not part of the patient's anatomy. Artifacts can contribute significantly to the total repeat rate; therefore, a thorough knowledge of artifacts and their possible causes is necessary so that corrective action can be taken.

Film/Screen Radiography

Image artifacts found in film/screen radiography can be placed into one of three categories: processing artifacts, exposure artifacts, and handling and storage artifacts.

Processing Artifacts

Processing artifacts are caused by or occur during the processing of diagnostic images.

Emulsion Pickoff. In emulsion pickoff, the emulsion is removed from or "picked off" of the film base. This occurs when two images are stuck together before or during processing and then pulled apart afterward. It also occurs with single sheets of film that are processed in underreplenished developer that results in glutaraldehyde failure. Because glutaraldehyde is the weak hardener added to the developer solution that keeps the film from sticking to the rollers, failure of this ingredient will cause the emulsion to be removed from the film and deposited on the rollers.

Gelatin Buildup. Emulsion that has been removed from earlier images and either stuck on processor rollers or dissolved in the developer solution can be deposited on subsequent images. The primary cause is underreplenished developer solution or failure of the developer circulation system filter.

Curtain Effect. Solution dripping on, or "running down," a film can form patterns on the film that resemble a lace curtain (Fig. 10-3). This is more common in manually processed images but can occur in automatically processed images if the wash water is dirty or if a film has jammed and must be removed from the processor before passing through the dryer section.

Chemical Fog. Chemical fog is an overdevelopment of the film that results in excessive base + fog and minimum diameter (D_{min}) values with sensitometry images and excessive optical density with radiographic images (Fig. 10-4). The main cause is developer temperature, time, pH, or concentration above the manufacturer's specifications. It also may occur with overreplenishment of the developer solution.

and patient population is considered. Any departments with repeat rates exceeding 10% to 12% should be examined seriously because these departments are inefficient and contribute to a high patient dose.

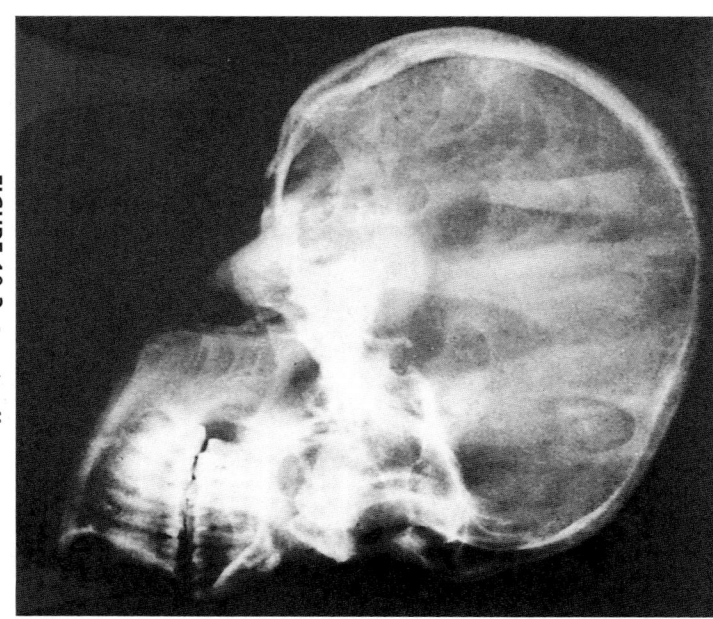

FIGURE 10-3 Curtain effect.

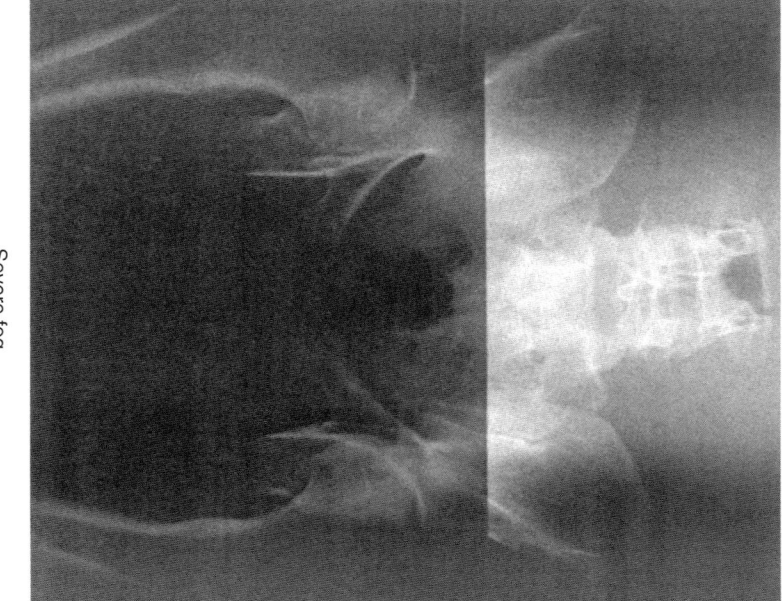

Severe fog   Normal fog

FIGURE 10-4 Chemical fog.

Guide Shoe Marks. Guide shoe marks are scratches on images made by the jagged edges of the guide shoes because they may be bent, worn, damaged, incorrectly installed, or incorrectly adjusted. They also may occur with improperly seated transport racks or rollers (Fig. 10-5). Guide shoe

CHAPTER 10   Outcomes Assessment of Radiographic Images

that this information be derived for mammographic procedures. From this information, the values of accuracy, sensitivity, and specificity; **prevalence; positive predictive value;** and **negative predictive value** can be obtained.

Accuracy

Accuracy is the percentage or fraction of cases that are diagnosed correctly; it can be determined by the following equation:

$$\text{Accuracy} = \frac{(N_{TP} + N_{TN})}{N_{Total}} \times 100$$

N designates the number of cases. For example, if 210 mammograms are performed in 1 month and the number of TNs is 167 and the number of TPs is 36, then the accuracy rate of the image diagnosis is 0.967, or 96.7%.

Sensitivity

Sensitivity also is referred to as the *TP fraction* and indicates the likelihood of obtaining a positive diagnosis in a patient with the disease (or the ability to detect disease). A sensitive test has a low FN rate. Sensitivity is determined by the following equation:

$$\text{Sensitivity} = \frac{N_{TP}}{(N_{TP} + N_{FN})}$$

If a department demonstrates 36 TPs and 3 FNs, then the sensitivity is 0.92, or 92%.

Specificity. Specificity is also known as the *TN fraction* and indicates the likelihood of a patient obtaining a negative diagnosis when no disease is present. A specific test has a low FP rate. Specificity is determined by the following equation:

$$\text{Sensitivity} = \frac{N_T}{(N_{TN} + N_{FP})}$$

A department receiving 167 TNs and 4 FPs has a specificity of 0.97, or 97%.

Positive Predictive Value. The positive predictive value is the probability of having the disease given a positive test and is determined by the following equation:

$$\frac{N_{TP}}{(N_{TP} + N_{FP})}$$

A department having 36 TPs and 4 FPs will have a positive predictive value of 0.9 or 90%.

Negative Predictive Value

The negative predictive value is the probability of not having the disease given a negative test and is determined by the following equation:

$$\frac{N_{TN}}{(N_{TN} + N_{FN})}$$

A department having 167 TNs and 3 FNs will have a negative predictive value of 0.98 or 98%.

The ideal for all of the previous values is 100%. In general, the diagnostic performance will depend on the disease prevalence, which is determined by the following equation:

$$\frac{[N_{TP} + N_{FN}]}{[N_{TP} + N_{FP} + N_{TN} + N_{FN}]}$$

A diagnostic imaging department is responsible for establishing its own threshold of acceptability for each value, with both internal and external factors being considered (see Chapter 1). Departments that want to improve accuracy, sensitivity, and specificity can use special statistical phantoms for radiographic, mammographic, and fluoroscopic analysis (Fig. 10-27). These specialized phantoms allow for the position of the phantom components (e.g., test wires, simulated bone fragments, low-contrast objects) to be moved to different parts of the phantom each time it is used. This can eliminate the problem of "familiarity," whereby the observer is familiar with the phantom test pattern and begins to expect or predict that the objects are appearing at the appropriate location. By varying the location each time, the observer has to actually "see" the object at its location for the phantom testing to be valid. Many diagnostic imaging departments also use "double read" as a method to improve accuracy. With this method, two radiologists separately read the same case, and if their diagnoses differ from each other, they confer and decide conclusively.

Receiver Operator Characteristic Curve

A receiver operator characteristic curve (ROC, also known as a *relative operator characteristic curve*) is a plot of the true-positive probability or sensitivity versus the false-positive probability, which also can be described as (1-specificity) (Fig. 10-28). An ideal image would yield a true-positive probability of 1 (100%) and a false-positive probability of 0. Data points that would fall toward the upper left-hand corner of an ROC curve would indicate an accurate diagnosis. If data points fall on a line that is at a 45° angle within the graph, it would indicate random guessing by the observer. The area under the ROC curve is a measure of overall imaging performance and has a maximum value of 1 (100%). As image quality and performance improve, the curve will move toward the upper left-hand corner, which increases the area under the curve. The area under the random guessing line is 0.5 (50%).

SUMMARY

Implementing a quality management program requires more than just equipment monitoring and maintenance. The outcomes assessment of diagnostic images also

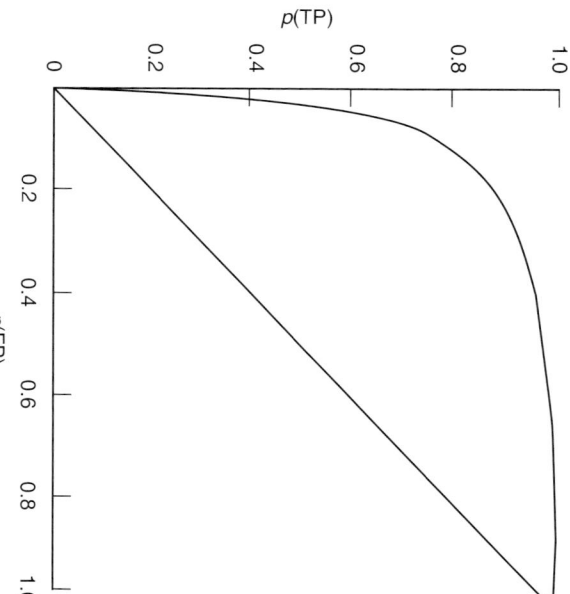

FIGURE 10-28 ROC curve. The 45° diagonal line in the graph indicates pure guesswork by the observer. The curve on the left hand side of the graph depicts an accurate imaging procedure. ROC, receiver operating characteristic.

REVIEW QUESTIONS

1. In departments with a quality management program in place, the greatest number of repeat images is due to which of the following?
   a. Equipment problems
   b. Image fog
   c. Patient motion
   d. Positioning error

2. If a department performs 1160 views during a 1-month period and 132 are repeated, the department repeat rate is which of the following?
   a. 9.5%
   b. 10.7%
   c. 11.4%
   d. 14.8%

3. Any repeat rate exceeding _____ should be seriously examined.
   a. 2% to 4%
   b. 4% to 6%
   c. 6% to 8%
   d. 10% to 12%

4. Which of the following processing artifacts run in the same direction as film travel?
   a. Pi lines
   b. Guide shoe marks
   c. Hesitation marks
   d. Chemical fog

5. Which of the following artifacts can occur in both CR and film/screen radiography?
   a. Static electricity
   b. Wet-pressure sensitization
   c. Moiré pattern
   d. Water spots

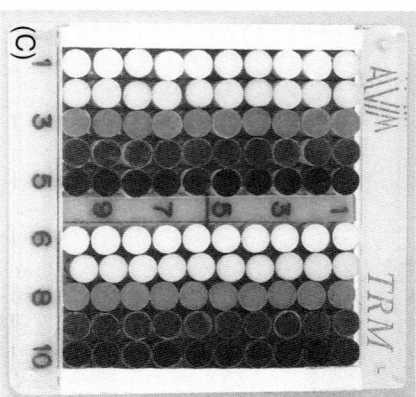

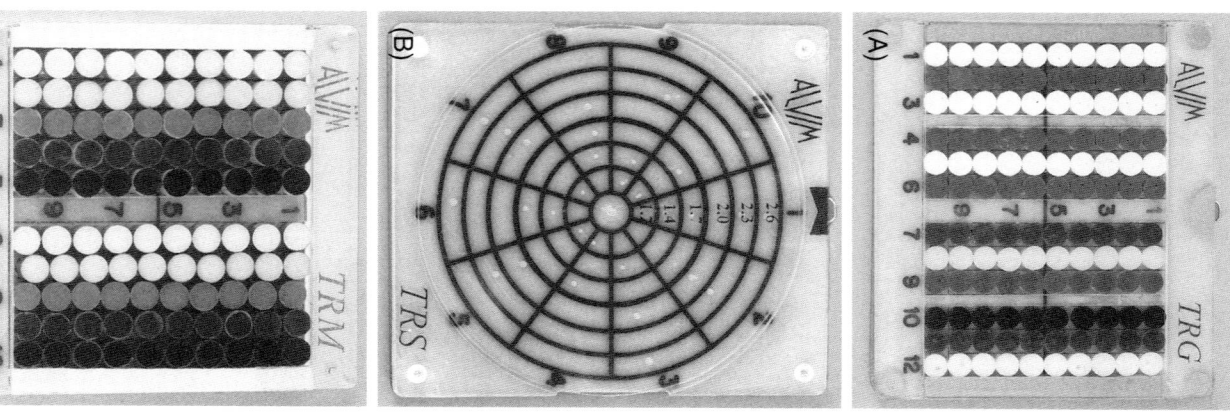

FIGURE 10-27 Statistical phantoms for (A) radiographic; (B) mammographic; and (C) fluoroscopic images. (*Courtesy Nuclear Associates, Carle Place, NY.*)

must be performed to evaluate the success of the procedure. In this way, future problems may be avoided by analyzing current causes of repeat images and artifacts. Continuous improvement of image quality and customer satisfaction can occur when diagnostic image quality and diagnostic accuracy are monitored on a routine basis.

Refer to the Evolve Website at https://evolve.elsevier.com for Student Experiment 10.1: Reject-Repeat Analysis.

CHAPTER 10 Outcomes Assessment of Radiographic Images

6. The types of static artifacts include (1) tree, (2) crown, and (3) smudge:
   a. 1 and 2
   b. 2 and 3
   c. 1 and 3
   d. 1, 2, and 3

7. Which of the following terms best describes the likelihood of obtaining a positive diagnosis in a patient with the disease actually present?
   a. Sensitivity
   b. Specificity
   c. Variance
   d. Frequency

8. Data for determining repeat rates should include at least _____ patients to obtain a statistical sample large enough for valid results.
   a. 100
   b. 150
   c. 250
   d. 500

9. Which of the following terms also is referred to as the TP fraction?
   a. Accuracy
   b. Sensitivity
   c. Specificity
   d. None of the above

10. Which of the following artifacts occurs as a result of patient motion during exposure?
    a. A processing artifact
    b. An exposure artifact
    c. A handling artifact
    d. No artifact

CHAPTER 11

Mammographic Quality Standards

KEY TERMS

Adverse event
Annotations and measurements
Beryllium window
Compression
Consumer
Emission spectrum
Extended processing
Gray-scale processing
Image inversion
Magnification
Mammography Quality Standards Act
Postprocessing
Serious adverse event
Serious complaint
Target composition
Tissue equalization
Tomosynthesis
Workflow

OBJECTIVES

At the completion of this chapter, the reader should be able to do the following:

- Explain the difference between dedicated mammography equipment and conventional equipment
- Describe the composition of the X-ray tube target in mammographic equipment
- Discuss the advantages of compression during mammographic procedures
- Describe the image receptor systems currently used in mammography
- Describe the basic differences between film/screen mammography and full-field digital mammography
- Indicate the quality control tasks relating to the radiologist and the medical physicist
- Describe the quality control duties of the mammographer on a daily, weekly, quarterly, and semiannual basis
- Describe the various components of a Food and Drug Administration/Mammography Quality Standards Act inspection

OUTLINE

Dedicated Mammographic Equipment
   X-ray Generator
   X-ray Tube
      X-ray Tube Window
      Target Composition
      Focal Spot Size
      Source-to-Image Distance and Target Angle
   Compression
   Grids
   Image Receptors
   Film Processors
   Magnification Mammography
Digital Mammography Systems
Stereotactic Localization
Mammographic Quality Assurance
MQSA and the Mammography Quality Standards Reauthorization Act
Quality Control Responsibilities
   Radiologist (Interpreting Physician)
   Medical Physicist
   Film/Screen Systems
   Digital Mammography Systems
   Radiologic Technologist (Mammographer)
Film/Screen Systems
   Daily Duties
   Weekly Duties
   Monthly Duties
   Quarterly Duties
   Semiannual Duties
   Full-Field Digital Mammography Systems
Inspection by the Food and Drug Administration
   Equipment Performance
   Records
   Inspection Report
Summary

CHAPTER 11 Mammographic Quality Standards

Mammography is soft tissue radiography of the breast. It requires different equipment and techniques from conventional radiography because of the close similarities among anatomic structures (low subject contrast). Low kilovolt (peak) (kVp) in the 20- to 30-kVp range must be deployed to maximize the amount of photoelectric effect and to enhance differential absorption. The side effect of using lower kilovolt (peak) exposure factors is correspondingly higher milliampere-second (mAs) values, which increase the total radiation dose to the patient. The American College of Radiology recommends the average glandular dose for a 4.2-cm thick breast should be less than 300 mrad (3 mGy) per view for film/screen image receptors used with a grid. If no grid is used, the average glandular dose should be less than 100 mrad (1 mGy) per view. Because the glandular tissue of the breast is inherently radiosensitive, care must be taken to minimize radiation exposure through dedicated equipment and quality control procedures.

DEDICATED MAMMOGRAPHIC EQUIPMENT

X-ray Generator

The X-ray generators used in mammographic studies should be dedicated solely to mammographic imaging (Fig. 11-1). All current mammographic imagers are high-frequency X-ray generators (see Chapter 7) that are smaller in size and less expensive than earlier single- and three-phase mammographic units. High-frequency X-ray generators also provide exceptional exposure reproducibility, which is essential for consistent image quality. The kilovolt (peak) range available on most units is between 20 kVp and 35 kVp, and typical X-ray tube currents are about 80 to 200 mA. Exposure times are usually about 1 second but can be as long as 4 seconds for dense or thick breasts, or for those with implants. For a normal compressed breast (4.5 cm), a typical X-ray tube voltage is 25 kVp with a milliampere-exposure time combination of about 120 mAs. All systems with film/screen image receptors must be equipped with an automatic exposure control (AEC) system that consists of two to three sensors to regulate the optical density (OD) of the resulting image. Each film/screen system should provide an AEC mode that is operable in all combinations of equipment configuration provided (for example, grid, nongrid, magnification, nonmagnification, and various target-filter combinations). The positioning or selection of the detector permits flexibility in the placement of the detector under the target tissue. The size and available positions of the detector must be clearly indicated at the X-ray input surface of the breast compression paddle. The system also must provide a means for the operator to vary the selected OD from the normal (zero) setting. The X-ray tube/image receptor assembly must be capable of being fixed in any position and not undergo any unintended motion or fail in the event of power interruption.

X-ray Tube

Modern mammographic X-ray units use rotating anode X-ray tubes just as conventional radiographic units do. However, some significant differences exist, including the X-ray tube window, target composition, focal spot size, and source-to-image distance (SID) and target angle.

X-ray Tube Window. X-ray tubes used in conventional radiographic, fluoroscopic, and computed tomographic units incorporate a window made primarily of glass (which is essentially silicon with an atomic number of 14). Because relatively high kilovolt (peak) exposure factors are used in these studies, absorption of lower energy X-rays in the window material is acceptable and actually desired. Mammographic X-ray tubes use a thinner glass window or a **beryllium window** (atomic number of 4), which is less likely to absorb the low kilovolt (peak) X-rays used in mammographic procedures. The inherent filtration of the beryllium is about 0.1 mm aluminum (Al) equivalent compared with 0.5 mm Al equivalent for standard radiographic tubes.

Target Composition. Conventional radiographic X-ray tubes use a **target composition** of a tungsten–rhenium alloy. A mixture of X-rays produced by both Bremsstrahlung (the slowing down of the projectile electron, causing a wide range of X-ray energies) and characteristic radiation (X-rays created by electron transitions

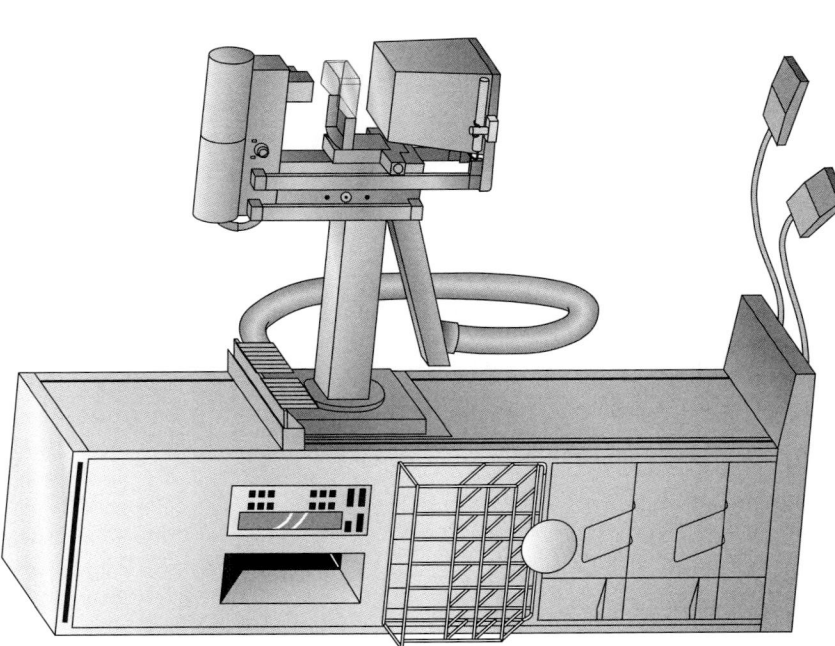

FIGURE 11-1 Dedicated mammographic unit.

between orbits resulting in specific or discrete energies) exists in the X-ray beam created with these X-ray tubes. This effect can be demonstrated with an X-ray **emission spectrum** graph (Fig. 11-2). This wide band of energies may be desirable in conventional radiography but is not desirable in mammography because of the low subject contrast. Factors affecting the X-ray emission spectrum graph include milliamperes, kilovolts (peak), added filtration, target material, and voltage waveform/ripple.

Milliamperes. The factor of milliamperes changes the amplitude of the curve (height of the y-axis) but not the shape of the curve (Fig. 11-3).

Kilovolts (Peak). The factor of kilovolts (peak) changes both the amplitude and the position of the spectrum curve. An increase in kilovolts (peak) shifts the spectrum to the right, indicating greater energy values (Fig. 11-4).

Added Filtration. Because filtration affects X-ray quality, the effect on the X-ray emission spectrum is similar to that of kilovolts (peak). If filtration is increased, the amplitude decreases and the spectrum shifts slightly to the right (Fig. 11-5).

Target Material. The amplitude and shape of the emission spectrum graph vary with any changes in the atomic number of the target material. If the atomic number increases, the continuous portion of the spectrum (Bremsstrahlung) increases slightly in amplitude, especially to the high-energy side, whereas the discrete portion of the spectrum (characteristic X-rays) shifts to the right (Fig. 11-6). The target materials used in mammographic X-ray tubes include tungsten, molybdenum, rhodium, or a combination of them.

Tungsten (Atomic Number 74). Tungsten produces a wide band of X-ray energies, including some that are not useful in mammographic imaging. The emission spectrum is then shaped with filters made of aluminum, molybdenum, or rhodium.

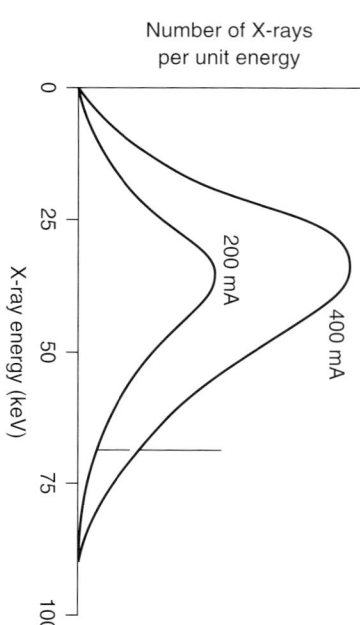

FIGURE 11-2 Emission spectrum for tungsten-rhenium target. keV, kiloelectron volt.

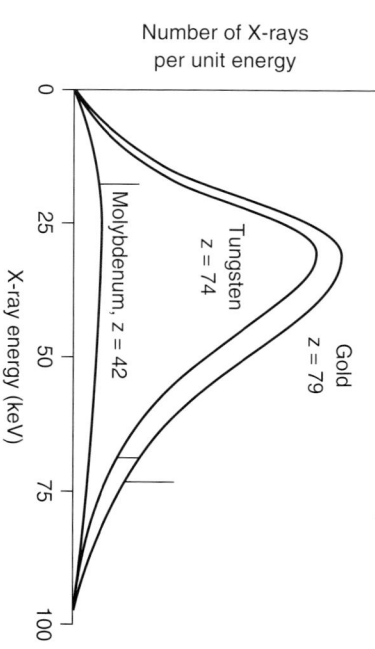

FIGURE 11-3 Effect of milliamperes on emission spectrum. keV, kiloelectron volt; mA, milliampere.

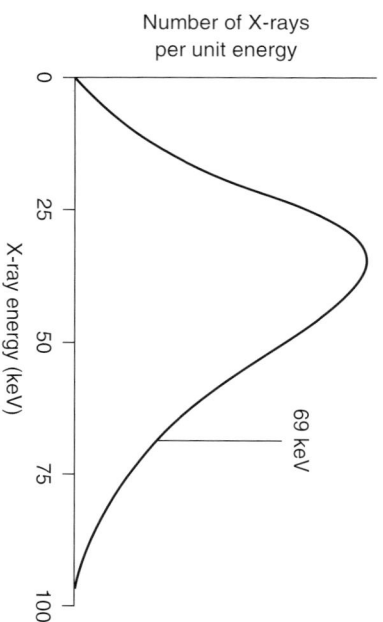

FIGURE 11-4 Effect of kilovolts (peak) on emission spectrum. keV, kiloelectron volt; kVp, kilovolt (peak).

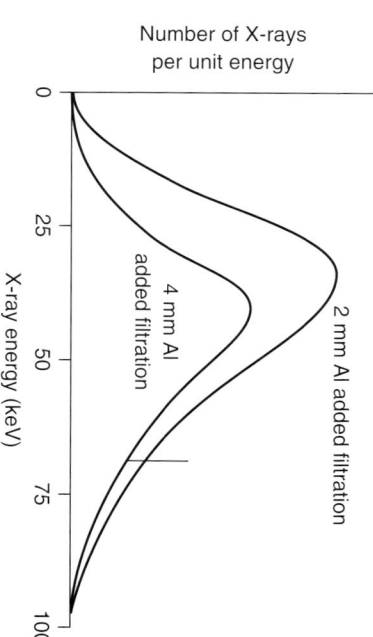

FIGURE 11-5 Effect of added filtration on emission spectrum. Al, aluminum; keV, kiloelectron volt.

FIGURE 11-6 Effect of target material on emission spectrum. keV, kiloelectron volt; z, atomic number.

CHAPTER 11 Mammographic Quality Standards

Molybdenum (Atomic Number 42). The lower atomic number reduces the number of Bremsstrahlung X-rays significantly, so virtually all the X-rays exiting the X-ray tube housing are characteristic X-rays of 17.9 kiloelectron volts (keV) and 19.5 keV (well within the K-edge of the image receptor being used). A 30- to 50-μm molybdenum filter is added to eliminate any additional Bremsstrahlung X-rays (which improves subject contrast). This target material is commonly used for normal or fatty breast composition.

Rhodium (Atomic Number 45). Rhodium creates an emission spectrum similar to that of molybdenum. The characteristic X-rays have an energy of 20.2 keV and 22.7 keV (slightly greater than molybdenum, making it better for more dense breast tissue), and more Bremsstrahlung X-rays are created. A 50-μm rhodium filter is used.

Molybdenum–Rhodium–Tungsten Alloy. Molybdenum–rhodium–tungsten alloy target material exhibits a mixed-emission spectrum with characteristics of each element. With the selection of either an aluminum, rhodium, or molybdenum filter, the emission spectrum can be shaped to fit the image receptor used. When more than one target material is available with the mammographic unit, the system must indicate, before exposure, the preselected target material.

Voltage Waveform/Ripple. Three-phase and high-frequency X-ray generators create X-rays with a greater average energy (quality) and in greater numbers (quantity) than single-phase X-ray generators; therefore, the amplitude and relative position of the spectrum are different. With three-phase and high-frequency generators, the increasing amplitude and the right-shifting spectrum indicate greater average energy (Fig. 11-7).

Focal Spot Size. The spatial resolution required in mammographic images is greater than that of conventional radiography because of the need to demonstrate microcalcifications, which is accomplished with a small focal spot ranging from 0.1 to 0.3 mm. When more than one focal spot is available on the unit, the system must indicate, before exposure, which focal spot is selected. Some manufacturers tilt the X-ray tube toward the cathode side (about 25°), which reduces the effective focal spot size even more. Most mammographic X-ray tubes use a circular focal spot rather than the rectangular focal spots found in conventional radiographic X-ray tubes. Circular focal spots provide better geometric sharpness but have a lower heat capacity because of less surface area of the anode under bombardment by the projectile electrons. Mammographic x-ray tubes often utilize the heel effect (increase in radiation toward the cathode side of the x-ray field) by placing the cathode side of the tube toward the chest wall (not all units allow for rotation of the X-ray tube). However, because geometric "unsharpness" is also greater toward the cathode side of the X-ray field, any suspicious areas near the chest wall are often reimaged with the anode side closer to the chest wall.

Source-to-Image Distance and Target Angle. The SID used in dedicated mammographic units ranges from 50 to 80 cm, with 65 cm being typical. Because of this relatively short SID, a larger target angle is necessary for mammographic X-ray tubes (22 to 24° compared with 7 to 13° angles for standard radiographic X-ray tubes) to create an X-ray field size large enough to cover the image receptor.

Compression

All modern mammographic units must be equipped with a compression device, usually made of radiolucent plastic. The amount of X-ray transmission through these devices is about 80% at 30 kVp. The function of these devices is to compress the breast tissue gently with a force of between 25 lb and 45 lb (111 N and 200 N). An automatic adjust-and-release mechanism is found on most systems. Effective October 28, 2002, each mammographic system must provide (1) an initial power-driven compression activated by hands-free controls operable from both sides of the patient and (2) fine adjustment compression controls operable from both sides of the patient. The chest wall edge of the compression paddle should be straight and parallel to the edge of the image receptor. The advantages of breast compression are shown in Box 11-1. The principal disadvantage of compression is patient discomfort.

Mammographic systems also must be equipped with various-size compression paddles that match the sizes of all full-field image receptors provided for the system. The compression paddle should be flat and parallel to the

---

BOX 11-1 **Advantages of Breast Compression**

1. Because of the part's immobilization, motion blur is reduced.
2. Part thickness is more uniform, which manifests as more uniform optical densities in the final image.
3. Bringing all object structures closer to the image receptor reduces geometric "unsharpness" and improves spatial resolution.
4. Because the part is thinner, patient dose and scattered radiation are reduced.

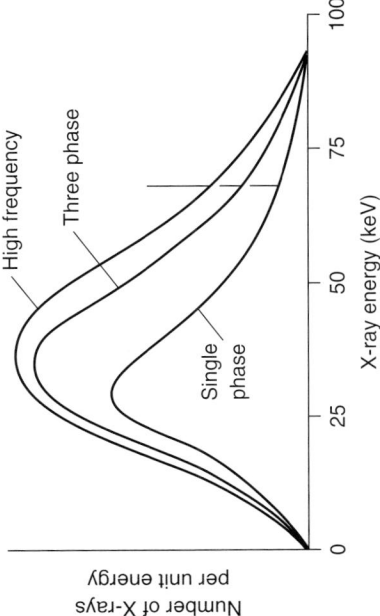

FIGURE 11-7 Effect of voltage waveform on emission spectrum. keV, kiloelectron volt.

Grids

The presence of scattered radiation in a diagnostic image always reduces or lowers image contrast. Because mammographic images have an inherently low subject contrast, it is imperative that scattered radiation be reduced as much as possible. Carbon fiber interspaced grids are often used to reduce scattered radiation (and therefore help to increase image contrast). The grid ratios range from 3:1 to 5:1, and the grid frequency can range from 30 to 50 lines/cm. The mammographic grids also are focused to the X-ray source and move during the exposure to eliminate grid lines. Uniformity of construction and motion is paramount for proper image quality. A new type of crosshatch grid, called the *high transmission cellular* (HTC) grid, has been developed for mammographic systems. Crosshatch grids are superior at removing scattered radiation (compared with focused or parallel linear grids) but require significantly greater milliampere-second exposure because of increased absorption of primary radiation. For alleviation of this problem, the HTC mammographic grid uses copper as the grid strip material (compared with lead in conventional grids) and air as the interspace material. The grid ratio of the HTC mammographic grid is 3.8:1. Systems with film/screen image receptors should be equipped with moving grids matched to all image receptor sizes provided. Systems used for magnification procedures should be capable of operating with the grid removed from between the X-ray source and the image receptor. Some studies have suggested that a grid can be omitted from mammographic examinations performed with full-field digital mammography (FFDM) for breasts less than 5 cm thick when compressed to decrease patient dose, because postprocessing of the digital images can maintain contrast despite the lack of a grid.

Image Receptors

In the past, most mammographic examinations that have been performed have used film/screen combinations as the primary image receptor. The film is most often single emulsion (to eliminate any parallax and crossover effects) and is matched spectrally to the screen. Mammographic films in general have a high average gradient (more than three) to deliver high inherent contrast, but consequentially have a low or narrow exposure latitude (meaning technique selection must be precise). The use of an AEC system and having a working technique chart available (Fig. 11-8) helps obtain precise techniques. The

---

breast support table, and should not deflect from parallel by more than 1 cm at any point on the surface of the compression paddle when compression is applied.

Mammography Phototimer Technique Chart
Room No. _____ Unit _____

Compressed Breast Thickness	Fatty Breast				50% Fatty-50% Dense				Dense breast			
	Target	Filter	kVp	Density	Target	Filter	kVp	Density	Target	Filter	kVp	Density
<3 cm												
3 to 5 cm												
5 to 7 cm												
>7 cm												

Techniques based upon proper photocell placement under the densest portion of the breast, screen-film combinations, and processing. Taut compression should be used for all patients except where noted.

Focal Spot size for:
Nonmagnification Technique: _____ mm
Magnification Technique: _____ mm

Special Techniques

Implant Displaced Views
Phototiming same as above chart

Manual Techniques for Implant Views

Breast size	Target	Filter	kVp	mAs
Small				
Medium				
Large				

Specimens: (Manual Technique Only)

Breast size	Target	Filter	kVp	mAs
Small				
Medium				
Large				

Apply minimal compression—enough to prevent motion. Specimens must be compressed.

FIGURE 11-8 Technique chart for mammographic imaging with an automatic exposure control system.

single-emulsion film is used with a single-screen image receptor. Mammographers must take special care to ensure the emulsion side of the film faces the intensifying screen. Double-screen image receptors used with duplitized film also are available. Rare earth phosphors (often containing yttrium or gadolinium) are used in the intensifying screens to help reduce patient dose and increase image contrast. The absorption efficiency of these screens can be as much as 70%, because low-energy X-ray photons are used. The main sources of image noise in film/screen mammography are quantum mottle and film granularity. It is also critical for film/screen image receptors to be kept clean to minimize artifacts. Mammographic systems with screen-film image receptors should provide, at a minimum, for operation with image receptors of 18 × 24 cm and 24 × 30 cm. Full-field digital and computed radiographic (CR) mammographic systems have replaced film/screen image receptors in many facilities and are discussed later in this chapter.

Film Processors

Film/screen mammographic images should have a dedicated film processor for conversion of the latent image to a manifest image. Mammographic films tend to have a relatively thick single emulsion, making them much more sensitive to processor artifacts. Mammographic images require ODs of between 1.5 and 2, which is a more narrow range than conventional radiography (OD range, 0.5 to 2.5). A common option for processing mammographic images is **extended processing**, which extends the standard cycle of a 20-second developing time to a cycle of 40 seconds and longer. The developer temperature, concentration, and composition remain unchanged. The main advantages of extended processing are greater image contrast (approximately 15%), increased image receptor sensitivity (about 30%), and reduced patient dose (about 30%). These improvements are seen only when single-emulsion films are used.

Magnification Mammography

Magnification studies are common during mammographic procedures to investigate small microcalcifications or lesions that may appear ambiguous at normal size. According to the Food and Drug Administration (FDA), mammographic systems used to perform noninterventional, problem-solving procedures should have radiographic magnification capability available for use by the operator. These systems should provide, at a minimum, at least one magnification value within the range of 1.4 to 2. This magnification factor is determined by the ratio of the image size compared with the object size or by the ratio of SID to source-to-object distance (SOD). Magnification of the image is achieved by increasing the object-to-image distance (OID), which reduces the SOD (typically 35 cm in magnification studies). Because this increase also reduces image sharpness, it is essential that the effective focal spot size for magnification studies not exceed 0.1 mm. However, the small focal spot can only tolerate low tube currents (25 mA), which can result in long exposure times of several seconds. The air gap created by the increased OID normally eliminates the need for a grid, thereby reducing the required milliampere-seconds.

Digital Mammography Systems

Computed radiographic (CR) and digital radiographic (DR) systems have become relatively common imaging systems for conventional radiography. However, early versions of these systems tended to have less spatial resolution than film/screen imaging systems and a greater capital cost, which slowed their application into mammographic imaging. On January 28, 2000, the FDA approved the Senographe 2000D Full Field Digital Mammography FFDM system for marketing and immediate use in facilities certified for film/screen imaging systems according to the **Mammography Quality Standards Act (MQSA)**. As of the writing of this edition, several additional digital mammographic systems have been approved by the FDA (with other systems pending). They include the following:

- Giotto Image 3D/3DL FFDM on November 2, 2012
- Agfa CR Mammography System on September 4, 2012
- Konica Minolta Xpress CR System on April 19, 2012
- Fuji Aspire HD FFDM system on April 10, 2012
- Fuji Aspire CR System on December 8, 2011
- GE Senographe Care FFDM on September 1, 2011
- Planmed Nuance Excel FFDM on October 7, 2011
- Planmed Nuance FFDM on September 23, 2011
- Siemens Mammomat Inspiration Pure FFDM on August 16, 2011
- Hologic Selenia Encore FFDM on June 15, 2011
- Philips (Sectra) Microdose L30 FFDM on April 28, 2011
- Hologic Selenia Dimensions Digital Breast Tomosynthesis on February 11, 2011
- Carestream Health Directview CR System on November 19, 2010
- Hologic Selenia Dimensions 2D FFDM on February 11, 2009
- Hologic Selenia S FFDM on February 11, 2009
- Siemens Mammomat Novation S FFDM on February 11, 2009
- Hologic Selenia FFDM System with a Tungsten target on November 1, 2007
- Fuji Computed Radiography Mammography Suite on July 10, 2006
- GE Senographe Essential FFDM system on April 11, 2006
- Siemens Mammomat Novation DR FFDM system on August 20, 2004

- GE Senographe DS FFDM System on February 19, 2004
- Lorad/Hologic Selenia FFDM System on October 2, 2002
- Lorad Digital Breast Imager FFDM System on February 15, 2002
- Fischer Imaging SenoScan FFDM System on September 25, 2001

The GE and Fischer (now owned by Hologic) systems are indirect conversion systems with cesium iodide coupled to either a thin film transistor (TFT) assembly (GE) or a charge-coupled device (CCD) assembly (Fischer). The Siemens, Lorad/Hologic, Fuji Aspire HD Plus, Giotto, and Planmed systems use a direct conversion system with amorphous selenium coupled to a TFT assembly. Philips MicroDose uses a crystalline silicon detector with photon counting technology. The Fuji Aspire, Agfa, and Carestream systems are based on CR technology used in radiography. The typical matrix size in digital mammographic systems is 4096 × 6144 pixels, with pixel sizes ranging from about 24 to 100 μm.

The spatial resolution for these systems is on the order of 5 to 11 line pairs (lp)/mm, compared with 11 lp/mm or more for film/screen mammography systems. This means that film/screen mammography may be better at detecting subtle tissue changes such as microcalcifications, which could indicate early cancer. However, a dual-energy subtraction technique that subtracts background objects from the image in digital systems could enable these systems to detect lesions that were masked previously by overlying structures. The limiting spatial resolution for digital mammography is about 10 lp/mm, which is inferior to film/screen systems, which can reach 20 lp/mm. However, digital images produce better contrast resolution (especially in dense breast tissues), have a greater dynamic range (3200 gray shades are available for imaging breast structures versus fewer than 100 gray shades for film/screen systems), and have a greater detective quantum efficiency than film/screen image receptor systems, which can be even more important in mammographic images. In digital mammography, the X-ray generator–X-ray tube combination is the limiting factor in determining the dynamic range. These images may be read directly from the monitor (soft-copy review) or from hard-copy images created by a laser camera or dry laser printer. These hard-copy images provide better contrast resolution and better visibility of detail than images from traditional film/screen mammography. The dry laser printer, with a maximum density (D_{max}) of 3.5 or greater, a base + fog level of less than 0.25, and 16-bit images with at least 12-bit gray levels, is recommended for printing hard-copy digital mammographic images. They should support true-size printing, and images should be justified so that the chest wall is printed as close to the edge of the film as possible by the printer. In addition, film artifacts are eliminated virtually completely. The Digital Mammographic Imaging Screening Trial, which was sponsored by the National Cancer Institute and coordinated by the American College of Radiology Imaging Network, demonstrated that digital mammographic systems are as effective as analog systems as a screening tool. For some women (such as those with dense breasts) digital mammography is more effective than film/screen in finding cancer.

A major advantage of digital imaging is postprocessing of the image, which can improve lesion visibility in underexposed or overexposed regions. **Postprocessing** is a manipulation of the image data in the memory of the computer, before the image is displayed on a monitor. Postprocessing functions available with FFDM and CR systems may include the following:

1. **Tissue equalization**—image processing that compensates for varying breast tissue densities so the entire breast (from the chest wall to the skin line) can be visualized in a single image
2. **Magnification**—electronic digital zoom with software manipulation that can reduce the need to take additional magnification views, as with film/screen mammography
3. **Image inversion**—conversion of a negative image (standard radiographic image) to a positive image (meaning, a reverse of the negative image, where white areas on the negative image are black on the positive image and vice versa)
4. **Grayscale processing**—manipulation of grayscale values displayed in the image, including windowing (or window width), which controls image contrast, and leveling (or window level), which controls image brightness (comparable with OD in film/screen imaging)
5. **Annotations and measurements**—software manipulation allowing electronic annotation on the image, and electronic measurement tools for calculating sizes and volumes

Improved **workflow** (the number of patients imaged per hour) can be another advantage of FFDM and CR mammography. A report published by the London-based Center for Evidence-based Purchasing looked at an average of 16,000 screening mammograms per year between 2002 and 2006 and found the following times to produce four mammographic images:

Film/screen: 3.5 to 6.5 minutes
CR: 2.5 to 4 minutes
FFDM: 1.3 to 4.7 minutes

Another advantage of digital systems is the use of scanning software (known as *computer-aided detection*, or CAD) to help radiologists locate suspicious areas in the images. Initial studies have shown this type of software has sensitivities as much as 90%, so they can help increase the accuracy of mammographic diagnoses. Film/screen mammographic images can also use CAD software, but the image must first be digitized with a scanner (discussed in Chapter 9).

Patient dose in digital mammography is the same or less (up to 50% less in some studies) than that obtained with film/screen systems. Also contributing to lower patient dose is fewer recalls for additional imaging with digital mammography.

Patient convenience/satisfaction also is considered an advantage for digital mammography because less time is required to perform mammographic procedures, especially with FFDM. This procedure is shorter because the image is available in less than a minute with digital systems, compared with 3.5 to 6.5 minutes with film/screen mammography.

A new application of digital mammography is tomosynthesis, which requires multiple images from many angles to generate tomographic slices that can eliminate overlapping structures. Playback of the sequence of slices is via a cine loop, similar to that used in computed tomographic scanning. These images can be used ultimately with three-dimensional visualization software to create three-dimensional images of breast structure. An emerging application of digital mammography is dual-energy subtraction imaging (similar to the type being used in chest imaging), which can enhance certain structures by subtracting background structures from the region of interest.

The main disadvantages of digital systems are possible lower spatial resolution (mentioned previously), greater capital cost for the equipment (currently about three to five times the cost of a film/screen system), greater maintenance costs, and greater adjunct costs (such as 5-megapixel primary viewing monitors that can cost up to $40,000 and last about 2 years). Because reimbursement of mammographic services by private insurance companies and the federal government (Medicare, Medicaid) is relatively low, it has been difficult for healthcare organizations to recover their investment in these systems. Technological issues also pose problems, such as file storage issues (the file size of digital mammograms may be as large as 200 MB) and remote viewing (person accessing the image also must have a 5-megapixel high-resolution monitor to be able to diagnose the image). Therefore, PACS systems must be able to store as much as 40 GB of image data per month just for mammographic images and must have a 5-megapixel monitor available to view the images for diagnosis, increasing both the cost and operational difficulties of these systems. For Picture Archiving and Communication System(s) (PACS) to transmit digital mammographic images, lossless compression capability is essential. Magnification studies may also be of concern in digital mammography. Film/screen mammography uses geometric magnification, such as increased OID and/or decreased SID, to obtain magnification studies. Digital systems can use electronic magnification, which usually increases pixel size to magnify the image. This results in less exposure to the patient and a shorter examination time, but greatly decreases the spatial resolution compared with those studies using geometric magnification.

Stereotactic Localization

Stereotactic localization is a method that has been developed to perform core needle biopsies using mammographic imaging. As with the old process of stereoradiography, two views of the breast are acquired, with the central ray at a different angle for each view (usually within 15° of normal). Images of the lesion shift by an amount depending on lesion depth, which permits a three-dimensional localization of the lesion. A biopsy needle gun is positioned at the correct location and then fired to obtain a core sample of the tissue. This type of biopsy is quick, accurate, and less invasive than other methods, with less scarring of the breast tissue. Full-field digital systems are better suited than film/screen systems for this technique because image acquisition is faster (no film processing is required), and the computer software can align the two images for optimum visualization.

MAMMOGRAPHIC QUALITY ASSURANCE

The importance of mammography to an early diagnosis of breast cancer has been well demonstrated. Breast cancer can be detected by means of mammograms as early as 2 years before a lump can be felt during a manual examination. For breast cancer detection to be accomplished successfully, the images must be of the highest quality, and the interpreting physician must be highly trained. This means a detailed quality management program must be in place to minimize any variations, which are even more detrimental to image quality in mammography because of the low subject contrast.

MQSA and the Mammography Quality Standards Reauthorization Act

Before 1992, quality standards for mammography were the responsibility of individual state agencies. The American College of Radiology (ACR) began a voluntary Mammography Accreditation Program in 1987 that required specific quality control and quality assurance procedures for equipment and personnel. Approximately 30% of facilities that initially applied for ACR accreditation failed on their first attempt. Because so few facilities sought and obtained ACR accreditation voluntarily, concern of mammographic image quality prompted the U.S. Senate Committee on Labor and Human Resources to hold hearings on breast cancer in 1992. This committee discovered many problems with mammographic procedures in the United States, including poor-quality equipment, a lack of quality assurance procedures, poorly trained interpreting physicians, and no consistent oversight or facility inspections. These discoveries led to the enactment of Public

CHAPTER 11 Mammographic Quality Standards

Law 102-539 (the MQSA), which passed on October 27, 1992. This law required all facilities (except for those of the Department of Veterans Affairs) to be accredited by an approved accrediting body and certified by the Secretary of Health and Human Services to provide mammography services legally after October 1, 1994. The Secretary of Health and Human Services delegated the authority to approve accreditation bodies and to certify facilities to the FDA or by the states of Illinois, Iowa, or South Carolina. These state agencies use the same certification requirements as the FDA. The MQSA has been superseded by the Mammography Quality Standards Reauthorization Act (MQSRA) of 1998. As part of the new law, final FDA regulations regarding mammographic procedures became effective on April 28, 1999, replacing interim regulations that were used during the original law. In 2002, the amended final regulations were published with new subparts that included addressing alternatives such as digital mammographic systems. The final regulations emphasize performance objectives rather than specify the behavior and manner of compliance.

The main provisions of MQSA and MQSRA include the following:

- Accreditation of mammography facilities by private, nonprofit organizations (such as the ACR) or state agencies that have met the standards established by the FDA (including Iowa, Arkansas, and Texas) and have been approved by the FDA
- An annual mammography facility physics survey, consultation, and evaluation performed by a qualified medical physicist
- Annual inspection of mammography facilities performed by FDA–certified federal and state inspectors
- Establishment of initial and continuing qualification standards for interpreting physicians, radiologic technologists, medical physicists, and mammographic facility inspectors
- Specification of boards or organizations eligible to certify the adequacy of training and experience of mammography personnel
- Establishment of quality standards for mammographic equipment and practices, including quality assurance and quality control programs
- Establishment of infection control policies and procedures for cleaning and disinfecting mammographic equipment after contact with blood or other potentially infectious materials
- Standards governing the final assessment of findings in the evaluation of mammographic; provision in the final report of overall final assessment findings, classified as one of the following categories:
  1. Negative—nothing on which to comment (if the interpreting physician is aware of clinical findings or symptoms, despite the negative assessment, these should be explained)
  2. Benign—also a negative assessment
  3. Probably benign—findings have a high probability of being benign
  4. Suspicious—findings without all the characteristic morphology of breast cancer but indicating a definite probability of being malignant
  5. Highly suggestive of malignancy—findings have a high probability of being malignant
  6. Incomplete/additional imaging evaluation needed—assigned in cases in which no final assessment category can be determined because of an incomplete workup; reasons for a nonassessment must be stated by the interpreting physician
- Communication of mammography results to the patient. Each facility should send each patient a summary of the mammography report written in lay terms within 30 days of the mammographic examination. If assessments are "suspicious" or "highly suggestive of malignancy," the facility should make reasonable attempts to ensure the results are communicated to the patient as soon as possible.
- Record keeping. Each facility that performs mammograms should maintain mammographic images and reports in a permanent medical record of the patient for a period of not less than 5 years or not less than 10 years if no additional mammograms of the patient are performed at the facility, or a longer period of time if mandated by state or local law. This storage may be in either digital data or hard-copy films. Each facility should, on request or on behalf of the patient, transfer permanently or temporarily the original mammograms (hard-copy films) and copies of the patient's reports to a medical institution or to a physician or healthcare provider of the patient, or to the patient directly.
- Specific regulations for accrediting bodies
- General facility provisions—such as requirements for the content and terminology in the mammography report, specific guidelines for mammography personnel, review of mammography medical outcomes data every 12 months, and standards for examinees with breast implants—and the requirement of facilities to develop a system for collecting and resolving serious complaints
- Personnel regulations for interpreting physicians, medical physicists, and mammographers. Facilities should maintain records to document the qualifications of all personnel who worked at the facility as interpreting physicians, radiologic technologists, or medical physicists. These records must be available for review for MQSA inspectors. Records of personnel no longer employed by the facility should not be discarded until the next annual inspection has been completed and the FDA has determined that the facility is in compliance with MQSA personnel requirements.

CHAPTER 11 Mammographic Quality Standards

MEDICAL PHYSICIST'S MAMMOGRAPHY QC TEST SUMMARY
(Siemens, continued)

Evaluation of Technologist QC Program

New units: Medical physicists ***must*** review the technologist QC ***within 45 days of installation*** and complete this section. The facility is required to submit the entire Mammography Equipment Evaluation report (including this form) along with their testing materials for accreditation.

Existing units: Medical physicists ***must*** complete this section as part of the unit's annual survey.

Relocating units: This section is ***not*** required if the medical physicist does ***not*** conduct a complete annual survey after relocation.

	FREQUENCY	PASS/FAIL
1. Phantom Image Quality	Daily	
2. Detector Calibration	Novation-Weekly; Inspiration-Quarterly	
3. Artifact Detection	Weekly	
4. SNR and CNR Measurements	Weekly	
5. Repeat Analysis	Quarterly	
6. Compression Force	Semi-annually	
7. Film Printer Check	Daily, when images printed	
8. Review Workstation QC-Overall *(NA if only hardcopy read)*	See FDA guidance	

Medical Physicist's Recommendations for Quality Improvement

Important:
1. The facility's "quality assurance program shall be ***substantially the same*** as the quality assurance program recommended by the ***image receptor [digital detector] manufacturer***." This is required by the FDA.
2. Use the QC manual version provided by the manufacturer **for the digital system surveyed**.
3. If the RWS or printer is FDA-cleared for FFDM, their **QC manual** is considered to be ***"substantially the same"*** and may be followed. (Check with the RWS or printer manufacturers for their clearance status and QC manual.)
4. If the RWS or printer is not cleared by the FDA for FFDM, ***follow the QC manual provided by the image receptor manufacturer.*** (Check with the image receptor manufacturer for their required tests.)
5. All tests must be evaluated for the facility's ***on and off-site*** equipment. If the evaluation was done on a different day than the survey date, note the date above.
6. See the FDA-approved alternative standard for Siemens FFDM regarding corrective action periods when components fail QC. However, if these tests are performed as part of a Mammography Equipment Evaluation (e.g., for a new system), corrective action must be taken before mammographic images are acquired.

FIGURE 11-15, cont'd

MEDICAL PHYSICIST'S MAMMOGRAPHY QC TEST SUMMARY
Full-Field Digital – Fuji CR

Site Name			Report Date	
Address			Survey Date	
Medical Physicist's Name			Signature	
X-Ray Unit Manufacturer			Model	
Date of Unit Installation			Room ID	
CR Image Receptor Mfr			CR Model	

QC Manual Version #: _____ (use version applicable to unit tested; contact mfr if questions)

Accessory Equipment	Manufacturer	Model	Location	QC Manual Version #
Review Workstation*			☐ On-site ☐ Off-site	
Film Printer*	Fuji		☐ On-site ☐ Off-site	

Survey Type   ☐ Mammo Eqpt Evaluation of new unit (include MQSA Rqmts for Mammo Eqpt checklist)   ☐ Annual Survey

*FDA **recommends** that only monitors and printers specifically cleared for FFDM use by FDA's Office of Device Evaluation (ODE) be used. See FDA's Policy Guidance Help System www.fda.gov/CDRH/MAMMOGRAPHY/robohelp/START.HTM

Medical Physicist's QC Tests

("Pass" means all components of the test pass; indicate "Fail" if any component fails. Tests must be done for both on and off-site equipment.)

		PASS/FAIL
1.	**S Value Confirmation** (≤ 120 ± 20% [96 ≤ corrected S value ≤ 144])	
2.	**System Resolution** (8 lp/mm ± 2 lp/mm in both directions)	
3.	**CR Reader Scanner Performance**	
4.	**Mammography Unit Assembly Evaluation**	
5.	**Collimation Assessment**	
	Chest wall edge of X-ray field extends to edge of IR	
	Deviation between X-ray field and light field ≤2% of SID	
	X-ray field does not extend beyond any side of the IR by more than 2% of SID	
	Paddle chest wall edge not beyond IR by more than 1% of SID or appear on the image	
6.	**Automatic Exposure Control (AEC) System Performance Assessment** Test date if different from above: _____	
	AEC density control function meets Fuji performance criteria	
	Reproducibility (CV) for either exposure or mAs is ≤0.05	
	Image mode tracking meets Fuji performance criteria	
	CNR per object thickness meets Fuji performance criteria	
7.	**System Artifact Evaluation**	
8.	**Phantom Image Quality Evaluation**	

	Fibers	Specks	Masses
Phantom IQ (printed images)			
Phantom IQ (softcopy)			

(at least 4 fibers, 3 speck groups & 3 masses)

	Other tests meet Fuji performance criteria (mAs, OD & DD for hardcopy, S value for soft copy)	
9.	**Dynamic Range**	
10.	**Primary Erasure (Additive and Multiplicative Lag Effects)**	
11.	**Inter-Plate Consistency** (variation of mAs within ± 10%; SNR within ± 15%)	
12.	**kVp Accuracy and Reproducibility** Test date if different from above: _____	
	Measured average kVp within ±5% of indicated kVp	
	kVp coefficient of variation ≤0.02	
13.	**Dose** (average glandular dose for average breast is ≤ 3 mGy [300 mrad]) Test date if different from above: _____ mrad	
14.	**Beam Quality Assessment & HVL Measurement** Test date if different from above: _____	
	HVL ≥kVp/100 mm Al	
15.	**Radiation Output** Test date if different from above: _____	
	Radiation output rate is ≥800 mR/sec (7.0 mGy/sec) at 28 kVp with Mo/Mo	
16.	**Viewing and Viewing Conditions**	
	Room illuminance ≤20 lux or as recommended by the monitor manufacturer	
17.	**Review Workstation (RWS) Tests** (for all RWS, even if located offsite; NA if only hardcopy read)	
18.	**Film Printer Tests** (for all printers used for mammography, even if located offsite)	

*** **YOUR MEDICAL PHYSICIST MUST SUMMARIZE HIS/HER RESULTS ON THIS FORM** ***

FIGURE 11-16 American College of Radiology Physicist's Mammography QC Test Summary for Fuji FCR$_m$.

CHAPTER 11 Mammographic Quality Standards

MEDICAL PHYSICIST'S MAMMOGRAPHY QC TEST SUMMARY
(Fuji CR, continued)

Evaluation of Technologist QC Program

New units: Medical physicists ***must*** review the technologist QC ***within 45 days of installation*** and complete this section. The facility is required to submit the entire Mammography Equipment Evaluation report (including this form) along with their testing materials for accreditation.

Existing units: Medical physicists ***must*** complete this section as part of the unit's annual survey.

Relocating units: This section is ***not*** required if the medical physicist does ***not*** conduct a complete annual survey after relocation.

	FREQUENCY	PASS/FAIL
1. CNR Weekly Check	Weekly	
2. Phantom Image	Weekly	
3. Visual Checklist	Monthly	
4. Repeat Analysis	Quarterly	
5. Compression	Semi-annually	
6. Imaging Plate (IP) Fog	Semi-annually	
7. Film Printer QC	See FDA guidance	
8. Review Workstation QC-Overall *(NA if only hardcopy read)*	See FDA guidance	

Medical Physicist's Recommendations for Quality Improvement

Important:
1. The facility's "quality assurance program shall be ***substantially the same*** as the quality assurance program recommended by the ***image receptor [digital detector] manufacturer***." This is required by the FDA.
2. Use the QC manual version provided by the manufacturer ***for the digital system surveyed***.
3. Fuji specifies that the ***printer and monitor manufacturers' QC program must be followed***; if no manufacturer-provided QC is available, the Fuji manual includes testing information.
4. All tests must be evaluated for the facility's ***on and off-site*** equipment. If the evaluation was done on a different day than the survey date, note the date above.
5. See the FDA-approved alternative standard for Fuji FFDM regarding corrective action periods when components fail QC. However, if these tests are performed as part of a Mammography Equipment Evaluation (e.g., for a new system), corrective action must be taken before mammographic images are acquired.

FIGURE 11-16, cont'd

MEDICAL PHYSICIST'S MAMMOGRAPHY QC TEST SUMMARY
Full-Field Digital – Fuji Aspire HD (FDR)

Site Name		Report Date	
Address		Survey Date	
Medical Physicist's Name		Signature	
X-Ray Unit Manufacturer	Fuji	Model	Aspire HD (FDR)
Date of Installation		Room ID	

QC Manual Version # (use version applicable to unit tested; contact mfr if questions)

Accessory Equipment	Manufacturer	Model	Location	QC Manual Version #
Review Workstation*			☐ On-site ☐ Off-site	
Film Printer*			☐ On-site ☐ Off-site	

*FDA recommends that only monitors and printers specifically cleared for FFDM use by FDA's Office of Device Evaluation (ODE) be used. See FDA's Policy Guidance Help System www.fda.gov/CDRH/MAMMOGRAPHY/robohelp/START.HTM.

Survey Type ☐ Mammo Eqpt Evaluation of new unit (include MQSA Rqmts for Mammo Eqpt checklist) ☐ Annual Survey

Medical Physicist's QC Tests

("Pass" means all components of the test pass; indicate "Fail" if any component fails. Tests must be done for both on and off-site equipment.)

PASS/FAIL

1. **1Shot PhantomM**
   - Missed Tissue on Chest Wall Edge
   - CNR *(Mammography Equipment Evaluation only)*
   - 1 Shot Phantom Sensitivity Constancy *(Mammography Equipment Evaluation only)*
   - Geometric Distortion *(Mammography Equipment Evaluation only)*
   - System Artifact Evaluation *(Mammography Equipment Evaluation only)*
   - Uniformity *(Mammography Equipment Evaluation only)*
   - Dynamic Range *(Mammography Equipment Evaluation only)*
   - Spatial Resolution (SR) *(Mammography Equipment Evaluation only)*
   - Low Contrast Detectability (LCD) *(Mammography Equipment Evaluation only)*
   - Linearity/Beam Quality Constancy *(Mammography Equipment Evaluation only)*

2. **ACR Phantom** *(Mammography Equipment Evaluation only)*

	Fibers	Specks	Masses
Phantom IQ Test on AWS			
Phantom IQ Test on RWS			

3. **Image Basic Test**
4. **Compression Device Confirmation**
5. **Viewbox Maintenance**
6. **Monitor Quality Control (Secondary/AWS)**
7. **Additive Lag Effects**
8. **Multiplicative Lag Effects (Ghost)**
9. **Visual and Functional Test**
10. **Spatial Resolution (Magnification)**
11. **kVp Accuracy and Reproducibility**
12. **Half Value Layer (HVL)**
13. **Collimation Assessment**
14. **Radiation Output**
15. **AEC Reproducibility**
16. **CNR Mode 1**
17. **AGD Mode 1**
18. **AGD-ACR Phantom**

Average glandular dose for average breast is ≤3 mGy (300 mrad) _____ mrad

19. **Review Workstation QC-Overall**
20. **Film Printer QC-Overall**

*** YOUR MEDICAL PHYSICIST MUST SUMMARIZE HIS/HER RESULTS ON *THIS FORM* ***

FIGURE 11-17 American College of Radiology Physicist's Mammography QC Test Summary for Fuji Aspimre.

MEDICAL PHYSICIST'S MAMMOGRAPHY QC TEST SUMMARY
(Fuji Aspire HD (FDR), continued)

Evaluation of Technologist QC Program

New units: Medical physicists *must* review the technologist QC *within 45 days of installation* and complete this section. The facility is required to submit the entire Mammography Equipment Evaluation report (including this form) along with their testing materials for accreditation.

Existing units: Medical physicists *must* complete this section as part of the unit's annual survey.

Relocating units: This section is *not* required if the medical physicist does *not* conduct a complete annual survey after relocation.

	FREQUENCY	PASS/FAIL
1. 1Shot PhantomM	Weekly	
2. Good Practice	Weekly	
3. ACR Phantom	Weekly	
4. Monitor Quality Control (Secondary/AWS)	Weekly	
5. Repeat Analysis	Quarterly	
6. Compression Device Confirmation	Semi-annually	
7. Review Workstation QC-Overall	See FDA guidance	
8. Film Printer QC	See FDA guidance	

Medical Physicist's Recommendations for Quality Improvement

Important:
1. The facility's "quality assurance program shall be ***substantially the same*** as the quality assurance program recommended by the ***image receptor [digital detector] manufacturer***." This is required by the FDA.
2. Use the QC manual version provided by the manufacturer ***for the digital system surveyed***.
3. If the RWS or printer is FDA-cleared for FFDM, their ***QC manual*** is considered to be ***"substantially the same"*** and may be followed. (Check with the manufacturers for the QC manual and clearance status of their products.)
4. If the RWS or printer is not cleared by the FDA for FFDM, ***follow the QC manual provided by the image receptor manufacturer***. (Check with the image receptor manufacturer for their required tests.)
5. All tests must be evaluated for the facility's ***on and off-site*** equipment. If the evaluation was done on a different day than the survey date, note the date above.

FIGURE 11-17, cont'd

MEDICAL PHYSICIST'S MAMMOGRAPHY QC TEST SUMMARY
Full-Field Digital – Carestream CR

Site Name		Report Date	
Address		Survey Date	
Medical Physicist's Name		Signature	
X-Ray Unit Manufacturer		Model	
Date of Unit Installation		Room ID	
CR Image Receptor Mfr	Carestream Health Inc.	CR Model	

QC Manual Version # _____ (use version applicable to unit tested; contact mfr if questions)

Accessory Equipment	Manufacturer	Model	Location
Review Workstation*			☐ On-site ☐ Off-site
Film Printer*			☐ On-site ☐ Off-site

*FDA **recommends** that only monitors and printers specifically cleared for FFDM use by FDA's Office of Device Evaluation (ODE) be used. See FDA's Policy Guidance Help System www.fda.gov/CDRH/MAMMOGRAPHY/robohelp/START.HTM

Survey Type ☐ Mammo Eqpt Evaluation of new unit (include MQSA Rqmts for Mammo Eqpt checklist) ☐ Annual Survey

Medical Physicist's QC Tests

("Pass" means all components of the test pass; indicate "Fail" if any component fails. Tests must be done for both on and off-site equipment.)

	PASS/FAIL
1. Cassette Exposure Response Test	
2. Cassette/Phosphor Screen Artifact Test	
3. Erased Screen Test	
4. Scanner Uniformity Test	
5. Scanner Response Linearity Test	
6. Spatial Frequency Response Test	
7. Geometric Accuracy Test	
8. Image Plate Fog Test	
9. AEC System Performance/Constancy Test	
AEC Function with Breast Thickness	
AEC Density Control Function	
CNR Tracking with Breast Thickness	
10. Mammography Unit Assembly Evaluation	
11. Mammographic Unit Collimation Assessment	Test date if different from above:
X-ray Field to Light Field Alignment	
X-ray Field to Image Plate Alignment	
Alignment of Chest Wall Edge of Compression Paddle to Image Plate	
12. Beam Quality and Half-Value Layer	Test date if different from above:
13. kVp Accuracy and Reproducibility	Test date if different from above:
Measured average kVp within ±5% of indicated kVp	
kVp coefficient of variation ≤0.02	
14. Breast Entrance Exposure, Dose and Radiation Output	
Average glandular dose for average breast is below 3 mGy (300 mrad)	
Average glandular dose to a 4.2-cm-thick breast on your unit is	
Radiation output rate is ≥800 mR/sec (7.0 mGy/sec) at 28 kVp with Mo/Mo	
15. Phantom Image Quality Evaluation	(at least 4 fibers, 3 speck groups & 3 masses)

	Fibers	Specks	Masses

16. Review Workstation (RWS) Tests (for all RWS, even if located offsite; NA if only hardcopy read)	
Phantom IQ (printed images)	
Phantom IQ (softcopy)	
17. Film Printer Test (for all printers, even if located offsite)	

*** *YOUR MEDICAL PHYSICIST MUST SUMMARIZE HIS/HER RESULTS ON* <u>THIS</u> *FORM* ***

FIGURE 11-18 American College of Radiology Physicist's Mammography QC Test Summary for Carestream CR systems.

MEDICAL PHYSICIST'S MAMMOGRAPHY QC TEST SUMMARY
(Carestream, continued)

Evaluation of Technologist QC Program

New units: Medical physicists ***must*** review the technologist QC ***within 45 days of installation*** and complete this section. The facility is required to submit the entire Mammography Equipment Evaluation report (including this form) along with their testing materials for accreditation.

Existing units: Medical physicists ***must*** complete this section as part of the unit's annual survey.

Relocating units: This section is ***not*** required if the medical physicist does ***not*** conduct a complete annual survey after relocation.

	FREQUENCY	PASS/FAIL
1. Erase Cassettes	Daily	
2. Phantom Test	Weekly	
3. CNR Check	Weekly	
4. Cassette/Phosphor and CR System Visual Inspection and Cleaning	Monthly	
5. Mammography Unit Visual Checklist	Monthly	
6. Repeat Analysis	Quarterly	
7. Compression	Semi-annually	
8. Image Plate Fog Test	Semi-annually	
9. Film Printer QC	See FDA guidance	
10. Review Workstation QC-Overall	See FDA guidance	

Medical Physicist's Recommendations for Quality Improvement

Important:
1. The facility's "quality assurance program shall be **substantially the same** as the quality assurance program recommended by the **image receptor [digital detector] manufacturer.**" This is required by the FDA.
2. Use the QC manual version provided by the manufacturer **for the digital system surveyed.**
3. Carestream specifies that the **printer and monitor manufacturers' QC program must be followed**; if no manufacturer-provided QC is available, the Careteam manual includes testing information.
4. All tests must be evaluated for the facility's on and off-site equipment. If the evaluation was done on a different day than the survey date, note the date above.

FIGURE 11-18, cont'd

MEDICAL PHYSICIST'S MAMMOGRAPHY QC TEST SUMMARY
Full-Field Digital – Konica Minolta

Site Name		Report Date	
Address		Survey Date	
Medical Physicist's Name		Signature	
X-Ray Unit Manufacturer		Model	
Date of Installation		Room ID	
CR Image Receptor Mfr		CR Model	
QC Manual Version #		QC Manual Version #	

(use version applicable to unit tested; contact mfr if questions)

Accessory Equipment:	Manufacturer	Model	Location
Review Workstation*			☐ On-site ☐ Off-site
Laser Film Printer*			☐ On-site ☐ Off-site

*FDA recommends that only monitors and printers specifically cleared for FFDM use by FDA's Office of Device Evaluation (ODE) be used. See FDA's Policy Guidance Help System www.fda.gov/CDRH/MAMMOGRAPHY/robohelp/START.HTM.

Survey Type: ☐ Mammo Eqpt Evaluation of new unit (include MQSA Rqmts for Mammo Eqpt checklist) ☐ Annual Survey

Medical Physicist's QC Tests

("Pass" means all components of the test pass; indicate "Fail" if any component fails. Tests must be done for both on and off-site equipment.)

PASS/FAIL

1. **Physical Inspection**
2. **Tube Voltage Measurement and Reproducibility**
3. **Beam Quality**
4. **Radiation Output Rate**
5. **Average Glandular Dose**
   Average glandular dose for average breast is ≤3 mGy (300 mrad) [____] mrad
6. **View Boxes and Viewing Conditions**
7. **Monitor QC (CR Console Monitor)**
8. **Dark Noise**
9. **Ghost Image Evaluation**
10. **S value Response Indicator**
    S value variation: ±20%
11. **AEC Performance Checks**
    Stability and Reproducibility: mAs CV ≤5%
    Thickness Tracking: CNR (2cm) >100%, CNR (6cm) >75%, S value variation ≤20%
12. **Collimation Assessment**
13. **CR Reader Scanner Performance**
14. **Spatial Resolution**
15. **Artifact Evaluation**
16. **Inter-Plate Consistency**
    SNR variation: ±15%
    S value variation: ±15%
17. **Phantom Image Quality**
    Phantom image scores: Fibers [____] Specks [____] Masses [____]
    Density Check: S value variation ±20%; background density change ±20;
    density difference change ±0.05
    Thickness Check: ±0.5 cm
18. **Review Workstation QC-Overall**
19. **Film Printer QC-Overall**

*** *YOUR MEDICAL PHYSICIST MUST SUMMARIZE HIS/HER RESULTS ON THIS FORM* ***

FIGURE 11-19 American College of Radiology Physicist's Mammography QC Test Summary for Konica-Minolta systems.

MEDICAL PHYSICIST'S MAMMOGRAPHY QC TEST SUMMARY
(Konica Minolta, continued)

Evaluation of Technologist QC Program

New units: Medical physicists ***must*** review the technologist QC ***within 45 days of installation*** and complete this section. The facility is required to Mammography Equipment Evaluation report (including this form) along with their testing materials for accreditation.

Existing units: Medical physicists ***must*** complete this section as part of the unit's annual survey.

Relocating units: This section is ***not*** required if the medical physicist does ***not*** conduct a complete annual survey after relocation.

	FREQUENCY	PASS/FAIL
1. Daily Operational Checks	Daily	
2. View Boxes and Viewing Conditions	Weekly	
3. Monitor QC (CR Console Monitor)	Weekly	
4. CNR Check	Weekly	
5. Phantom Image Quality	Weekly	
6. Visual Inspection	Monthly	
7. Repeat Analysis	Quarterly	
8. Compression Force Test	Semi-annually	
9. Image Plate Fog	Semi-annually	
10. Review Workstation QC*	See FDA guidance	
11. Film Printer QC*	See FDA guidance	

Medical Physicist's Recommendations for Quality Improvement

Important:
1. The facility's "quality assurance program shall be ***substantially the same*** as the quality assurance program recommended by the ***image receptor [digital detector] manufacturer***." This is required by the FDA.
2. Use the QC manual version provided by the manufacturer ***for the digital system surveyed***.
3. If the RWS or printer is FDA-cleared for FFDM, their ***QC manual*** is considered to be ***"substantially the same"*** and may be followed. (Check with the manufacturers for the QC manual and clearance status of their products.)
4. If the RWS or printer is not cleared by the FDA for FFDM, ***follow the QC manual provided by the image receptor manufacturer.*** (Check with the image receptor manufacturer for their required tests.)
5. All tests must be evaluated for the facility's ***on and off-site*** equipment. If the evaluation was done on a different day than the survey date, note the date above.
6. See the FDA-approved alternative standard for Konica Minolta FFDM regarding corrective action periods when components fail QC. However, if these tests are performed as part of a Mammography Equipment Evaluation (e.g., for a new system), corrective action must be taken before mammographic images are acquired.

FIGURE 11-19, cont'd

MEDICAL PHYSICIST'S MAMMOGRAPHY QC TEST SUMMARY
Full-Field Digital – Philips (Sectra)

Site Name		Report Date	
Address		Survey Date	
Medical Physicist's Name		Signature	
X-Ray Unit Manufacturer	Philips (Sectra)	Model	
Date of Installation		Room ID	

QC Manual Version # ☐ (use version applicable to unit tested; contact mfr if questions)

Accessory Equipment	Manufacturer	Model	Location	QC Manual Version #
Review Workstation*			☐ On-site ☐ Off-site	
Film Printer*			☐ On-site ☐ Off-site	

*FDA recommends that only monitors and printers specifically cleared for FFDM use by FDA's Office of Device Evaluation (ODE) be used. See FDA's Policy Guidance Help System www.fda.gov/CDRH/MAMMOGRAPHY/robohelp/START.HTM.

Survey Type   ☐ Mammo Eqpt Evaluation of new unit (include MQSA Rqmts for Mammo Eqpt checklist)   ☐ Annual Survey

Medical Physicist's QC Tests

("Pass" means all components of the test pass; indicate "Fail" if any component fails. Tests must be done for both on and off-site equipment.)

PASS/FAIL

1. **X-ray Tube Output** (air kerma)   ☐
2. **Air Kerma Reproducibility**   ☐
3. **Half Value Layer**   ☐
4. **AEC System: Breast Thickness and Exposure**   ☐
5. **AEC System: Density Compensation**   ☐
6. **Image Quality Evaluation**   ☐
   Phantom image scores: Fibers ☐   Specks ☐   Masses ☐
   Average glandular dose for average breast is ≤1 mGy (100 mrad)
7. **Contrast-to-Noise Ratio Reference Level**   ☐
   CNR (value) ☐
8. **Tube Voltage**   ☐
9. **Image Field and X-Ray Field Agreement**   ☐
10. **Missed Tissue at Chest Wall**   ☐
11. **Viewing Conditions**   ☐

*** *YOUR MEDICAL PHYSICIST MUST SUMMARIZE HIS/HER RESULTS ON <u>THIS</u> FORM* ***

FIGURE 11-20 American College of Radiology Physicist's Mammography QC Test Summary for Philips FFDM systems.

CHAPTER 11 Mammographic Quality Standards 227

MEDICAL PHYSICIST'S MAMMOGRAPHY QC TEST SUMMARY
(Philips (Sectra), continued)

Evaluation of Technologist QC Program

New units: Medical physicists ***must*** review the technologist QC ***within 45 days of installation*** and complete this section. The facility is required to submit the entire Mammography Equipment Evaluation report (including this form) along with their testing materials for accreditation.

Existing units: Medical physicists ***must*** complete this section as part of the unit's annual survey.

Relocating units: This section is ***not*** required if the medical physicist does ***not*** conduct a complete annual survey after relocation.

	FREQUENCY	PASS/FAIL
1. Daily Quality Control	Daily	
2. Full Calibration	Weekly	
3. Mammographic Accreditation Phantom	Weekly	
4. Contrast-to-Noise Ratio	Weekly	
5. Display QC-AWS	Weekly	
6. Spatial Resolution	Monthly	
7. Visual Checklist	Monthly	
8. Repeat Analysis	Quarterly	
9. Thickness Indication	Semi-annually	
10. Compression	Semi-annually	
11. Film Printer QC	See FDA Guidance	
12. Review Workstation QC-Overall (NA if only a hard copy read)	See FDA Guidance	

Medical Physicist's Recommendations for Quality Improvement

Important:
1. The facility's "quality assurance program shall be ***substantially the same*** as the quality assurance program recommended by the ***image receptor [digital detector] manufacturer.***" This is required by the FDA.
2. Use any QC manual version that is applicable to the Philips (Sectra) model surveyed.
3. If the RWS or printer is FDA-cleared for FFDM, their ***QC manual*** is considered to be ***"substantially the same"*** and may be followed. (Check with the RWS or printer manufacturers for clearance status and QC manual.)
4. If the RWS or printer is not cleared by the FDA for FFDM, ***follow the QC manual provided by the image receptor manufacturer.*** (Check with the image receptor manufacturer for their required tests.)
5. All tests must be evaluated for the facility's ***on and off-site*** equipment. If the evaluation was done on a different day than the survey date, note the date above.
6. See the FDA-approved alternative standard for Philips (Sectra) FFDM regarding corrective action periods when components fail QC. However, if these tests are performed as part of a Mammography Equipment Evaluation (e.g., for a new system), corrective action must be taken before mammographic images are acquired.

FIGURE 11-20, cont'd

MEDICAL PHYSICIST'S MAMMOGRAPHY QC TEST SUMMARY
Full-Field Digital – Planmed

Site Name		Report Date	
Address		Survey Date	
Medical Physicist's Name		Signature	
X-Ray Unit Manufacturer	Planmed	Model	
Date of Installation		Room ID	

QC Manual Version # _____ (use version applicable to unit tested; contact mfr if questions)

Accessory Equipment	Manufacturer	Model	Location	QC Manual Version #
Review Workstation*			☐ On-site ☐ Off-site	
Film Printer*			☐ On-site ☐ Off-site	

*FDA recommends that only monitors and printers specifically cleared for FFDM use by FDA's Office of Device Evaluation (ODE) be used. See FDA's Policy Guidance Help System www.fda.gov/CDRH/MAMMOGRAPHY/robohelp/START.HTM.

Survey Type ☐ Mammo Eqpt Evaluation of new unit (include MQSA Rqmts for Mammo Eqpt checklist) ☐ Annual Survey

Medical Physicist's QC Tests

("Pass" means all components of the test pass; indicate "Fail" if any component fails. Tests must be done for both on and off-site equipment.)

PASS/FAIL

1. **Monitor Cleaning (AWS and RWS)** *(Mammography Equipment Evaluation only)*
2. **Monitor Quality (AWS) - TG-18 QC test phantom** *(Mammography Equipment Evaluation only)*
3. **Phantom Image Quality (AWS and RWS)** *(Mammography Equipment Evaluation only)*

	Fibers	Specks	Masses
Phantom IQ Test on AWS			
Phantom IQ Test on RWS			

4. **Viewbox and Viewing Conditions** *(Mammography Equipment Evaluation only)*
5. **Signal Homogeneity** *(Mammography Equipment Evaluation only)*
6. **Uncorrected Defective Elements (DEL)** *(Mammography Equipment Evaluation only)*
7. **Large Focus Calibration** *(Mammography Equipment Evaluation only)*
8. **Small Focus Calibration (for mags only)** *(Mammography Equipment Evaluation only)*
9. **Signal-to-Noise (SNR)** *(Mammography Equipment Evaluation only)*
10. **Contrast-to-Noise Ratio (CNR)** *(Mammography Equipment Evaluation only)*
11. **Visual Checklist** *(Mammography Equipment Evaluation only)*
12. **Repeat Analysis** *(Mammography Equipment Evaluation only)*
13. **Defect Acceptance Test** *(Mammography Equipment Evaluation only)*
14. **System Fault Report** *(Mammography Equipment Evaluation only)*
15. **Review Workstation QC-Overall** *(Mammography Equipment Evaluation only)*
16. **Film Printer QC** *(Mammography Equipment Evaluation only)*
17. **Ghosting**
18. **Modulation Transfer Function (MTF)**
19. **Linearity/Noise Linearity**
20. **AEC**
21. **Compression Force**
22. **Mammographic Unit Assembly**
23. **Beam Quality Assessment - HVL Measurement**
24. **Breast Entrance Exposure and Average Glandular Dose**

Average glandular dose for average breast is ≤3 mGy (300 mrad) _____ mrad

*** *YOUR MEDICAL PHYSICIST MUST SUMMARIZE HIS/HER RESULTS ON <u>THIS</u> FORM* ***

FIGURE 11-21 American College of Radiology Physicist's Mammography QC Test Summary for Planmed systems.

CHAPTER 11 Mammographic Quality Standards

MEDICAL PHYSICIST'S MAMMOGRAPHY QC TEST SUMMARY
(Planned, continued)

Evaluation of Technologist QC Program

New units: Medical physicists ***must*** review the technologist QC ***within 45 days of installation*** and complete this section. The facility is required to submit the entire Mammography Equipment Evaluation report (including this form) along with their testing materials for accreditation.

Existing units: Medical physicists ***must*** complete this section as part of the unit's annual survey.

Relocating units: This section is ***not*** required if the medical physicist does ***not*** conduct a complete annual survey after relocation.

	FREQUENCY	PASS/FAIL
1. Monitor Cleaning (AWS and RWS)	Daily	
2. Monitor Quality (AWS) - TG-18 QC test phantom	Daily	
3. Phantom Image Quality (AWS and RWS)	Daily	
4. Viewbox and Viewing Conditions	Weekly	
5. Signal Homogeneity	Weekly	
6. Uncorrected Defective Elements (DEL)	Weekly	
7. Large Focus Calibration	Weekly	
8. Small Focus Calibration (for mags only)	Weekly	
9. Signal-to-Noise (SNR)	Monthly	
10. Contrast-to-Noise Ratio (CNR)	Monthly	
11. Visual Checklist	Monthly	
12. Repeat Analysis	Quarterly	
13. Defect Acceptance Test	Semi-annually	
14. Compression Force	Semi-annually	
15. System Fault Report	When needed	
16. Review Workstation QC-Overall	See FDA guidance	
17. Film Printer QC	Weekly	

Medical Physicist's Recommendations for Quality Improvement

Important:
1. The facility's "quality assurance program shall be ***substantially the same*** as the quality assurance program recommended by the ***image receptor [digital detector] manufacturer***." This is required by the FDA.
2. Use the QC manual version provided by the manufacturer ***for the digital system surveyed***.
3. If the RWS or printer is FDA-cleared for FFDM, their ***QC manual*** is considered to be "***substantially the same***" and may be followed. (Check with the manufacturers for the QC manual and clearance status of their products.)
4. If the RWS or printer is not cleared by the FDA for FFDM, ***follow the QC manual provided by the image receptor manufacturer***. (Check with the image receptor manufacturer for their required tests.)
5. All tests must be evaluated for the facility's ***on and off-site*** equipment. If the evaluation was done on a different day than the survey date, note the date above.
6. See the FDA-approved alternative standard for Planned FFDM regarding corrective action periods when components fail QC. However, if these tests are performed as part of a Mammography Equipment Evaluation (e.g., for a new system), corrective action must be taken before mammographic images are acquired.

FIGURE 11-21, cont'd

MEDICAL PHYSICIST'S MAMMOGRAPHY QC TEST SUMMARY
Full-Field Digital – Agfa CR

Site Name		Report Date	
Address		Survey Date	
Medical Physicist's Name		Signature	
X-Ray Unit Manufacturer		Model	
Date of Installation		Room ID	
CR Image Receptor Mfr	Agfa	CR Model	

QC Manual Version # _____ (use any version applicable to model; contact mfr if questions)

Accessory Equipment	Manufacturer	Model	Location	QC Manual Version #
Review Workstation*			☐ On-site ☐ Off-site	
Film Printer*			☐ On-site ☐ Off-site	

Survey Type   ☐ Mammo Eqpt Evaluation of new unit (include MQSA Rqmts for Mammo Eqpt checklist)   ☐ Annual Survey

*FDA recommends that only monitors and printers specifically cleared for FFDM use by FDA's Office of Device Evaluation (ODE) be used. See FDA's Policy Guidance Help System www.fda.gov/CDRH/MAMMOGRAPHY/robohelp/START.HTM.

Medical Physicist's QC Tests

("Pass" means all components of the test pass; indicate "Fail" if any component fails. Tests must be done for both on and off-site equipment.)

                                                            PASS/FAIL

1. **Mechanical Inspection**
2. **AEC Thickness Compensation**
3. **Mean Glandular Dose**
4. **Phantom Image**
       Mean glandular dose for average breast is ≤3 mGy (300 mrad) _____ mrad
       Phantom Image on Modality Workstation
       Phantom Image on Printer

Fibers	Specks	Masses

5. **Spatial Resolution (High Contrast)**
6. **Signal Linearity**
7. **Artifact Analysis**
8. **Ghosting Evaluation**
9. **Interplate Absorption and Sensitivity**
10. **Missed tissue**
11. **View Box Luminance and Room Illuminance**
        Room illuminance ≤20 lux or as recommended by the monitor manufacturer
12. **Monitor Check - Modality Workstation**
13. **Radiologic Technologist's QC program**
14. **Collimation Assessment**
15. **Radiation Output Rate Inspection**
16. **kVp Accuracy and Reproducibility**
17. **Beam Quality Assessment (HVL)**
18. **Density Step Control and AEC Reproducibility**
19. **Diagnostic Review Workstation (RWS) QC** (for all RWS, even if located offsite; NA if only hardcopy read)
20. **Film Printer QC**

*** *YOUR MEDICAL PHYSICIST MUST SUMMARIZE HIS/HER RESULTS ON __THIS__ FORM* ***

FIGURE 11-22 American College of Radiology Physicist's Mammography QC Test Summary for Agfa CR systems.

CHAPTER 11 Mammographic Quality Standards

MEDICAL PHYSICIST'S MAMMOGRAPHY QC TEST SUMMARY
(Agfa, continued)

Evaluation of Technologist QC Program

New units: Medical physicists *must* review the technologist QC *within 45 days of installation* and complete this section. The facility is required to submit the entire Mammography Equipment Evaluation report (including this form) along with their testing materials for accreditation.

Existing units: Medical physicists *must* complete this section as part of the unit's annual survey.

Relocating units: This section is *not* required if the medical physicist does *not* conduct a complete annual survey after relocation.

	FREQUENCY	PASS/FAIL
1. Viewbox/Monitor Cleanliness and Viewing Conditions	Weekly	
2. Phantom Image	Weekly	
3. AEC and CNR Consistency	Weekly	
4. Monitor Check - Modality Workstation	Weekly	
5. Mechanical Inspection	Monthly	
6. Artifact Evaluation	Monthly	
7. Repeat Analysis	Quarterly	
8. Compression Check	Semi-annually	
9. Diagnostic Review Workstation QC *(NA if only hardcopy read)*	See FDA Guidance	
10. Film Printer QC	See FDA Guidance	

Medical Physicist's Recommendations for Quality Improvement

Important:
1. The facility's "quality assurance program shall be *substantially the same* as the quality assurance program recommended by the *image receptor [digital detector] manufacturer*." This is required by the FDA.
2. Use the QC manual version provided by the manufacturer *for the digital system surveyed*.
3. If the RWS or printer is FDA-cleared for FFDM, their *QC manual* is considered to be *"substantially the same"* and may be followed. (Check with the manufacturers for the QC manual and clearance status of their products.)
4. If the RWS or printer is not cleared by the FDA for FFDM, *follow the QC manual provided by the image receptor manufacturer*. (Check with the image receptor manufacturer for their required tests.)
5. All tests must be evaluated for the facility's *on and off-site* equipment. If the evaluation was done on a different day than the survey date, note the date above.
6. See the FDA-approved alternative standard for Agfa CR regarding corrective action periods when components fail QC. However, if these tests are performed as part of a Mammography Equipment Evaluation (e.g., for a new system), corrective action must be taken before mammographic images are acquired.

FIGURE 11-22, cont'd

MEDICAL PHYSICIST'S MAMMOGRAPHY QC TEST SUMMARY
Full-Field Digital – Giotto

Site Name		Report Date	
Address		Survey Date	
Medical Physicist's Name		Signature	
X-Ray Unit Manufacturer	Giotto	Model	
Date of Installation		Room ID	

QC Manual Version # _____ (use any version applicable to model; contact mfr if questions)

Accessory Equipment	Manufacturer	Model	Location	QC Manual Version #
Review Workstation*			☐ On-site ☐ Off-site	
Film Printer*			☐ On-site ☐ Off-site	

*FDA recommends that only monitors and printers specifically cleared for FFDM use by FDA's Office of Device Evaluation (ODE) be used. See FDA's Policy Guidance Help System www.fda.gov/CDRH/MAMMOGRAPHY/robohelp/START.HTM.

Survey Type ☐ Mammo Eqpt Evaluation of new unit (include MQSA Rqmts for Mammo Eqpt checklist) ☐ Annual Survey

Medical Physicist's QC Tests

("Pass" means all components of the test pass; indicate "Fail" if any component fails. Tests must be done for both on and off-site equipment.)

PASS/FAIL

1. Collimation Assessment ☐
2. Artifact Evaluation ☐
3. Automatic Exposure Control (AEC), Signal-To-Noise Ratio (SNR) & Contrast-To-Noise Ratio (CNR) ☐
   SNR (value) [____] ≥40
   CNR (value) [____] (Required for both new unit Mammography Equipment Evaluations and Annual Surveys)
   CNR should not vary by more than ±20% (NA for Equipment Evaluation)
4. AEC Reproducibility ☐
5. ACR Phantom Image Quality ☐
   Phantom image scores: Fibers [____] Specks [____] Masses [____]
6. Ghost Factor ☐
7. Inactive Border at Chest Wall Edge ☐
8. Flat Field Homogeneity ☐
9. Detector Response Function and Noise Evaluation ☐
10. Spatial Resolution ☐
11. kVp Accuracy and Reproducibility ☐
12. Tube Output ☐
13. Exposure Time ☐
14. Beam Quality (HVL) ☐
15. Mean Glandular Dose (MGD) ☐
    Average glandular dose for average breast is ≤3 mGy (300 mrad) [____] mrad
16. Viewbox Luminance ☐
17. Diagnostic Review Workstation (RWS) QC (for all RWS, even if located offsite; NA if only hardcopy read) ☐
18. Film Printer QC ☐

*** *YOUR MEDICAL PHYSICIST MUST SUMMARIZE HIS/HER RESULTS ON <u>THIS</u> FORM* ***

FIGURE 11-23 American College of Radiology Physicist's Mammography QC Test Summary for Giotto systems.

CHAPTER 11 Mammographic Quality Standards

PROCEDURE

1. Take a mammographic phantom and film/screen image receptor into the mammographic examination room.
2. Place the image receptor into the image receptor holder of the mammographic unit.
3. Place the mammographic phantom on top of the image receptor holder and position the edge of the phantom with the chest wall side of the image receptor. Place the compression device in contact with the phantom.
4. Make an exposure appropriate for a 4- to 4.5-cm compressed breast using either the manual technique or an AEC device. If using AEC, be sure to use the same sensor as all previous phantom images. The exposure should produce an OD of between 1.2 and 1.5.
5. Bring the image receptor into the darkroom and place the film on the loading bench with the emulsion side up under the safelight. All lights (including the safelight) should be off at this time. Cover half the phantom image with cardboard or opaque paper. The cardboard or opaque paper should be perpendicular to the chest wall edge of the film.
6. Turn on all safelights, let the film lie on the countertop for 2 minutes, then process the film.
7. Using a densitometer, measure the OD of both the covered and uncovered sides of the film. Do not obtain any readings where there are test objects. The difference between the two values should not exceed an OD value of 0.05. If the difference does exceed this value, corrective action must be taken.

Mammography Repeat-Reject Analysis

From _____ To _____

Reason for Reject	Projection Repeated (mark one for each repeated film)						Number of Films	% of Repeats
	Left CC	Right CC	Left MLO	Right MLO	Left Other	Right Other		
1. Positioning								
2. Patient Motion								
3. Light Films								
4. Dark Films								
5. Black Films								
6. Static, Artifacts								
7. Fog								
8. Incorrect ID or Double Exposure								
9. Mechanical								
10. Miscellaneous								
11. Good Films (No apparent reason)								
12. Clear Film								
13. Wire Localization								
14. Q.C.								

Total Films Used _____

Repeats (1-11) Number _____ _____ %

Rejects (All; 1-14)

Remarks: _____

Corrective Action: _____

FIGURE 11-29 American College of Radiology repeat-reject analysis chart.

240 CHAPTER 11 Mammographic Quality Standards

Film/Screen Contact. Mammographic image receptors must provide a spatial resolution of at least 11 lp/mm, which is significantly greater than that of conventional image receptors (2–5 lp/mm). For this level of spatial resolution to be maintained, the contact between the film and the screen must be as close as possible. A mammography film/screen contact test tool consisting of a copper screen with 40 wires/in is required (Fig. 11-31) and is usually laminated in plastic, with the equivalent density of 4 cm of acrylic.

PROCEDURE

1. Place the contact tool over the cassette, move the compression device as close as possible to the X-ray tube, and expose at 28 kVp and enough milliamperes-seconds to produce an OD between 0.7 and 0.8 when measured over the mesh area near the chest wall side of the film.
2. After processing, place the film on a viewbox and look for clarity and nonuniformity in OD. Dark or "fuzzy" areas indicate poor film/screen contact. Areas that are larger than 1 cm, or more than two areas of less than 1 cm should not be tolerated.

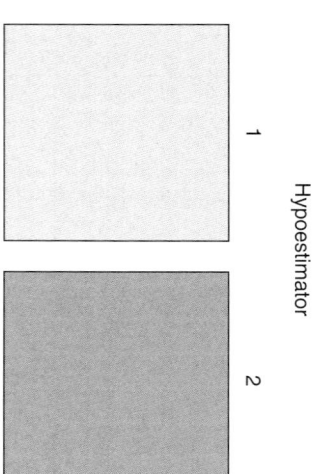

FIGURE 11-30 Hyporetention estimator test strip.

Compression. For adequate compression of the breast, the compression force should range from at least 111 N (25 lb) to a maximum of 200 N (45 lb) in both manual and power-drive modes. Compression should be held for at least 15 seconds, and can be evaluated with a scale placed directly under the compression device. A bathroom scale is acceptable; however, commercially available mammography compression scales are available and are more accurate (Fig. 11-32). Any compression of more than 200 N (45 lb) is dangerous to the patient. If the power drive fails to cease compression when more than 200 N (45 lb) is measured, a service engineer is required to repair the system. A checklist for documentation of monthly, quarterly, and semiannual testing for film/screen systems is shown in Fig. 11-33.

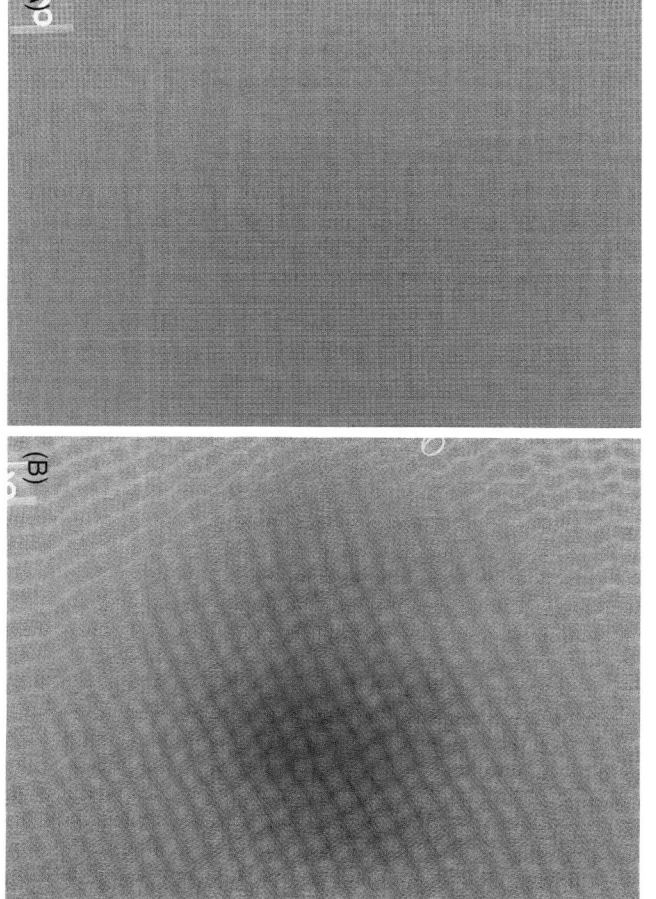

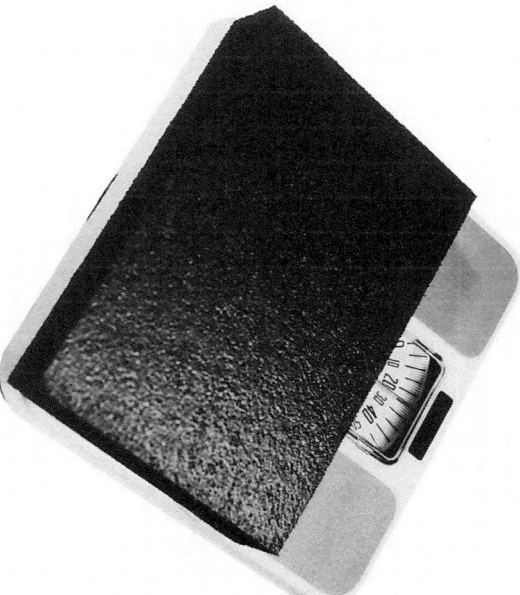

FIGURE 11-31 Wire mesh test images showing good **(A)** and poor **(B)** film screen contrast. *Courtesy Sharon Glaze; from Bushong SC: Radiologic science for technologists, ed 6, St Louis, 1997, Mosby.*

FIGURE 11-32 Mammographic compression scale. *Courtesy Nuclear Associates, Carle Place, N.Y.*

CHAPTER 11 Mammographic Quality Standards

Full-Field Digital Mammography Systems

Daily Duties. As with film/screen systems, mammographers have daily responsibilities for FFDM systems as well. However, each system manufacturer lists slightly different duties. In general, these duties include monitor cleaning and testing, darkroom cleanliness and processor quality control (if applicable), and laser imager quality testing. The manufacturer's quality control manual and the medical physicist should be consulted for the exact procedure to perform these duties.

Weekly Duties. The weekly duties performed by mammographers for FFDM systems again vary by manufacturer but generally include phantom image testing, detector flat-field calibration, viewbox and viewing conditions, SNR and CNR measurements, and MTF measurements. The manufacturers' quality control manuals and a medical physicist should be consulted for the exact procedure to perform these duties.

The quality control checklists for daily and weekly duties for FFDM and CR systems are shown in Figs. 11-34 through 11-44.

Monthly Duties. Again, these duties vary by manufacturer but include, in general, visual checks using a checklist, system resolution, detector alignment, scan speed uniformity, and monitor calibration check. The manufacturer's quality control manual and the medical physicist should be consulted for the exact procedure to perform these duties.

Quarterly Duties. The quarterly duties are essentially the same as those for film/screen systems and include repeat analysis and hyporetention analysis (laser cameras only).

Semiannual Duties. Semiannual duties for FFDM systems also are essentially the same as those of film/screen systems and include the compression force test and darkroom fog test (laser cameras only). Fuji CR systems require an imaging plate fog test be performed semiannually.

The quality control checklists for monthly, quarterly, and semiannual tests for FFDM and CR systems are presented in Figs. 11-45 through 11-54.

After completion of the required quality control tests, the facility should compare the test results with the corresponding specified action limits or, for nonscreen/film modalities, with the manufacturer's recommended

Mammography Quality Control Checklist

Department of Diagnostic Radiology

Monthly, Quarterly, and Semiannual Tests
(date, initial, and enter number where appropriate)

Year Month	JAN	FEB	MAR	APR	MAY	JUN	JUL	AUG	SEP	OCT	NOV	DEC
Visual checklist (Monthly)												
Repeat Analysis (≤2% change) (quarterly)												
Fixer (≤0.05 gm/m²) (quarterly)												
Darkroom Fog (≤0.05) (semiannually)												
Screen-film contact (semiannually)												
Compression (25-45 lb) (semiannually)												

Date: _____ Test: _____

Comments: _____

FIGURE 11-33 American College of Radiology mammographer quality control checklist for monthly, quarterly, and semiannual duties for film/screen systems.

MAMMOGRAPHY QUALITY CONTROL CHECKLIST – FULL-FIELD DIGITAL
GENERAL ELECTRIC MODEL (circle all that apply): 2000D   DS   Essential Care

Daily and Weekly

Year																															
Month																															
Date																															
Initials																															
Monitor Cleaning *(daily)*																															
Darkroom Cleanliness *(daily, if app)*																															
Processor QC *(daily, if app)*																															
Flat Field *(weekly)*																															
Phantom Image Quality *(weekly)*																															
CNR *(weekly)*																															
Viewbox and Viewing Conditions *(weekly)*																															
MTF *(DS/Essential/Care-weekly)*																															
Laser Film Printer QC *(printer mfr rec)*																															
Review Workstation QC *(See QC Manual)*																															

Year																															
Month																															
Date																															
Initials																															
Monitor Cleaning *(daily)*																															
Darkroom Cleanliness *(daily, if app)*																															
Processor QC *(daily, if app)*																															
Flat Field *(weekly)*																															
Phantom Image Quality *(weekly)*																															
CNR *(weekly)*																															
Viewbox and Viewing Conditions *(weekly)*																															
MTF *(DS/Essential/Care-weekly)*																															
Laser Film Printer QC *(printer mfr rec)*																															
Review Workstation QC *(See QC Manual)*																															

FIGURE 11-34 American College of Radiology mammography quality control checklist for daily and weekly tests for GE full-field digital mammography systems.

MAMMOGRAPHY QUALITY CONTROL CHECKLIST – FULL-FIELD DIGITAL FISCHER MODEL: _____

Monthly, Quarterly, and Semi-Annual
(date, initial and enter number where appropriate)

Year / Month	JAN	FEB	MAR	APR	MAY	JUN	JUL	AUG	SEP	OCT	NOV	DEC
System Resolution (Detector Alignment/Scan Speed Uniformity) (monthly)												
System Operation (monthly)												
Reject/Repeat Analysis (≤2% change) (quarterly)												
Compression Force Test (25-45 lb) (semi-annually)												
Review Workstation QC (See QC Manual)												

Date: _____   Test: _____   Comments: _____

FIGURE 11-47 American College of Radiology mammography quality control checklist for monthly, quarterly, and semiannual duties for Fischer full-field digital mammography systems.

FULL-FIELD DIGITAL MAMMOGRAPHY QUALITY CONTROL CHECKLIST

SIEMENS MODEL: _____

Monthly, Quarterly, and Semi-Annual Tests
(date, initial and enter number where appropriate)

Year Month	JAN	FEB	MAR	APR	MAY	JUN	JUL	AUG	SEP	OCT	NOV	DEC
Repeat Analysis (quarterly)												
Detector Calibration (Inspiration-quarterly)												
Compression Force (25-45 lb) (semiannually)												
Review Workstation QC (See QC Manual)												

Date: _____   Test: _____   Comments: _____

_____
_____
_____
_____
_____
_____
_____
_____
_____
_____

FIGURE 11-48 American College of Radiology mammography quality control checklist for monthly, quarterly, and semiannual duties for Siemens full-field digital mammography systems.

CHAPTER 11 Mammographic Quality Standards

MAMMOGRAPHY QUALITY CONTROL CHECKLIST – FULL-FIELD DIGITAL FUJI FCRm

Monthly, Quarterly, and Semi-Annual
(date, initial and enter number where appropriate)

Year Month	JAN	FEB	MAR	APR	MAY	JUN	JUL	AUG	SEP	OCT	NOV	DEC
Visual Checklist *(monthly)*												
Repeat Analysis (≤2% change) *(quarterly)*												
Compression (25-45 lb) *(semi-annually)*												
Imaging Plate Fog *(semi-annually)*												
Review Workstation QC *(See QC Manual)*												

Date:

Test:

Comments:

FIGURE 11-49 American College of Radiology mammography quality control checklist for monthly, quarterly, and semiannual duties for Fuji systems.

MAMMOGRAPHY QUALITY CONTROL CHECKLIST – FULL-FIELD DIGITAL AGFA MODEL: _____

Monthly, Quarterly, and Semi-Annual
(date, initial and enter number where appropriate)

Year Month	JAN	FEB	MAR	APR	MAY	JUN	JUL	AUG	SEP	OCT	NOV	DEC
Mechanical Inspection *(monthly)*												
Artifact Evaluation *(monthly)*												
Repeat Analysis (≤2% change) *(quarterly)*												
Compression Check (25-45 lb) *(semi-annually)*												
Diagnostic Review Workstation QC *(See QC Manual)*												
Film Printer QC *(See QC Manual)*												

Date: _____   Test: _____   Comments: _____

FIGURE 11-50 American College of Radiology mammography quality control checklist for monthly, quarterly, and semiannual duties for Agfa computed radiographic systems.

CHAPTER 11 Mammographic Quality Standards

FULL-FIELD DIGITAL MAMMOGRAPHY QUALITY CONTROL CHECKLIST – CARESTREAM

Monthly, Quarterly, and Semi-Annual Tests
(date, initial and enter number where appropriate)

Year Month	JAN	FEB	MAR	APR	MAY	JUN	JUL	AUG	SEP	OCT	NOV	DEC
Cassette/Phosphor and CR System Visual Inspection and Cleaning *(monthly)*												
Mammography Unit Visual Checklist *(monthly)*												
Repeat Analysis (≤2% change) *(quarterly)*												
Compression (25-45 lb) *(semi-annually)*												
Image Plate Fog Test *(quarterly)*												
Printer QC *(see FDA guidance)*												
Review Workstation QC *(see FDA guidance)*												

Date: _____ Test: _____ Comments: _____

FIGURE 11-51 American College of Radiology mammography quality control checklist for monthly, quarterly, and semiannual duties for Fuji Carestream computed radiographic systems.

MAMMOGRAPHY QUALITY CONTROL CHECKLIST – FULL-FIELD DIGITAL GIOTTO MODEL: _____

Monthly, Quarterly, and Semi-Annual
(date, initial and enter number where appropriate)

Year Month	JAN	FEB	MAR	APR	MAY	JUN	JUL	AUG	SEP	OCT	NOV	DEC
Repeat/Reject Analysis (≤2% change) (quarterly)												
Automatic Exposure Control System (AEC) (semi-annually)												
Compression Force (25-45 lb) (semi-annually)												
Diagnostic Review Workstation QC (See QC Manual)												
Film Printer QC (See QC Manual)												

Date: _____ Test: _____ Comments: _____

FIGURE 11-52 American College of Radiology mammography quality control checklist for monthly, quarterly, and semiannual duties for Giotto systems.

CHAPTER 11 Mammographic Quality Standards

with the MQSA. Proper documentation of these procedures is essential for a facility to remain accredited to perform mammographic procedures.

Refer to the Evolve Website at https://evolve.elsevier.com for Student Experiment 11.1: Daily Mammographic Quality Control, and 11.2: Phantom Image and Visual Inspection.

BOX 11-2 Definitions by the Food and Drug Administration

1. **Consumer**—an individual who chooses to comment or complain in reference to a mammographic examination, including the patient or representative of the patient (for example, a family member or referring physician)
2. **Adverse event**—an undesirable experience associated with mammographic activities within the scope of the Mammography Quality Standards Reauthorization Act. Adverse events include but are not limited to poor image quality, the failure to send mammographic reports to the referring physician within 30 days or to the self-referred patient in a timely manner, or the use of unqualified personnel (those who do not meet the applicable requirements of 21 Code of Federal Regulations Part 900, Section 12[a]).
3. **Serious adverse event**—an adverse event that may compromise clinical outcomes significantly or an adverse event for which a facility fails to take appropriate corrective action in a timely manner
4. **Serious complaint**—a report of a serious adverse event

Courtesy Code of Federal Regulations.

Inspection Report. After the inspection, a report summarizing the inspection findings is sent to the institution. The findings belong to one of the following categories.

Level 1. A Level 1 finding is a deviation from MQSA standards that may seriously compromise the quality of mammographic services offered by a facility. For example, a Level 1 finding for the phantom image test exists when the score is less than three fibers, less than two speck groups, or less than two masses, or if the raw score is less than six. A Level 1 finding also is issued if the interpreting physician is not certified by a board, has not had the initial (2 or 3 months) training in mammography, or has never had a valid license to practice medicine. A warning letter is sent if a Level 1 finding exists to allow the facility to correct the problem before any enforcement action is implemented.

Level 2. A Level 2 finding is not as serious a deviation from MQSA standards as a Level 1 finding, but it still may compromise the quality of a facility's mammographic program and should be corrected as soon as possible. Facilities with these findings are rated "acceptable," but they must submit an acceptable corrective action plan to the FDA.

Level 3. A Level 3 finding is a minor deviation from MQSA standards. Facilities with a Level 3 finding are rated "satisfactory," but should institute policies and procedures to correct these conditions.

No Findings. A report of no findings shows the facility has met all requirements of the MQSA.

SUMMARY

Quality control and quality assurance of mammographic equipment and procedures are mandatory for compliance

REVIEW QUESTIONS

1. What kilovolt (peak) range should be used during film/screen mammography?
   a. 15 to 20 kVp
   b. 20 to 28 kVp
   c. 30 to 40 kVp
   d. 40 to 50 kVp

2. Which of the following value ranges is the correct focal spot size for most mammographic X-ray tubes?
   a. 0.1 to 0.6 mm
   b. 0.6 to 1 mm
   c. 1 to 1.5 mm
   d. 1.5 to 2.5 mm

3. Which type of filter material should be used with a molybdenum target X-ray tube?
   a. Aluminum
   b. Copper
   c. Rhodium
   d. Molybdenum

4. Which of the following does not change the shape of the X-ray emission spectrum?
   a. Milliampere
   b. Kilovolt (peak)
   c. Exposure time
   d. Target material

5. What is the usual range of force for mammographic system compression devices?
   a. 5 to 20 lb
   b. 15 to 30 lb
   c. 25 to 45 lb
   d. 45 to 60 lb

6. Which of the following is not an advantage of extended film processing in mammography?
   a. Greater image contrast
   b. Increased image receptor sensitivity
   c. Reduced patient dose
   d. Increased recorded detail

7. The light field/X-ray field alignment for mammographic units must be accurate to within ± ____ % of the source-to-image distance.
   a. 2
   b. 3
   c. 4
   d. 5

8. The base + fog value of a mammographic sensitometry film should not vary by more than ± _____ from the initial control value.
   a. 0.02
   b. 0.03
   c. 0.05
   d. 0.1

9. The contrast indicator, or density difference, of mammographic sensitometry films should not vary by more than ± _____ from the initial control value.
   a. 0.03
   b. 0.05
   c. 0.1
   d. 0.15

10. At a minimum, how often should phantom images with an American College of Radiology accreditation phantom be obtained?
    a. Daily
    b. Weekly
    c. Monthly
    d. Yearly

CHAPTER 12

Quality Control in Computed Tomography

Lorrie Kelley*

KEY TERMS

Acceptance testing
Action or control limit
Computed tomography dose index (CTDI)
Contrast scale
High-contrast spatial resolution
Linearity
Low-contrast resolution
Mean CT number
Noise
Phantoms
Region of interest
Standard deviations
Volume computed tomography dose index ($CTDI_{vol}$)

OBJECTIVES

At the completion of this chapter, the reader will be able to do the following:

- Differentiate between high- and low-contrast resolution
- Describe how basic quality control tests for computed tomography are conducted
- Describe the selection factors for quality control measurements
- Identify the parameters under the technologist's control that influence noise and spatial resolution

OUTLINE

Acceptance Testing
Routine Testing
  Alignment Light Accuracy
  Image Quality
    High-Contrast (Spatial) Resolution
    Low-Contrast Resolution
    Image Uniformity
    Noise
    Computed Tomography Number Accuracy
    Test–Computed Tomography Number Accuracy
American College of Radiology Acceptance Criteria
  Slice Thickness
  Linearity
  Patient Dose
American College of Radiology Computed Tomography Technologist's Quality Control Testing Requirements
  Water Computed Tomography Number and Standard Deviation (Noise)
Artifact Evaluation
Wet Laser Printer Quality Control
Visual Checklist
Hard Copy Image Quality Control of Dry Laser Printers
Gray Level Performance of Computed Tomography Scanner Display Monitors
Summary

The goal of any quality control (QC) program is to ensure that the imaging equipment is producing the best possible image quality with a minimal radiation dose to the patient. The image quality in computed tomography (CT) can be difficult to maintain because of the complex nature of image acquisition and display. A contemporary CT system is composed of numerous electronic parts and computers that generate and process huge amounts of data. Because of the system's complexity, a quality assurance program is essential to ensure optimal system performance and image quality with the least amount of radiation dose to the patient. Quality assurance programs

---

*The author and publisher wish to acknowledge the previous edition's contributor.

ACCEPTANCE TESTING

Typically, the installation of most CT units is immediately followed by extensive acceptance testing by qualified medical physicists. The purpose of the acceptance tests is to ensure that the equipment is performing according to the manufacturer's specifications before it is released for clinical use. **Acceptance testing** consists of measuring radiologic and electromechanical performance, analyzing image performance, and evaluating the system components. The results of the acceptance tests are used to identify system components that may need only slight adjustments and defective parts that should be replaced. At the end of the acceptance testing, scans are taken of standard objects so that their images, CT numbers, and **standard deviations** can be recorded as a baseline for future measurements of the system's performance.

ROUTINE TESTING

To provide more consistency in the performance measurements of CT scanners, federal performance standards state that the vendors of CT systems manufactured after September 1985 are required to supply the following: instructions for performing QC tests, a schedule for testing, allowable variations for the indicated parameters, a method to store and record the quality assurance data, and dose information in the form of a CT dose index. In addition, each vendor is required to supply **phantoms** capable of testing the following parameters: **contrast scale**, noise, slice thickness, spatial resolution capabilities for both high- and low-contrast objects, and the **mean CT number** for water or other reference material. Many routine QC tests can be performed by a CT technologist. In most instances, vendors specify the test conditions for evaluating their system's performance; therefore, specific procedures for evaluating a system's performance may vary among manufacturers. Also, there is some disagreement among manufacturers about the proper monitoring frequency for high- and low-contrast resolution, alignment, contrast scale, and slice thickness. Until standards for monitoring frequency can be agreed on, it is best to follow those recommended by the manufacturer. QC testing must also be completed after major repairs and before the first clinical scan after the repair. Major repairs include replacement or repair of any of the following subsystem components: X-ray tube, generator, collimator assembly, or X-ray detectors.

The performance of CT scanners is evaluated with a phantom as a test object. The phantoms that are supplied by the manufacturer can vary among vendors because of the differing requirements for performance evaluations and QC testing. However, a typical phantom used to assess the performance of a CT system is a multisectioned phantom, which enables the separate evaluation of different parameters (Figs. 12-1 and 12-2). In general, a phantom is constructed from plastic cylinders, with each section filled with water or other test objects to measure specific parameter performance. Some phantoms are designed so that numerous parameters can be evaluated with a single scan.

CT has undergone significant technologic advancements in recent years, resulting in new clinical applications and changes in clinical protocols in numerous CT departments across the United States. In 2002, in an effort to establish a reasonable standard of image quality, the American College of Radiology (ACR) approved the implementation of the CT Accreditation Program. This program was designed to evaluate the primary determinants of clinical image quality including the qualifications of the radiologists, medical physicists, and technologists; equipment performance; effectiveness of QC tests and measures; and clinical image quality and examination protocols. The ACR CT Accreditation Committee developed a specially designed CT phantom, along with test protocols for use in the accreditation process and for establishing quality assurance programs for clinical CT scanners. The multisectioned ACR CT accreditation phantom was designed to examine a wide variety of scanner parameters including: positioning accuracy, CT number accuracy, slice thickness, low-contrast resolution, high-contrast resolution, image uniformity and noise, distance measurement accuracy, section sensitivity profiles, and image artifacts. In the summer of 2008,

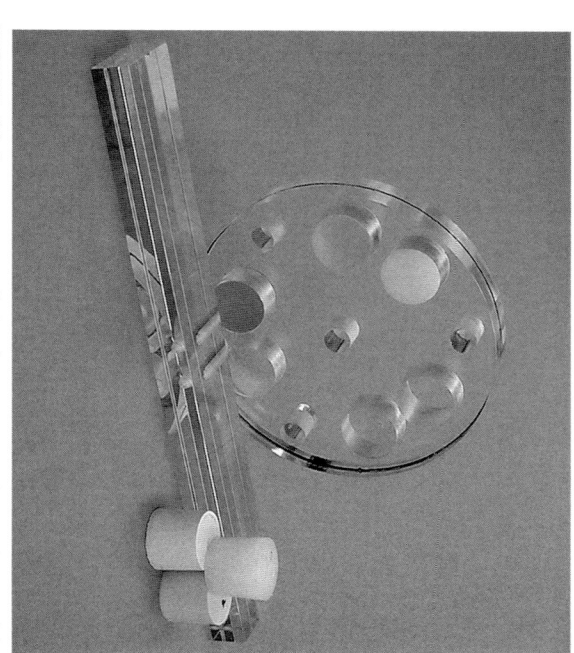

FIGURE 12-1 A version of the five-pin test object designed by the American Association of Physicists in Medicine. The attenuation coefficient for each pin is known precisely, and the computed tomography number is computed. (Courtesy Cardinal Health.) (From Bushong S: Radiologic science for technologists, ed 10, St Louis, 2012, Mosby.)

CHAPTER 12 Quality Control in Computed Tomography

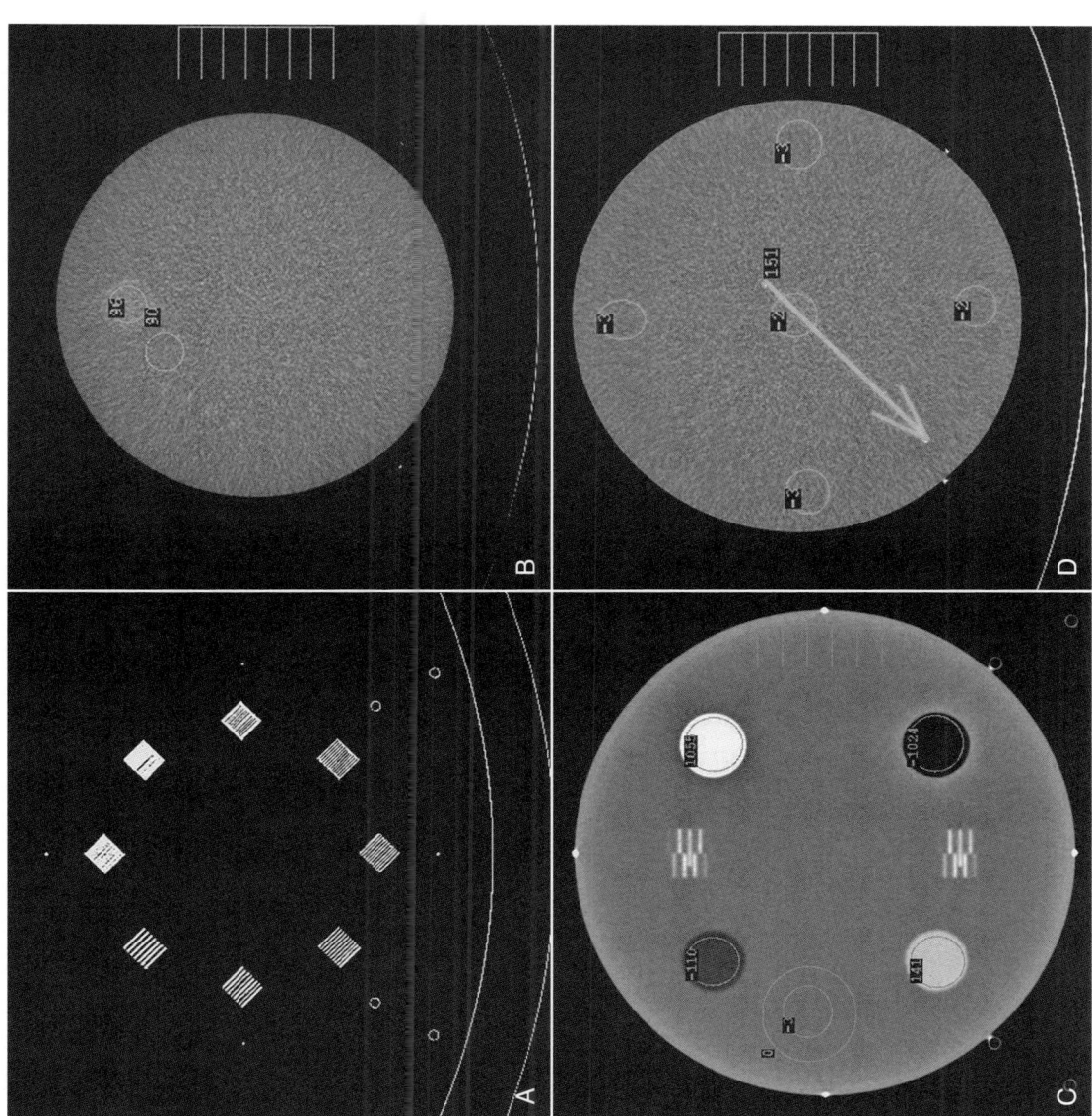

FIGURE 12-2 The phantom for evaluating computed tomography image quality contains test objects designed to measure spatial resolution (**A**), contrast resolution (**B**), linearity (**C**), and other image-quality factors (**D**). (*From Bushong S: Radiologic science for technologists, ed 10, Mosby, 2012, St Louis.*)

Congress passed the Medicare Improvements for Patients and Providers Act of 2008, which mandates that any nonhospital institution performing advanced diagnostic services (such as CT) must be accredited by a Centers for Medicare & Medicaid Services designated accrediting organization to receive federal funding (Medicare reimbursement). As of the writing of this edition, Centers for Medicare & Medicaid Services has approved three national accreditation organizations: the ACR, the Intersocietal Accreditation Commission, and The Joint Commission. This rule affects providers of magnetic resonance imaging, CT, positron emission tomography, and nuclear medicine imaging services for Medicare beneficiaries on an outpatient basis. The accreditation applies only to the suppliers of the images and not to the physician's interpretation of the image. The CARE bill (discussed in Chapter 1), if passed, would make similar requirements for hospital-based facilities. Therefore, accreditation programs are becoming mandatory for CT departments to succeed.

All QC tests described in this chapter should be performed according to the following three basic tenets of QC:

- The QC tests should be performed on a regular basis.
- All QC test measurements should be documented with the data form provided by the manufacturer (Fig. 12-3) or accrediting agency.
- The QC test should indicate whether the tested parameter is within specified guidelines known as **action** or **control limits**.

The material in this chapter follows the procedures recommended by the ACR, but the Intersocietal Accreditation Commission and The Joint Commission require

CHAPTER 12 Quality Control in Computed Tomography

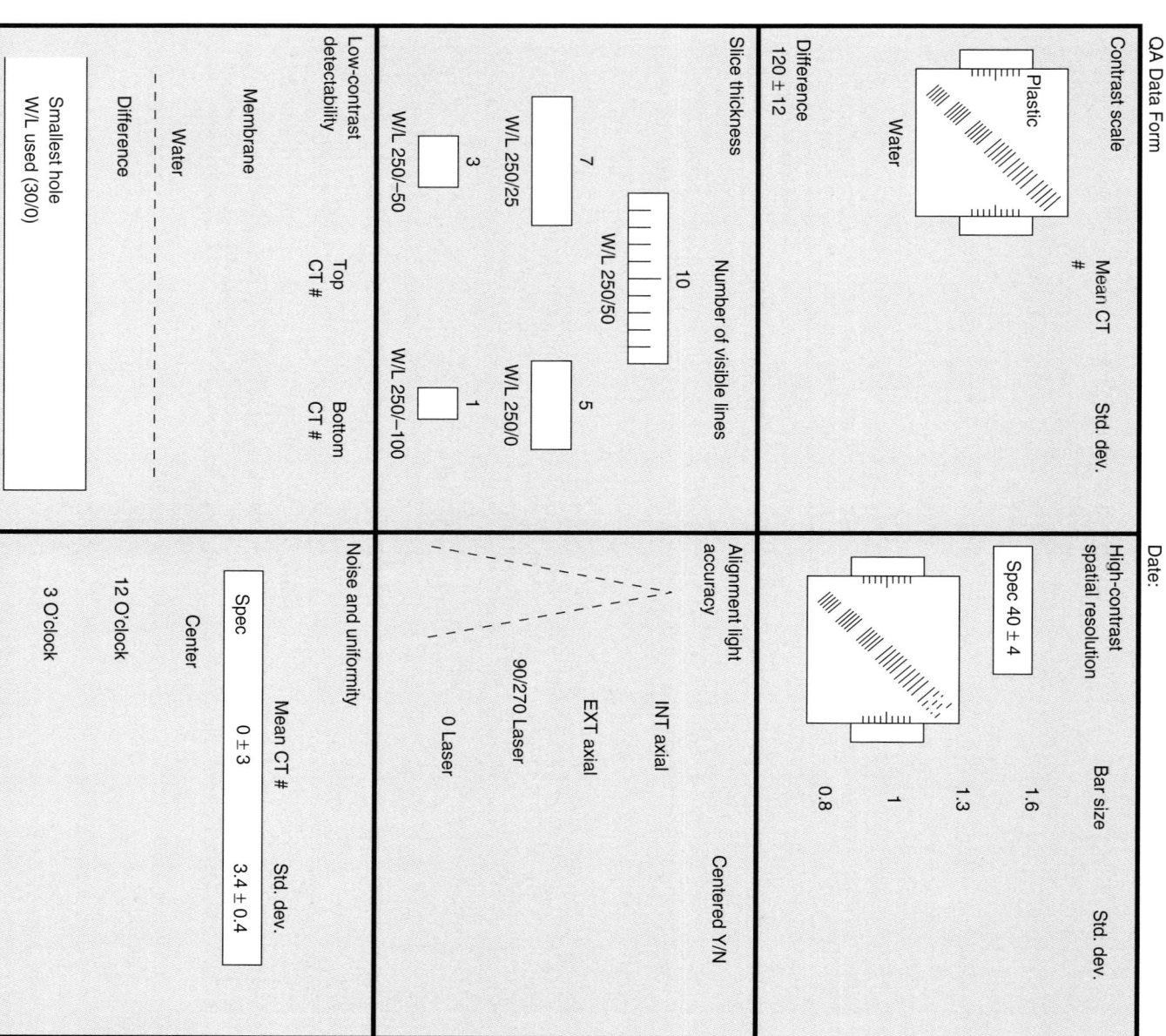

FIGURE 12-3 Sample quality assurance data form.

similar procedures. To maintain ACR CT accreditation status, the ACR states that a QC program must be implemented under the direction of a qualified medical physicist. The medical physicist is responsible for the annual performance evaluations of each CT unit as well as the establishment of a continuous QC program for implementation by a qualified CT technologist. The medical physicist will determine the frequency that each test must be performed on the basis of the facility and CT usage. The ACR recommends that a continuous QC program include, but not be limited to, evaluations of the following: alignment light accuracy, slice thickness, image quality, high-contrast resolution, low-contrast resolution, image uniformity, noise, artifact evaluation, CT number accuracy, and display devices.

The methodology of most of the following QC tests uses the ACR CT Accreditation Phantom and testing

CHAPTER 12 Quality Control in Computed Tomography

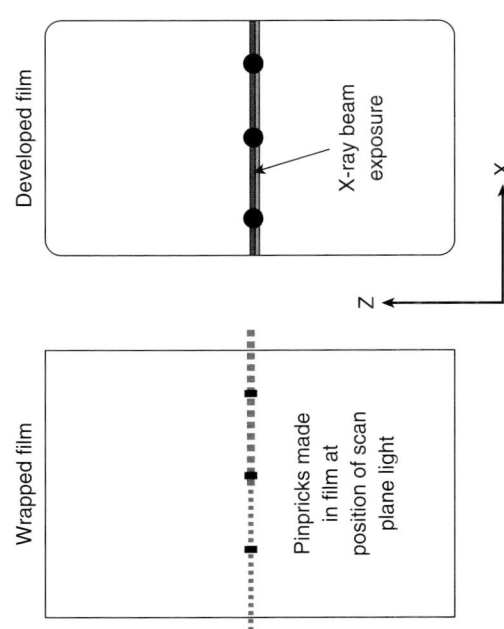

FIGURE 12-4 Technique for assessing laser light accuracy. (*Courtesy ImPACT, a Medical Devices Agency Evaluation Group, London, UK.*)

> **PROCEDURE**
>
> 1. Tape the unexposed X-ray film securely to the CT table.
> 2. To measure the accuracy of the internal laser lights, turn on the internal laser lights and poke two or three small holes through the wrapper and X-ray film at the exact location of the light field. The holes should be located near the right and left edges and center of the film.
> 3. Perform a scan through the location specified by the internal laser lights.
> 4. To measure the accuracy of the external laser lights, turn on the external laser lights and poke two small holes through either edge of the film at the exact location of the external light field.
> 5. Advance the table so that it is in position to scan, and perform a scan at that location.

criteria, but the same tests can be performed with phantoms supplied by the CT system's vendor. When using a vendor-supplied phantom, test measures should be compared with the limits specified by the vendor or during acceptance testing.

The ACR CT Accreditation Phantom is a solid phantom constructed primarily from a water-equivalent material. It consists of four contiguous modules, each 4 cm in width and 20 cm in diameter. Various test objects are embedded within the phantom in order to measure the various image quality parameters of a QC program.

Before starting any QC tests, it is important to complete a tube warm-up and daily system calibrations recommended by the manufacturer to optimize image quality.

Alignment Light Accuracy

Internal and external laser lights are used extensively for patient positioning and alignment. Accurate laser light performance is critical during stereotactic and interventional procedures.

Measurements to determine laser light accuracy can be made with the manufacturer's specific phantoms or a piece of covered, unexposed X-ray film.

After the X-ray film has been processed, the two sets of holes represent the internal and external light fields and the two dark bands from radiation exposure represent the radiation field. To measure the accuracy of the laser lights, one should check to see whether the dark bands of exposure fall directly over the associated holes (Fig. 12-4). For optimal performance, the light field should coincide with the radiation field to within 2 mm.

An alternative method to measure laser light accuracy is to scan the phantom and place a grid over the resultant image. The grid should line up accurately with the lines on the phantom.

Image Quality

High-Contrast (Spatial) Resolution. High-contrast spatial resolution is described as the minimum distance between two objects that allows them to be seen as separate and distinct. The parameters that influence the high-contrast spatial resolution of a CT scanner include the following:

1. Scanner design (focal spot size, detector size and spacing, magnification)
2. Image reconstruction (pixel size, reconstruction algorithm, slice thickness)
3. Sampling (number of rays per projection and number of projections)
4. Image display capabilities (display matrix)

Two procedures can be used to evaluate the spatial resolution capabilities of a CT scanner. In the first method, an edge is measured to determine the point spread function. The point spread function is then mathematically transformed to obtain the modulation transfer function. This process takes considerable time and is usually completed by the medical physicist. In the second method, a bar or hole pattern is used to determine the spatial resolution. This method is commonly performed by the CT technologist and is explained in the following procedure.

> **PROCEDURE**
>
> 1. Take a single scan through the test object.
> 2. On the resultant image, determine which row has the smallest set of holes in which all of the holes can be clearly identified. This is known as the *limiting resolution* of the CT scanner.

The ACR CT Accreditation Phantom contains eight bar-resolution patterns, which represent spatial frequencies corresponding to: 4, 5, 6, 7, 8, 9, 10, and 12 line pairs per centimeter (lp/cm), each fitting into a 15-mm × 15-mm square region on module 4.

Test—High-Contrast Resolution

1. Scan module 4 with adult abdomen and high-resolution chest protocols making sure to use the appropriate reconstruction algorithm.
2. Display the images with a window width of 100 and window level ≈ 1100.
3. Record the bar pattern for which the bars and spaces are distinctly visualized for both images.

American College of Radiology Acceptance Criteria

- The adult abdomen and high-resolution chest protocols must be used.
- Window width = 100.
- Window level ≈ 1100.
- The 5 lp/cm bar pattern must be clearly resolved for adult abdomen protocol.
- The 6 lp/cm bar pattern must be clearly resolved for adult high-resolution chest protocol.

The limiting high-contrast spatial resolution of a CT scanner is measured in line pairs per centimeter. Even though many modern scanners have the ability to resolve holes as small as 0.3 mm, the spatial resolution of CT scanners is still lower than that of conventional radiography. The results of this test can be compared with the baseline measurement of the scanner collected during optimal system performance or compared with the manufacturer's specifications. Comparative measurements over time provide an index of the performance reproducibility of the CT system.

Low-Contrast Resolution. Low-contrast resolution refers to the capability of the CT system to demonstrate subtle differences in tissue densities from one region of anatomy to another. Compared with conventional radiography, CT provides superior low-contrast resolution. Typically, contrast resolution is expressed in one of two ways: the smallest diameter of an object with a specific contrast that can be detected or the smallest difference in X-ray attenuation that can be discriminated for an object of a specific diameter.

A phantom consisting of test objects such as holes drilled into plastic is used for this test. The rows of holes should be of varying sizes and filled with a liquid that has a CT number different from the CT number for the plastic by approximately 0.6%.

PROCEDURE

1. Scan the phantom, and determine the smallest row of holes that can be seen clearly.
2. Current CT scanners are capable of displaying 3-mm objects with density differences of 0.5% or less.

The ACR CT Accreditation Phantom uses module 2 to assess low-contrast resolution. It consists of a series of cylinders of varying diameters with a 0.6% Hounsfield unit (HU) difference from the background material, which has a CT number of approximately 90 HU. Four cylinders exist for each of the following diameters: 2, 3, 4, 5, and 6 mm. The space between each cylinder is equal to the diameter of the cylinder. An additional 25-mm cylinder is used to verify the contrast between the cylinders and the background material.

Test—Low-Contrast Resolution

1. Scan module 2 with the adult abdomen and adult head protocols.
2. Display images with window width of 100 and window level of 100.
3. Record the diameter of the smallest set of cylinders for which all four cylinders can be resolved.
4. Place a 100-mm **region of interest (ROI)** within the 25-mm diameter cylinder and outside the cylinder over the background material. Record the mean CT number of each ROI and calculate the difference. Low contrast = 6 HU ± 0.5 HU (Fig. 12-5).

American College of Radiology Acceptance Criteria

- The adult abdomen and head protocols must be used.
- Window width = 100.
- Window level = 100.
- All four of the 6-mm cylinders must be clearly visible.

The primary factor limiting low-contrast resolution in CT is image noise caused by quantum mottle. As noise increases in an image, the edge definition of anatomic borders and subtle differences in attenuation between tissues decreases.

Image Uniformity. *Uniformity* refers to the ability of the CT scanner to yield the same CT number regardless of the location of the ROI within a homogenous object. A simple 20-cm water phantom can be used to measure noise and uniformity in CT. Module 3 of the ACR CT Accreditation Phantom is used to assess image uniformity. Module 3 consists of a uniform, tissue-equivalent material with two small BBs placed at known distances within the material for optional measurements of in-plane distance measurements (Fig. 12-6).

PROCEDURE

1. Take a scan through the water phantom and position a cursor over the resultant image in three different locations.
2. The cursor should be positioned in the center, at the top, and at the side of the image (see Fig. 12-6).
3. At each cursor location, take an ROI measurement and record the standard deviation and mean CT number. For noise measurements, the noise in a CT system should not exceed ± 10 HU. However, if the scanner is used for quantitative CT, tighter specifications might be necessary.

Test—Image Uniformity

1. Scan module 3 with adult abdomen protocol.
2. Display the image with a window width of 100 and window level of 0.

CHAPTER 12 Quality Control in Computed Tomography

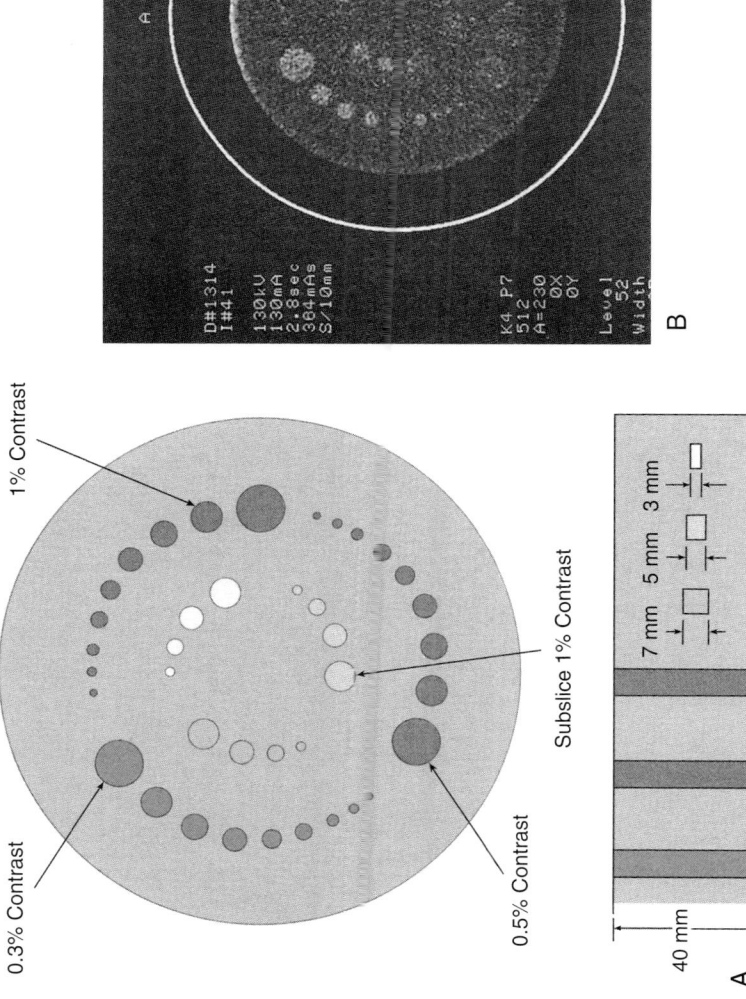

FIGURE 12-5 Schematic drawing (**A**) of a low-contrast computed tomography (CT) test object and (**B**) its image. This test object is designed especially for multislice helical CT. (*From Bushong S: Radiologic science for technologists, ed 10, St Louis, 2012, Mosby.*)

5. Determine the difference between the mean CT number of the center ROI to the mean CT numbers for all four edge ROIs (mean CT number of center ROI − mean CT number of edge ROI).
6. Assess the image for streaking or artifacts.

American College of Radiology Acceptance Criteria.

- Edge-to-center mean CT number difference must be less than 5 HU for all four edge positions.
- Correct size and location of ROIs.
- The center CT number must be between −7 and +7 HU (±5 HU preferred).
- Adult abdomen protocol must be used.
- Window width = 100.
- Window width = 0.
- No image artifacts.

Noise. Noise represents the portion of the CT image that contains no useful information. It is defined as the random variation of CT numbers about a mean value when an image of a uniform object is obtained. The contrast resolution of a CT system is primarily determined by the amount of noise in the images. Noise produces a "salt-and-pepper" appearance or grainy quality in the image. The sources of noise in a CT image include quantum (statistical) noise, electronic noise, object size, reconstruction algorithms, detector efficiency, and artifacts. Of these, the predominant source of noise is quantum noise, which is defined as the statistical variation in the number of photons detected.

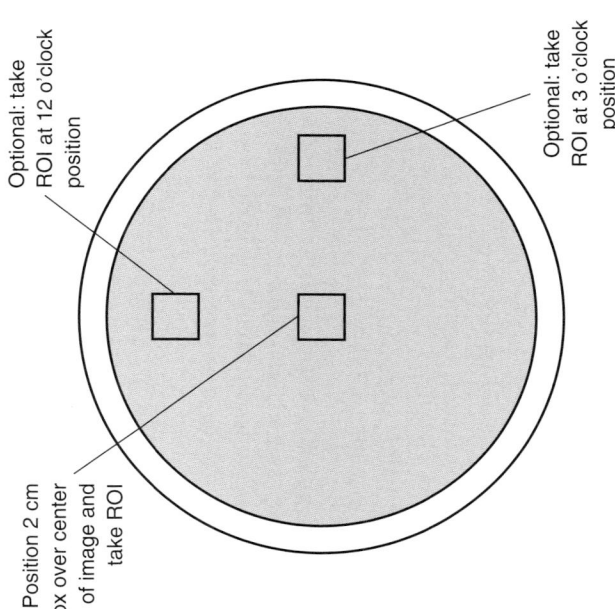

3. Place an ROI, approximately 400 mm in diameter, at the center of the image and record the HU and standard deviation.
4. Place the same size ROI at peripheral edges of the phantom at positions 12, 3, 6, and 9 o'clock. Record the HU and standard deviation for each ROI.

FIGURE 12-6 *Test for noise and uniformity.* ROI, Region of interest.

Factors under the influence of the technologist that affect the amount of noise in an image are pixel size, slice thickness, reconstruction algorithm, and technique factors. Simple methods to minimize noise and help provide uniform images include tube warm-ups and daily system calibrations. Because the amount of noise contained in an image is inversely proportional to the total amount of radiation absorbed, noise can be measured by obtaining the mean and standard deviation of the CT numbers within an ROI.

Test—Noise

1. Scan module 3 with adult abdomen protocol.
2. Display the image with a window width of 100 and window level of 0.
3. Place an ROI, approximately 20 mm in diameter, at the center of the image and record the HU and standard deviation.

American College of Radiology Acceptance Criteria. No value given, compare with manufacturer's specifications.

Computed Tomography Number Accuracy

CT numbers represent the attenuation values of different structures within the body according to their atomic number and physical density. The CT numbers are assigned a shade of gray corresponding with the attenuation value they represent. This constitutes the gray-scale or contrast scale of the displayed image. The contrast scale is determined by the CT numbers for air (−1000 HU) and water (0 HU). In CT, the scanner assigns CT numbers according to the attenuation values of X-rays passing through tissue. Water is the reference material used to determine CT numbers because it constitutes up to 90% of soft-tissue mass, is easy to obtain, and is completely reproducible. Because water has a CT number value of zero, tissues with densities greater than water have positive CT numbers and those with densities less than water have negative CT numbers (Fig. 12-7).

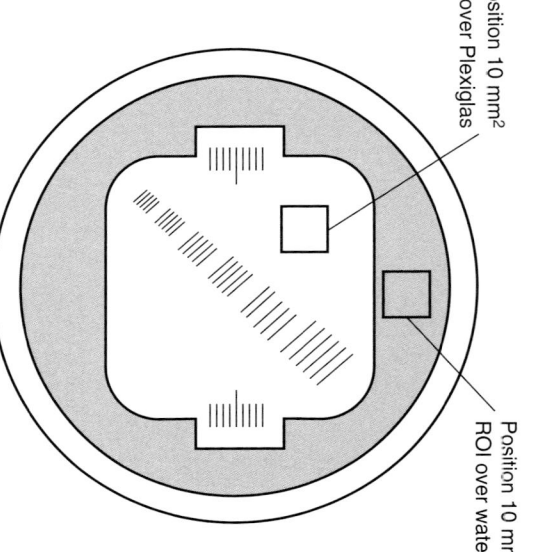

FIGURE 12-7 Test for contrast scale, ROI, Region of interest.

conditions in the image. Calculating the CT number of known materials is necessary to measure the accuracy of the CT numbers.

Test–Computed Tomography Number Accuracy

1. Align module 1 to lasers. Module 1 consists of water embedded with four cylinders of known reference materials (air, polyethylene, bone, and acrylic).
2. Scan with adult abdomen protocol and at all kilovolt (peaks) (kVps) available.
3. Place an ROI approximately 200 mm over the center of each cylinder and the water. Record all HUs.
4. Scan varying slice thicknesses and repeat step 3.

The contrast scale can vary with different X-ray energies; therefore, for QC testing, each test should be repeated at the same kVp setting and for each kVp setting that can be selected. For consistent results, the same cursor size and location should be used each time the test is performed.

American College of Radiology Acceptance Criteria

- ROIs must be placed within the cylinders.
- Polyethylene mean CT number must be between −107 and −87 HU.
- Water mean CT number must be between −7 and +7 HU (±5 HU preferred).
- Acrylic mean CT number must be between +110 and +130 HU.
- Bone mean CT number must be between +850 and +970 HU.
- Air mean CT number must be between −1005 and −970 HU.
- Image data are required for all selectable kVp settings.

Slice Thickness. The slice thickness in single-slice CT is determined primarily by the collimators. The position of the collimators determines the width of the slice that falls within the view of each detector. In multidetector CT, the slice thickness is determined by the width of the active detector elements. Another factor affecting slice thickness

PROCEDURE

1. Using a specific technique, take a single scan through the phantom.
2. On the reconstructed image, select a 2- to 3-cm area in the center of the phantom and measure the ROI (see Fig. 12-7).
3. From the pixels located within the ROI, calculate the two parameters, the mean CT number, and the standard deviation of the CT numbers.
4. On a monthly basis, move the cursor outside of the phantom on the reconstructed image and perform the ROI function over air.

This test is performed to determine if the scanner is assigning CT numbers that accurately correspond to the appropriate tissue. Many radiologists use CT numbers as quantitative parameters to identify suspected pathologic

CHAPTER 12 Quality Control in Computed Tomography

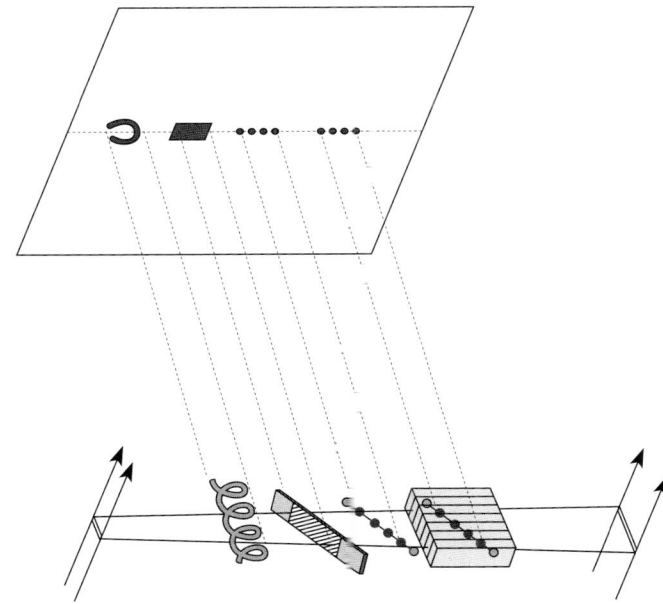

FIGURE 12-8 Test objects used for determining slice thickness. *(From Marshall C: The physical basis of computed tomography, St Louis, 1982, Warren H Green.)*

is the focal spot size. The focal spot size can influence the penumbra, or sharpness of the edge of the X-ray beam, which can cause the edge of the slice to spread. Focal spot size in CT is determined by the technique factors or algorithm selected for the scan parameters. Slice thickness is a primary factor of image quality and spatial resolution.

Measurements of slice thickness are determined with a phantom that includes a ramp, spiral, or step wedge in the test objects. The test objects have known measurements and provide a standard to compare with the scanner. Typically, the test objects are aligned obliquely to the scan plane (Fig. 12-8).

If it is 5 mm or more, the slice thickness should not vary more than ±1 mm from the intended slice thickness. If it is 5 mm or less, the slice thickness should not vary more than ±0.5 mm.

Module 1 of the ACR CT Accreditation Phantom is used to assess slice thickness. Embedded within module 1 are a series of discrete wires that are positioned on a ramp inclined with respect to the axial plane such that the spacing between them equals 0.5 mm along the z-axis.

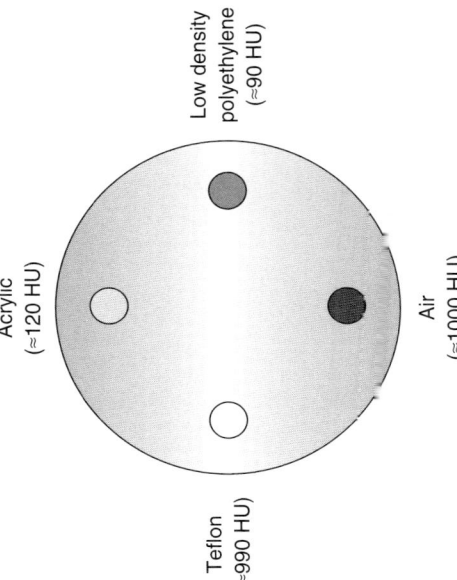

FIGURE 12-9 Phantom with known physical and X-ray absorption properties used for measuring linearity. HU, Hounsfield unit. *(Courtesy ImPACT, a Medical Devices Agency Evaluation Group, London, UK.)*

Test—Slice Thickness

1. Scan module 1 with 3, 5, and 7 mm and high-resolution chest slice thicknesses.
2. Use a WW (Window Width) = 400 and a WL (Window Level) = 0 to view images.
3. Count the number of wires visualized in each of the two slice thickness ramps at each slice thickness (count the number of wires in the top and bottom ramps separately).
4. Estimate the slice thickness by counting the number of well-visualized wires at the top and bottom of each slice and divide by two. For example, if you can visualize 11 wires, 11 ÷ 2 is 5.5 mm.

American College of Radiology Acceptance Criteria

- Image data is required for high-resolution chest, 3, 5, 7 mm slice thicknesses.
- The slice width must be within 1.5 mm of the prescribed width.

Linearity. Linearity refers to the relationship between CT numbers and the linear attenuation values of the scanned object with a particular kVp value. When linearity is present within an image, it is an indication that subject contrast is constant across the range of CT numbers within the image.

A standard phantom containing materials with known physical and X-ray absorption properties is used for this test (Fig. 12-9).

Over time, these values can vary because of changes in system components. Daily calibrations help maintain image quality by compensating for changes in detector channel variations and responses.

The plotted values should demonstrate a straight line between the average CT numbers and the linear attenuation coefficients (Fig. 12-10). Any deviation from the straight line can indicate that inaccurate CT numbers are being generated or the scanner is malfunctioning.

PROCEDURE

1. Perform three separate scans through the test object, each with a specified thickness (10, 5, and 1 mm).
2. Display the images using the manufacturer's recommendations.
3. If a ramp is used, the length of the resultant image gives the slice width. For a spiral test object, the resultant image contains an arc, with the arc length giving the slice width. When a step wedge is used, the slice width can be determined according to the number of steps that are imaged.

PROCEDURE

1. Take a single scan through the appropriate phantom.
2. Plot the average CT numbers as a function of the attenuation values corresponding to the materials within the phantom.

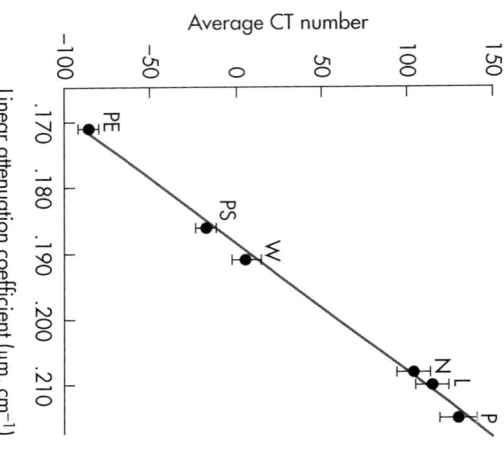

FIGURE 12-10 Graph showing computed tomography (CT) linearity. L, Lexan; N, nylon; P, Plexiglas; PE, polyethylene; PS, polystyrene; W, water. (From Bushong S: Radiologic science for technologists, ed 6, Mosby, 1997, St Louis.)

PROCEDURE

1. Along with a standard phantom, position the radiation-detecting device at the location and intervals of the desired radiation measurements.
2. Initiate the appropriate scans at the selected locations, and measure the resultant radiation dose. Some facilities prefer to take two scans at each location, but with a change in the technique factors to simulate the difference between head and body examinations. This gives a more reliable dose estimate for a particular CT examination.

Patient Dose. Personnel should monitor the amount of radiation to which patients and staff are exposed. It is equally important for a CT technologist to realize that the patient dose can increase with changes in slice thickness, kVp, and milliampere-seconds (mAs). In addition, if it is necessary for ancillary personnel to remain within the scan room, all CT technologists should be able to direct them to the safest location within the room to avoid unnecessary radiation exposure. Fig. 12-11 provides representative isodose curves for a typical CT scanner.

Specially designed ionization chambers or thermoluminescent dosimeters are used to measure the radiation dose. These specially designed radiation detectors are capable of providing measurements from which the dose can be calculated for the exposure factors used (slice thickness, mAs, and kVp).

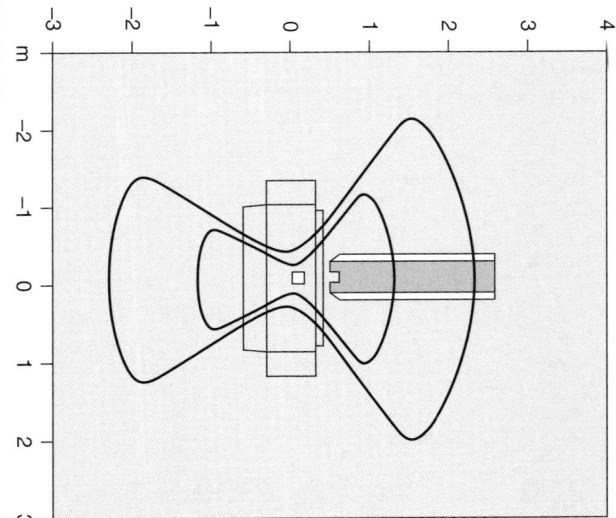

FIGURE 12-11 Isodose curves for a typical computed tomography (CT) scanner. (From Wegener OH: Whole body computed tomography, Cambridge, MA, 1992, Blackwell Scientific.)

No acceptable maximum levels of radiation are specified for the permissible dose to a patient during a CT procedure. In addition, the results can vary according to patient location and distance from the X-ray source. However, most experts agree that the values should remain within ±10% of the manufacturer's specifications when a fixed technique is used.

For ACR CT accreditation purposes, a medical physicist is required to perform **computed tomography dose index** (CTDI) testing on every CT unit at the clinical facility. This value is measured in a cylindrical acrylic phantom placed at the scanner isocenter and obtained by using a 100-mm-long pencil-shaped ionization chamber in one of two phantom sizes. A 16-cm phantom is used to calculate the CTDI for head examinations, and a 32-cm phantom is used to calculate the CTDI for body examinations. Because multislice CT units have become the prevalent system in CT departments, a more appropriate dose descriptor of **volume computed tomography dose index** ($CTDI_{vol}$) is now used. This value incorporates CTDI values measured at the both the center of the acrylic phantom and the slice thickness. For a given scanner and set of scanning parameters being used (i.e., kVp, mA, tube rotation time, beam width, and CT pitch), the $CTDI_{vol}$ is fixed and is not affected by patient size or scan length. This means that $CTDI_{vol}$ does not measure how much a specific patient receives but rather indicates the intensity of radiation that is being directed at that patient. For the CT unit to pass the phantom image quality tests, it has to be demonstrated that the scanner meets the ACR dose reference levels. The ACR has recently updated the ACR CT accreditation dose pass/fail criteria and reference levels (Table 12-1).

CHAPTER 12 Quality Control in Computed Tomography

TABLE 12-1 American College of Radiology CT Accreditation Dose Pass/Fail Criteria and Reference Levels

Examination	Pass/Fail Criteria CTDI$_{vol}$ (mGy)	Reference Levels CTDI$_{vol}$ (mGy)
Adult head	80	75
Adult abdomen	30	25
Pediatric head (1 year old)	40	35
Pediatric abdomen (40–50 lb)	20	15

American College of Radiology Computed Tomography Technologist's Quality Control Testing Requirements

In addition to the medical physicist's testing, the ACR also requires that CT technologists perform QC tests on a regular basis and that the test results are properly documented. These results should be reviewed with the medical physicist and radiologist regularly. The technologists QC tests include:

Procedure	Minimum Frequency	Approximate Time (min)
Water CT number and standard deviation	Daily	5
Artifact evaluation	Daily	5 or Less
Wet laser printer quality control (if film is used for primary interpretation)	Weekly	10
Visual checklist	Monthly	5
Dry laser printer quality control (if film is used for primary interpretation)	Monthly	10
Display monitor quality control	Monthly	5

PROCEDURE

1. Warm up the scanner's X-ray tube/s according to manufacturer recommendations.
2. Perform calibration scans (often called air-calibration scans) according to scanner manufacturer recommendations.
3. Place the QC phantom on the holder device provided. Center the phantom at the isocenter of the scanner using the laser alignment lights of the scanner and the alignment marks on the phantom surface.
4. Set up a scan of the QC phantom using the scanner's daily QC scan parameter settings. It is strongly recommended that the QC scan protocols be preprogrammed for consistency. Usually these scan protocols will follow the parameter settings recommended by the scanner manufacturer. Water mean and standard deviation values should be monitored for both axial and helical scan modes. If the scanner manufacturer specifies only one of these modes, the medical physicist should assist the QC technologist in establishing and preprogramming a similar scan protocol for the other mode.
5. While viewing the phantom image, place an ROI at the center of the image. If a group of images were obtained on a multislice CT scanner, select an image from the central portion of the group to analyze. If the size of this ROI is not specified by the manufacturer, use an area of about 400 mm^2. Record the value reported for the water mean and standard deviation on the Data Form for Daily CT Equipment Quality Control (Fig. 12-12).
6. Repeat the previous measurement for an image that is either at the leading or trailing edge of the fan beam during the acquisition (i.e., an image at the beginning or end of the stack).
7. Repeat steps 5 and 6 for image(s) acquired in the second scan mode.
8. The water values should be 0 ± 5 HU, but must be 0 ± 7 HU. The medical physicist will establish limit criteria for noise (standard deviation) for both axial and helical modes after consulting manufacturer's recommendations.
9. If either the mean CT number or the noise (standard deviation) is not within the criteria limit for 3 days in a row or 3 times within a 7-day period, corrective action should be taken by reporting the problem to service personnel.

Water Computed Tomography Number and Standard Deviation (Noise). This test is performed to ensure that the relative calibration of all CT numbers to water remains within acceptable limits and that quantum noise and electronic system noise do not increase (this would cause a decrease in low-contrast detectability). Images of the water phantom provided by the scanner manufacturer or the ACR CT phantom are obtained prior to the first clinical scan of the day (or the equivalent for scanners used around the clock). Images of the water phantom are acquired in both the axial and helical scan modes using predetermined scan techniques.

Artifact Evaluation. The images of the water phantom or ACR CT phantom obtained in the water number and standard deviation procedure should be reviewed daily to identify and correct artifacts in images before they become severe enough to be detected in patient images. Data are recorded on the Data Form for Daily CT Equipment Quality Control (Fig. 12-12).

Wet Laser Printer Quality Control. This test must be performed weekly if film is used for primary interpretation. For printers that are used infrequently (i.e., back-up printers), this test should be performed before clinical use. Equipment necessary for this test are a densitometer, Laser Film QC Chart (Fig. 12-13), and an SMPTE (Society of Motion Picture and Television Engineers) test pattern (see Chapter 9).

Visual Checklist. A visual checklist should be performed on a monthly basis (at minimum) to ensure the CT system's patient bed transport, alignment and system indicator lights, intercom, the emergency cart, room safety lights, signage, and monitors are present, working properly, and are mechanically and electrically stable. Results should be recorded on the Visual Checklist Form (Fig. 12-14). Items missing from the room should be replaced immediately. Malfunctioning equipment should be reported to the CT service engineer for repair or replacement as soon as possible.

DATA FORM FOR DAILY CT EQUIPMENT QUALITY CONTROL

CT Facility Name: _____   CT Scanner Identifier: _____

Date		Water HU	Limit	Water SD	Limit	Axial Artifacts	Notes
	Axial		Y/N		Y/N	Y/N	
	Helical		Y/N		Y/N	Y/N	
	Axial		Y/N		Y/N	Y/N	
	Helical		Y/N		Y/N	Y/N	
	Axial		Y/N		Y/N	Y/N	
	Helical		Y/N		Y/N	Y/N	
	Axial		Y/N		Y/N	Y/N	
	Helical		Y/N		Y/N	Y/N	
	Axial		Y/N		Y/N	Y/N	
	Helical		Y/N		Y/N	Y/N	
	Axial		Y/N		Y/N	Y/N	
	Helical		Y/N		Y/N	Y/N	
	Axial		Y/N		Y/N	Y/N	
	Helical		Y/N		Y/N	Y/N	
	Axial		Y/N		Y/N	Y/N	
	Helical		Y/N		Y/N	Y/N	
	Axial		Y/N		Y/N	Y/N	
	Helical		Y/N		Y/N	Y/N	
	Axial		Y/N		Y/N	Y/N	
	Helical		Y/N		Y/N	Y/N	
	Axial		Y/N		Y/N	Y/N	
	Helical		Y/N		Y/N	Y/N	
	Axial		Y/N		Y/N	Y/N	
	Helical		Y/N		Y/N	Y/N	
	Axial		Y/N		Y/N	Y/N	
	Helical		Y/N		Y/N	Y/N	
	Axial		Y/N		Y/N	Y/N	
	Helical		Y/N		Y/N	Y/N	
	Axial		Y/N		Y/N	Y/N	
	Helical		Y/N		Y/N	Y/N	
	Axial		Y/N		Y/N	Y/N	
	Helical		Y/N		Y/N	Y/N	
	Axial		Y/N		Y/N	Y/N	
	Helical		Y/N		Y/N	Y/N	
	Axial		Y/N		Y/N	Y/N	
	Helical		Y/N		Y/N	Y/N	
	Axial		Y/N		Y/N	Y/N	
	Helical		Y/N		Y/N	Y/N	

Reviewed by: _____   Qualified Medical Physicist
Date of Review: _____

FIGURE 12-12 American College of Radiology Data Form for Daily CT Equipment Quality Control.

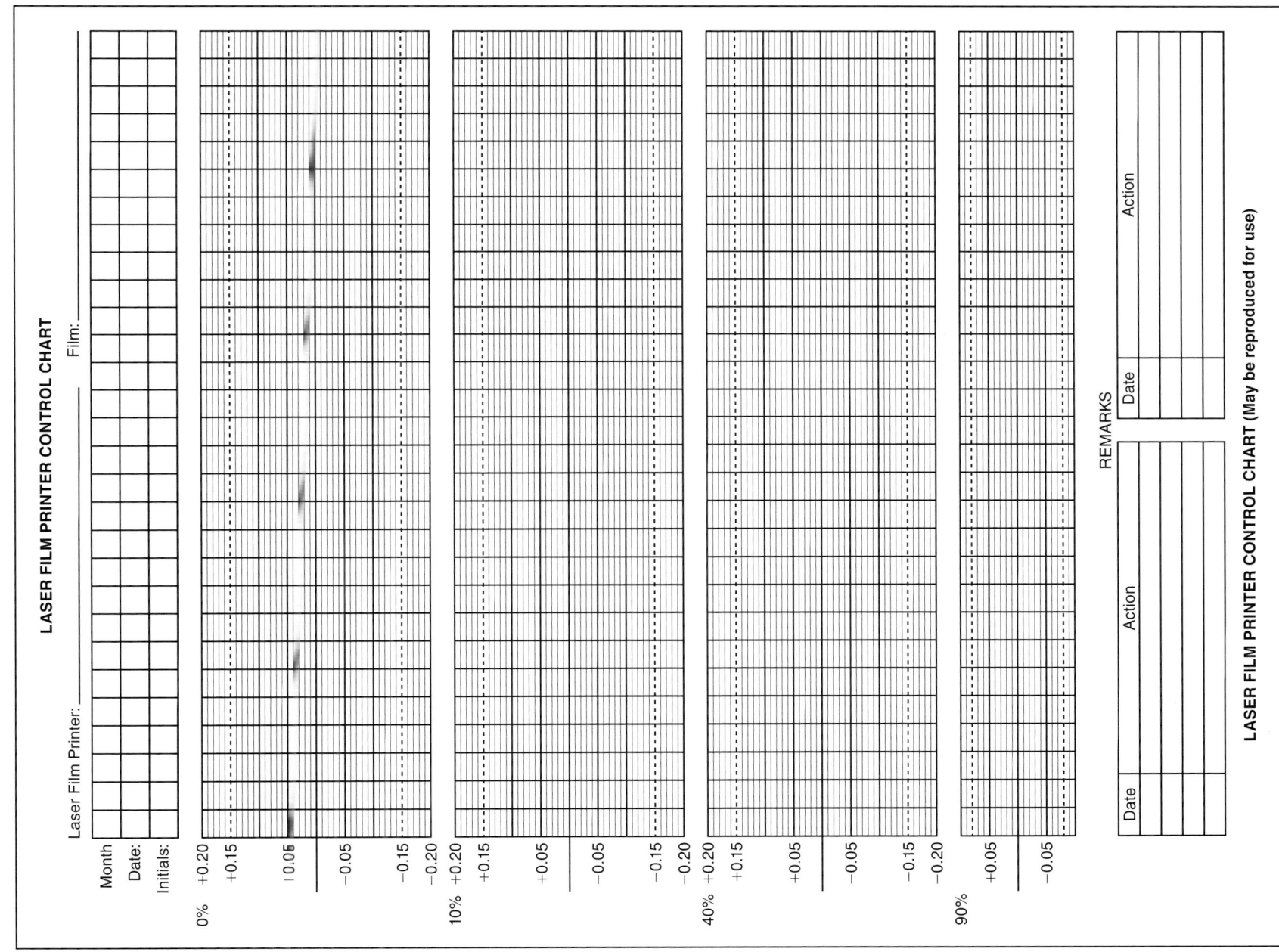

FIGURE 12-13 American College of Radiology Laser Film Printer Control Chart.

CT QUALITY CONTROL VISUAL CHECKLIST

Facility: _____   Room # _____

		Month:																												
		Date:																												
		Initials:																												
GANTRY	Table height indicator........																													
	Table position indicator.......																													
	Angulation indicator...........																													
	Laser localization light........																													
	High voltage cable/other cables.																													
	Smoothness of table motion....																													
CONTROL CONSOLE	Exposure switch placement.....																													
	View Window.................																													
	Panel switches/lights/meters...																													
	Protocols....................																													
	Door interlocks..............																													
	Warning labels...............																													
OTHER	Postings.....................																													
	Service records...............																													
	Exposure reports..............																													
OTHER	_____																													
	_____																													
	_____																													
	_____																													
	_____																													

PASS = P
FAIL = F
DOES NOT APPLY = NA

FIGURE 12-14 American College of Radiology.

PROCEDURE | ARTIFACT EVALUATION

1. View the images obtained in the water number and standard deviation procedure using the appropriate window width/level setting and scan for artifacts (additional images may be necessary). The artifact images should: (1) be the thinnest axial images possible on the scanner and (2) span the z-axis of the detector array on the scanner.
2. Look for rings in the image, which can be darker or lighter than the water portion. Also look for streaks, lines, etc. that should not be present in the image. Record the findings on the data form.
3. Ring artifacts typically indicate detector or data channel imbalance. Repeating the air-calibration procedure (Step 2 of the water number procedure) may smooth out these imbalances. If they are not corrected after performing several air-calibration procedures, service of the scanner should be arranged.

CHAPTER 12 Quality Control in Computed Tomography

PROCEDURE

1. Display the SMPTE test pattern on the filming console. Set the display window width/level to the manufacturer-specified values for the SMPTE pattern.
2. Film the SMPTE pattern. Use a 6-on-1 format and capture the pattern in all six frames.
3. Using a film densitometer, measure the optical density of the 0, 10%, 40%, and 90% gray-level patches of the SMPTE pattern in the upper left frame of the film.
4. Plot these optical densities in the appropriate places on the laser film QC chart. Circle any points that fall outside the control limit.

SMPTE Patch	Optical Density	Control Limits
0	3.00	±0.15
10%	2.20	±0.15
40%	1.15	±0.15
90%	0.30	±0.15

5. Put the film on a viewbox and inspect it for streaks, uneven densities, and other artifacts.
6. If optical densities fall outside of control limit or if artifacts are found, corrective action should be taken.

Hard Copy Image Quality Control of Dry Laser Printers. This test must be performed monthly if film is used for primary interpretation. For printers used infrequently (i.e., back-up printers), this test should be performed prior to clinical use. The equipment required and procedures are exactly the same as that used for the Wet Laser Printer Quality Control.

Gray Level Performance of Computed Tomography Scanner Display Monitors. This test must be performed monthly (or whenever a significant change is made to the imager's display monitors) to ensure that images on the monitors of the CT scanner display the entire range of gray shades produced by the CT scanner.

PROCEDURE

1. Display an SMPTE Test Pattern (or American Association of Physicists in Medicine TG 18QC Test Pattern) on the imaging console. Set the display window width/level to the manufacturer-specified values for the test pattern. The monitor should be positioned so that there is no glare from room lighting.
2. Examine the pattern to confirm that the gray level display on the imaging console is subjectively correct. The visual impression should indicate an even progression of gray levels around the ring of gray-level patches. Verify the following: (1) the 5% patch can be distinguished in the 0/5% patch; (2) the 95% patch can be distinguished in the 95/100% patch; and (3) all the gray-level steps around the ring of gray levels are distinct from adjacent steps.
3. If these conditions are not met, corrective action is needed. This may be as simple as reducing ambient light in the room. Otherwise, perform the manufacturer's recommended procedures for monitor contrast and brightness adjustment. If this still does not correct the problem, have the medical physicist or service engineer make adjustment.

SUMMARY

An effective quality assurance program provides a method for systematic monitoring of the CT system's performance and image quality. The collected data are beneficial in identifying specific problems or malfunctions. Increasingly, it is becoming the responsibility of the CT technologist to perform and document the routine QC tests. However, more extensive quality assurance procedures should be performed periodically by the department physicist or service engineer. As with all quality management and accreditation processes, documentation of all QC testing and maintenance of all records is imperative for program success.

Refer to the Evolve Website at https://evolve.elsevier.com for Student Experiment 12.1: Computed Tomography (CT) Quality Control.

REVIEW QUESTIONS

1. What is used as the reference material for CT number calibrations?
   a. Bone
   b. Liver
   c. Water
   d. Lung
2. Which of the following is the expected result of a CT number calibration test?
   a. 0 ± 5
   b. 1000 ± 5
   c. 0 ± 3
   d. 1000 ± 3
3. Which of the following is the primary determination of slice thickness?
   a. Spacing between detectors
   b. Collimators
   c. Focal spot size
   d. Field of view (FOV)
4. Which term describes the ability of a CT scanner to differentiate objects with minimal differences in attenuation coefficients?
   a. Spatial resolution
   b. Contrast resolution
   c. Linearity
   d. Modulation
5. Which of the following factors can affect the accuracy of a density (HU) measurement in a CT image?
   a. System calibration
   b. Window width setting
   c. Window level setting
   d. Display FOV

6. Increasing which of the following factors can improve spatial resolution?
   a. FOV
   b. Matrix
   c. Pixel size
   d. Slice thickness
7. Which of the following is the main limiting factor for contrast resolution?
   a. Noise
   b. Pixel depth
   c. Voxel volume
   d. Focal spot size
8. Which of the following is measured using the modulation transfer function method?
   a. Low-contrast resolution
   b. High-contrast spatial resolution
   c. Attenuation
   d. Section thickness
9. A contemporary CT system should be able to detect 3-mm objects with which of the following density differences?
   a. 0.05%
   b. 0.5%
   c. 1%
   d. 1.5%
10. What is the tolerance limit for noise in a CT image?
    a. ±3
    b. ±5
    c. ±10
    d. ±15

CHAPTER 13

Quality Control for Magnetic Resonance Imaging Equipment

*Lorrie Kelley**

KEY TERMS

Center frequency
Geometric accuracy
High-contrast resolution
Image intensity uniformity
Low-contrast resolution
Signal-to-noise ratio
Slice position accuracy
Transmit gain

OBJECTIVES

At the completion of this chapter the reader will be able to do the following:

- Describe the various types of phantoms used in magnetic resonance (MR) scanners
- Understand the frequency of quality control testing of various MR parameters
- Describe the concept of signal-to-noise ratio
- Understand the concept of center frequency
- Perform quality control testing for center frequency, transmit gain, geometric accuracy, and high- and low-contrast resolution

OUTLINE

Phantoms
QC Testing Frequency
Weekly Tests
  Setup and Table Positioning Accuracy
  Center (Resonance) Frequency
  Transmit Gain (Attenuation)
  Geometric Accuracy (Three Axes)
  High-Contrast Resolution (Spatial Resolution)
  Low-Contrast Resolution (Detectability)
  Artifact Analysis
  Hard Copy Quality Control
  Visual Inspection
Annual Tests
  Magnetic Field Homogeneity
  Slice Position Accuracy
  Slice Thickness Accuracy
  RF Coils
  Signal-to-Noise Ratio
  Interslice RF Interference
  Soft-Copy Display Devices
Optional Tests
  Signal-to-Noise Ratio Consistency
  Magnetic Fringe Field
  Summary

Quality assurance procedures for magnetic resonance imaging (MRI) equipment are designed to establish a standard of measurement for daily system performance and the documentation of any variance thereof. Although the definition of *standard* varies from scanner to scanner, the goal of quality control (QC) is the detection of any changes or potential changes in the system performance. Documentation of daily QC measurements is considered an essential part of the MRI QC program and must be done properly. The ultimate goal is to maintain high image quality and patient safety.

MRI is a relatively new imaging modality that has seen tremendous growth and technologic advancements in recent years. The rapid proliferation of new and used magnetic resonance (MR) units in conjunction with the older units still in place has contributed to increasing variation in MRI quality across the country. In an effort to address those concerns and to establish a reasonable

---

*The author and publisher wish to acknowledge the previous edition's contributor.

standard of image quality, the American College of Radiology (ACR) developed an MRI Accreditation Program. The MRI Accreditation Program was designed to review the qualifications of the radiologists, MR scientists/medical physicists and technologists as well as the clinical image quality and effectiveness of QC testing procedures of each site applying for accreditation. In November 1996, the ACR approved the MRI Accreditation Program for implementation. More information about the MRI accreditation process can be obtained by contacting the ACR (*www.acr.org*). In the summer of 2008, Congress passed the Medicare Improvements for Patients and Providers Act of 2008, which mandates that any nonhospital institution performing advanced diagnostic services (such as MRI) must be accredited by a Centers for Medicare & Medicaid Services (CMS)—designated accrediting organization to receive federal funding (Medicare reimbursement). As of the writing of this edition, CMS has approved three national accreditation organizations: the ACR, the Intersocietal Accreditation Commission, and The Joint Commission. This rule affects providers of MRI, computed tomography, positron emission tomography, and nuclear medicine imaging services for Medicare beneficiaries on an outpatient basis. The accreditation applies only to the suppliers of the images and not to the physician's interpretation of the image. The CARE bill (discussed in Chapter 1), if passed, would make similar requirements for hospital-based facilities. Therefore, accreditation programs are becoming mandatory for MRI departments to succeed.

PHANTOMS

Typically, the phantoms for routine QC tests are provided by the manufacturer of the MR system. A user's manual and charts for documenting standardized tests also are provided. Use of the equipment can be easily taught to the technologists during the site installation. Specific actions for obtaining and documenting QC results vary among manufacturers.

Generally, QC phantoms are paramagnetic materials in an oil or water solution. Ions such as copper, aluminum, manganese, and nickel often are used. The materials used are designed to mimic biologic tissues or to shorten T1 relaxation times for strong MR signals. The relaxation rates vary with each material, main magnetic field strength (B_0), and temperature. Other considerations for materials are minimal chemical shifts and thermal and chemical stability. For the sake of the scan time, when QC tests are performed, the T1 repetition time (TR) of the phantom material should be compatible with a short TR, and the T2 TR should be long enough for any echo-time (TE) value that can be obtained. Fig. 13-1 demonstrates a copper sulfate phantom used daily at a clinical site.

QC phantoms are designed with various shapes, sizes, and geometric variables. The same type of phantom may

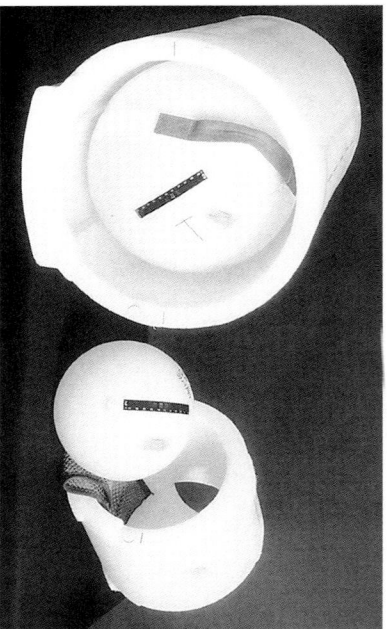

FIGURE 13-1 *Left,* Body coil phantom and holder. *Right,* Head coil phantom and holder.

be used for signal-to-noise ratio (SNR) and resonant frequency tests, whereas a different phantom is required for spatial resolution and linearity tests. Regardless of the type of test being performed, any QC phantom must be placed in the magnet at the isocenter, unless specified otherwise. The scanning parameters used (e.g., TR, TE, flip angle, slice thickness, matrix, and coil) should be documented.

The ACR MRI Accreditation Committee developed a specially designed MR phantom along with test protocols for use in establishing quality assurance programs for clinical MRI scanners. The ACR MRI Accreditation phantom is designed to examine several important instrument parameters within a single phantom, which means that each test can be accomplished in a reasonable amount of time. The phantom is a short, hollow cylinder constructed of acrylic plastic and is filled with a solution of nickel chloride and sodium chloride to simulate biologic tissue relaxation properties. Structures located within the phantom provide the tools necessary for quantitative assessment of seven important equipment performance parameters affecting image quality.

QC TESTING FREQUENCY

QC tests should be performed regularly by an MR technologist and/or service engineer under the supervision of a qualified MR scientist/medical physicist. Planning and preparing for the QC tests should be part of the site installation process. The ACR states that a qualified medical physicist must have the responsibility of overseeing the equipment QC program. The medical physicist, in conjunction with the service engineer, system manufacturer specialist, and site technologist, should discuss goals and potential outcomes for regular QC tests. It can then be decided which tests should be performed at certain intervals and by which personnel. Although all of the tests are important, not all are required at the same frequency. Testing can be thought of as monitoring essential fluids in a car: The windshield washer fluid may be checked infrequently, the oil checked more regularly, and the gasoline

CHAPTER 13 Quality Control for Magnetic Resonance Imaging Equipment

positioning, RF coil malfunctions, and improper use of image filters.

Typically, low-contrast resolution is expressed in one of two ways: the smallest diameter of an object with a specific contrast that can be detected or the smallest difference in signal intensity that can be discriminated for an object of a specific diameter. A phantom that contains objects of varying size and contrast should be selected. The ACR MRI Accreditation phantom consists of three rows of low-contrast objects that radiate from the center in a circular arrangement. Each row contains 10 holes of varying diameters (from 7 to 1.5 millimeter). Slices acquired from four locations within the phantom provide contrast values of 1.4%, 2.5%, 3.6%, and 5.1%.

PROCEDURE

1. When using the ACR phantom, measurements for this test are made by counting the number of complete spokes seen in each of the images.
2. Use slices 8–11 from the ACR phantom test series.
3. Starting with slice 11, adjust the window width and level display settings for best visibility of the objects (typically a narrow window width; Fig. 13-8).
4. Begin counting the number of complete spokes starting with the spokes with the largest diameter disks (positioned at 12 o'clock or just slightly to the right of 12 o'clock). Count clockwise from spoke 1 until a spoke is reached where one or more of the disks is not distinguishable from the background. The number of complete spokes counted is the score for the slice. Repeat the counting procedure with slices 8–10.
5. MR systems with field strengths less than 3 T should have a total score of at least nine spokes for each ACR series, and there should be a score of 37 spokes for MR systems with field strengths of 3 T.

Note: A spoke can only be counted as complete if all three of its disks are discernible.

According to the action limits of the ACR, an MR scanner with a field strength less than 3 T should be able to display nine spokes of holes from the low-contrast inserts and 3 T MR systems should be able to display 37 spokes. The ACR requires that an MR scanner pass on both of the ACR T1 and T2 series or on both of the site's T1 and T2 series.

Artifact Analysis

Various artifacts can occur during the routine QC testing procedures. Artifacts can vary according to imaging conditions, pulse sequence parameters, choice of RF coils, and with individual patients. The presence of artifacts can be an early indication of equipment failure. The MR technologist should become familiar with the common appearances of artifacts that are due to particular subsystems of the MR scanner. These include the RF system, gradient system, image and data processing, and magnetic field homogeneity.

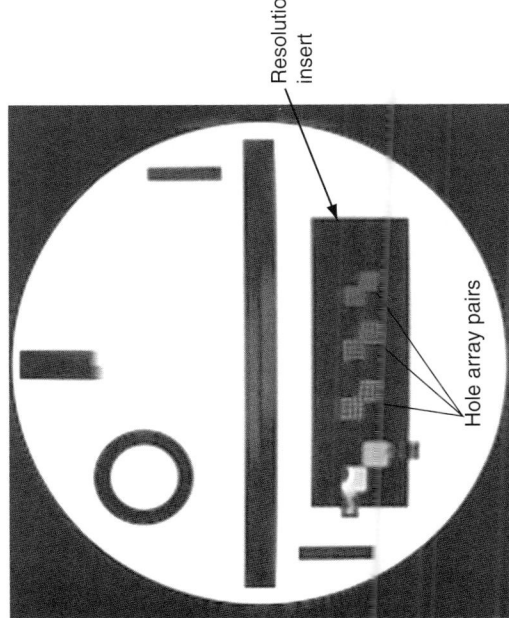

FIGURE 13-6 Slice 1 from American College of Radiology T2 series demonstrating resolution insert and hole array pairs. (*Courtesy St. Luke's Health System.*)

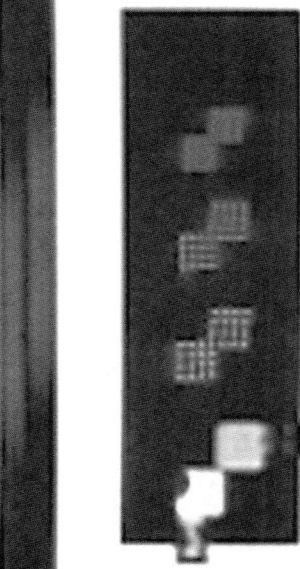

FIGURE 13-7 Magnified portion of slice 1 displayed for visual assessment of high-contrast resolution. (*Courtesy St. Luke's Health System.*)

The ACR standard is a measurement of 1 millimeter or better in both directions.

Although resolution is traditionally known as *lines pairs per millimeter*, here it is determined by the pixel size and what the human eye can resolve on the image. Resolution is determined by the smallest array element (e.g., a bar, rod) visible that is completely separated by distance from the adjacent element. The calculated pixel size is then compared with the smallest resolvable element.

This QC test may be routinely performed by the site engineer during the preventive maintenance of the system. This test is likely to fail in conjunction with the failure of the geometric accuracy test. The gradient amplitude, the gradient duty cycle, and reconstruction filters can easily affect the spatial resolution.

Low-Contrast Resolution (Detectability)

Low-contrast resolution is a measure of the MR system's ability to differentiate between adjacent tissues having minimal differences in signal intensities. Several factors can influence low-contrast resolution, including increased noise, ghosting artifacts, improper phantom

the gray scale between the monitor and hard copy is with a Society of Motion Picture and Television Engineers (SMPTE) test pattern.

ACR control limits for the SMPTE test pattern:

SMPTE Test Pattern	Control Limits
0	±0.15
10%	±0.15
40%	±0.15
90%	±0.8

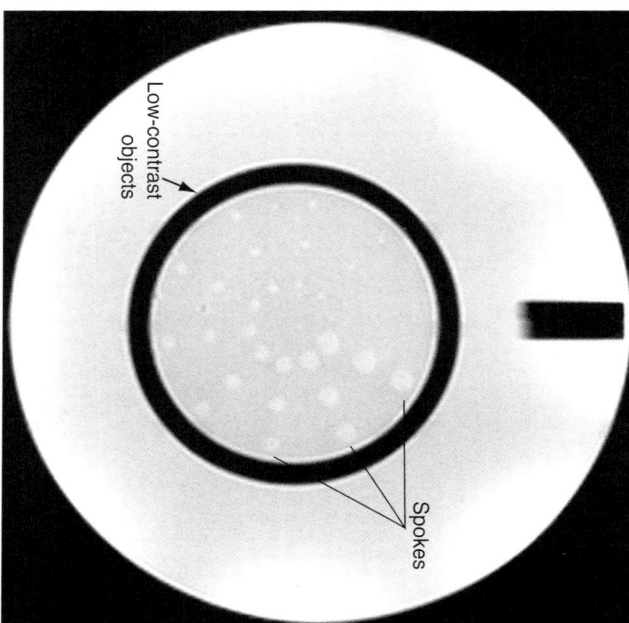

FIGURE 13-8 Slice 2 of American College of Radiology T1 series with the circle of low-contrast objects displayed. (*Courtesy St. Luke's Health System.*)

During each QC test, the MR technologist should be evaluating each image for signs of ghosting, geometric distortion, discrepancies in signal intensities, and any other interference with the known parameters of the image. The ACR requirement for assessment of image artifacts follows the following procedure:

1. Use the image slices from the ACR T1-weighted slices.
2. Adjust the display window width and window level to show the full range of pixel values for each image.
3. On each image validate the following: the phantom appears circular and is not distorted, there are no ghost images of the phantom, there are no streaks or spots, and there are no abnormal or new elements in the image.

Hard Copy Quality Control

Any digital modality is challenged to provide hard-copy images that match the gray-scale display of the system's monitor. One way to verify accurate representation of

PROCEDURE

1. Display SMPTE test pattern on the console's monitor. Be sure to use the manufacturer-specified window width and level for display settings.
2. Verify that 0/5% and 95/100% gray-level patches are visible and note any artifacts.
3. Film the SMPTE test pattern using a 6-on-1 format.
4. Use a film densitometer to plot the optical density of the 10%, 40%, and 90% gray-level patches.
5. Plot the optical densities on a QC chart (Box 13-2) and circle any points that fall outside the control limits.

Visual Inspection

The visual inspection is a method to quantitatively and qualitatively verify that all equipment is available and working properly. The inspection can be scanner specific depending on the use of the equipment. Items that are typically included in a visual inspection are the patient table smoothness of motion and stability, alignment lights, high tension cable/other cable integrity, monitors, RF door contacts, RF window-screen integrity, operator console switches/lights/meters, patient monitors, patient intercom, and room temperature and relative humidity. The visual inspection checklist should also include a section on facility safety that would include the emergency cart, safety warning signage, door indicator switch (if installed), cryogen level indicator, and oxygen monitor. Items that are missing or malfunctioning should be repaired or replaced as soon as possible. A visual inspection checklist can be provided by the equipment manufacturer or the facility's accreditation agency. Box 13-3 contains the ACR visual checklist form.

ANNUAL TESTS

As stated previously, all QC measurements are considered essential for overall system performance. Box 13-4 lists abbreviated definitions of tests that should be performed by a medical physicist or system engineer. These tests should be performed on a regular schedule and also whenever there are changes to the site scanner and environment such as hardware and software upgrades, magnet quench, or facility construction. The ACR requires that the following tests be performed on an annual basis to meet the ACR MRI Accreditation Standard. The ACR Form to document the results of the annual tests is found in Box 13-5.

Magnetic Field Homogeneity

The homogeneity of a system's magnetic field is an indication of the quality or uniformity of its field. Homogeneity is usually expressed in parts per million within a given spherical volume. A spherical volume is given as the diameter of a spherical volume (DSV). MRI system manufacturers provide specifications for their magnets, and values obtained from QC tests should be compared with those specified. The medical physicist can choose

CHAPTER 13 Quality Control for Magnetic Resonance Imaging Equipment

BOX 13-2 | ACR Laser Film Printer Control Chart

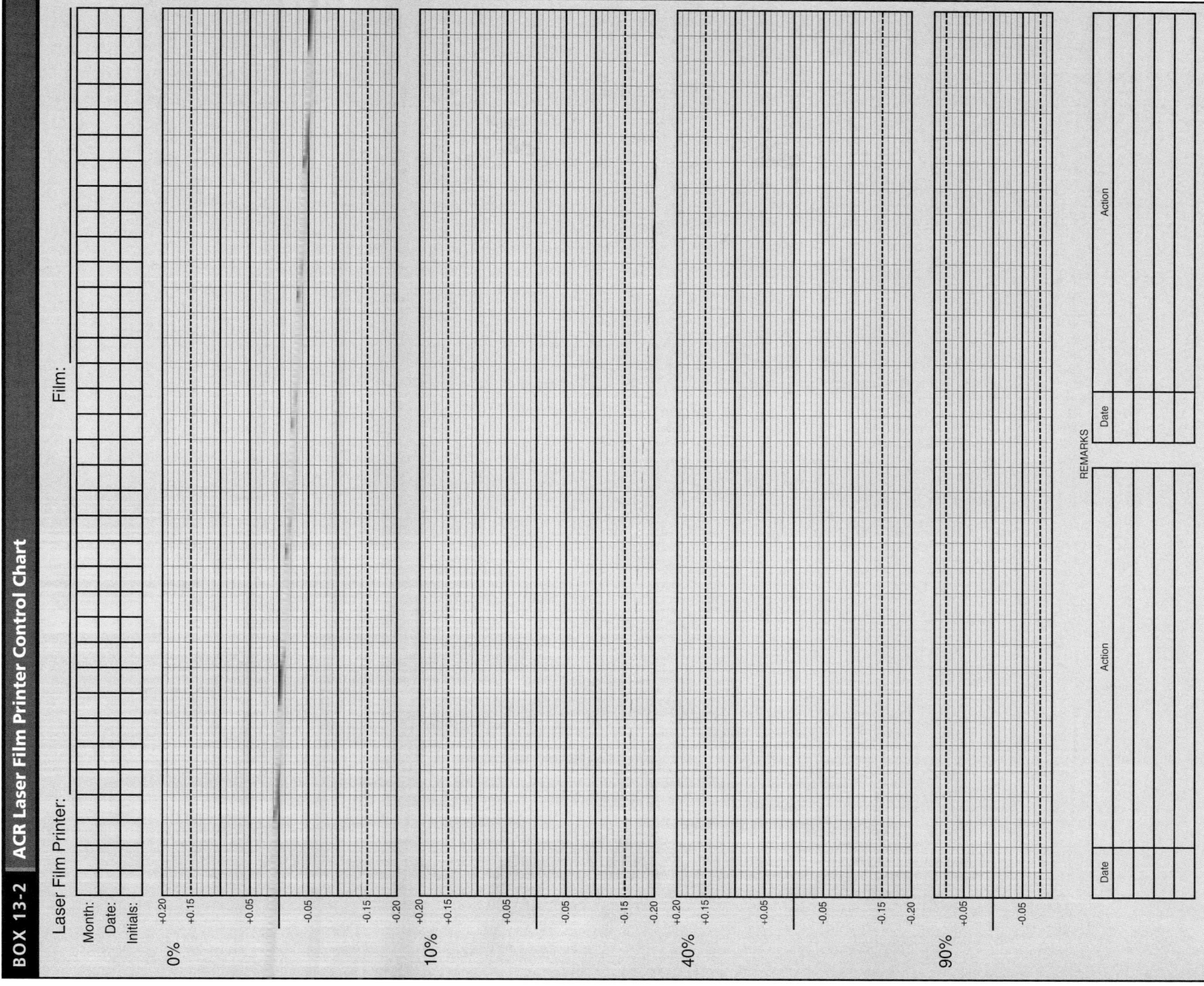

BOX 13-3 ACR MRI Facility Quality Control Visual Checklist

MRI FACILITY QUALITY CONTROL VISUAL CHECKLIST

MR Facility Name _____   MR Scanner Identifier _____

Category	Item	Date
Patient Transport & Magnet	Bed position and other lights	
	Alignment light	
	High tension cable/other cables	
	Horizontal smoothness of motion and stability	
	Vertical motion smoothness and stability	
Filming and Viewing	Laser Camera (cables, cassettes, lights)	
	Light Boxes (improper function)	
RF Integrity and Control Room	RF door contacts	
	RF window-screen integrity	
	Operator console switches/lights/meters	
	Patient monitors	
	Patient intercom	
	Room temperature/Room humidity	
Facility Safety	Emergency cart	
	Safety warning signage	
	Door indicator switch (if installed)	
	Cryogen level indicator	
	Oxygen monitor	
	Pass = ✓ Fail = F Does not apply = NA	Technologist's Initials

Reviewed by: _____   _____
Qualified Medical Physicist/MRI Scientist   Date of Review

CHAPTER 13 Quality Control for Magnetic Resonance Imaging Equipment

BOX 13-4 | Quality Control Tests Performed by a Medical Physicist or System Engineer

Receiver Gain (Attenuation): The receiver setting is the amount by which MR signals are amplified before digitization.

Transmitter Setting: The transmitter setting is a number expressed in decibels that influences the flip angle of each RF pulse.

Coil Q: Known as the quality factor, coil Q describes the performance of a coil used to receive MR signals.

Ghost Intensity: Ghost intensity is an expression of the intensity of background ghosts relative to the intensity of a phantom.

RF Shielding Effectiveness: The RF shielding effectiveness test verifies that the RF shield is attenuating radiowaves originating from outside the scan room.

Surface Coil Performance: For the surface coil performance to be checked, a separate test is done on each surface coil to determine the SNR and image uniformity.

Slice Thickness: Slice thickness is the FWHM of a slice profile, the region from which MR signals are emitted.

Maximum Gradient Strength: The maximum gradient strength determines if gradients are still achieving the maximum amplitude specified by the manufacturer and originally measured.

Specific Absorption Rate Monitor: The SAR monitor verifies that the imaging procedures do not cause excessive RF power to be deposited into a patient.

FWHM, Full width at half maximum; *MR,* magnetic resonance; *RF,* radio frequency; *SAR,* specific absorption rate; *SNR,* signal-to-noise ratio.

PROCEDURE

1. Use slices 1 and 11 of the ACR T1 and T2 phantom test series and magnify the images by a factor of 2 to 4, making sure to keep the vertical bars of the crossed wedges within the displayed image (Figs. 13-9 and 13-10).
2. Using a fairly narrow display window width, measure the difference in length between the left and right bars of the crossed wedges in each image.

Note: Because the crossed wedges have a 45° slope, the measured bar length difference is really twice the actual slice displacement, meaning that if the measurement of the bar length difference is 6.0 mm, the slice is displaced superiorly by 3.0 mm (Fig. 13-11).

The ACR MR Accreditation phantom uses crossed wedges from slices 1 and 11 as a reference. On slices 1 and 11, the crossed wedges appear as a pair of dark bars at the top of the phantom. The ACR criterion is that the absolute bar length difference should be equal to or less than 5 millimeter.

Slice Thickness Accuracy

Slice thickness is an important image-quality parameter. The accuracy of slice thickness is especially important for stereotactic and interventional procedures. The thickness of each slice is determined by both the transmit RF bandwidth and the amplitude of the slice select gradient. Factors that influence slice thickness include gradient calibration and the RF pulse profile. Inaccuracies in slice thickness can cause interslice interference (crosstalk) in multislice acquisitions and can alter the validity of SNR measurements in all pulse sequences. When the ACR MRI Accreditation phantom is used to perform this test, the lengths of two signal ramps located within the slice thickness insert in slice 1 are measured. To meet the ACR criteria, the measured slice thickness should be 5.0 mm ± 0.7 mm.

PROCEDURE

1. Use slice 1 of the ACR T1 and T2 phantom test series and magnify the images by a factor of 2 to 4, making sure the keep the slice thickness insert visible within the displayed image (Fig. 13-12).
2. Display the images with a narrow window level and window width to provide optimal visualization of the signal ramps.
3. Place a rectangular region of interest (ROI) at the middle of each signal ramp and note the mean signal values for both ROIs, then average the two values together (Fig. 13-13).
4. Lower the window level of the display to half of the average of the ramp signal calculated in step 3.
5. Measure the length of the top and bottom ramps and record their lengths (Fig. 13-14).

Note: The following formula is used to calculate slice thickness:

$$\text{slice thickness} = 0.2 \times (\text{top} \times \text{bottom}) / (\text{top} + \text{bottom})$$

from a couple of methods for measuring the magnetic field homogeneity. The spectral peak method uses a uniform, spherical phantom to measure the full width at half maximum of the spectral peak over the imaging volume. The other method uses a phase difference map to calculate the magnetic field inhomogeneity. Using phase-contrast images, a medical physicist can calculate the change in phase across images acquired from a uniformity phantom as proportional to the inhomogeneity of the magnetic field. For a superconducting magnet, typical values are 2 ppm over a 30- to 40-cm DSV. For MR systems with spectroscopy capabilities, the suggested value is less than or equal to 0.5 ppm at 35 cm DSV.

Poor homogeneity can result in poor image quality and artifacts. Changes in homogeneity can be due to ferromagnetic objects located within the bore of the magnet and external ferromagnetic structures that may be neighboring the magnetic field. Sometimes magnetic inhomogeneities can be improved with gradient adjustments or shimming.

Slice Position Accuracy

The slice position test is performed to ensure that the land-marking location is actually centered to the magnet bore. Misalignment can simply be due to mechanical problems with the table, positioning devices, or alignment light beams. Other causes of poor performance include operator error, gradient miscalibration, magnetic field inhomogeneities, and table positioning shift.

BOX 13-5 MRI Equipment Performance Evaluation Form

MRI Equipment Performance Evaluation Data Form

Site: _____ Date: _____

MRAP Number: _____ Serial Number: _____

Equipment:

MRI System Manufacturer: _____ Model: _____

Film Processor Manufacturer: _____ Model: _____

PACS Manufacturer: _____ Model: _____

ACR MRAP Phantom Number used: _____

1. Magnetic Field Homogeneity

Method Used (check one): ____ Spectral Peak ____ Phase Difference

____ Other (describe) _____

Measured Homogeneity: Diameter of Spherical Volume (cm) _____ Homogeneity (ppm) _____

2. Slice Position Accuracy

From Slice Positions #1 and #11 of the ACR Phantom:

Wedge (mm)

```
  =  -
  =  +
```

Slice Location #1 _____
Slice Location #11 _____

3. Slice Thickness Accuracy

From Slice Position #1 of the ACR Phantom:

Slice Thickness (fwhm in mm)   Top: _____   Bottom: _____   Calculated slice Thickness (mm): _____

4. RF Coil Performance Evaluation

A. Volume RF Coil—

RF coil description: _____ Date: _____

Phantom description: _____

Pulse sequence: _____ Type: _____ TR: _____ TE: _____ flip angle: _____ degrees

FOV: _____ cm² Matrix: _____ BW: _____ kHz; NSA: _____

Slice thickness: _____ mm; spacing: _____ mm

TX attenuation (or gain): _____

Data Collected:

Mean Signal	Maximum Signal	Minimum Signal	Background Signal	Noise Standard Deviation	Ghost Signal

Calculated Values: Max − Min = _____ ; Max + Min = _____

Signal-to-Noise Ratio	Percent Image Uniformity	Percent Signal Ghosting

B. Volume RF Coil—

RF coil description: _____

Phantom description: _____

Pulse sequence: _____ Type: _____ TR: _____ TE: _____ FOV: _____ cm²

Orientation: _____ Matrix: _____ BW: _____ kHz; NSA: _____

Slice thickness: _____ mm; spacing: _____ mm

Flip angle: _____ degrees TX attenuation (or gain): _____

BOX 13-5 MRI Equipment Performance Evaluation Form—cont'd

Maximum Signal	Noise Standard Deviation	Maximum Signal-to-Noise Ratio

Image uniformity distribution OK? _____
Image ghosting OK? _____
HARD COPY IMAGE: WINDOW WIDTH: _____ Window level: _____

5. Inter-slice RF Evaluation

Phantom description: _____
Pulse sequence: Type: _____ TR: _____ TE: _____ FOV: _____ cm^2
Matrix: _____ BW: _____ kHz, NCA: _____
Number of slices: _____ Flip angle: _____ degrees

Series Number	Slice Gap mm	Signal-to-Noise Ratio
1		
2		
3		
4		

Measured SNR: 100%, 90%, 80%, 70%
Inter-slice Gap (percent of slice thickness): 0, 25%, 50%, 75%, 100%

6. Soft Copy Displays

Luminance Meter Make/Model: _____ Cal expires: _____
Monitor Description: _____
Luminance measured: Cd m^{-2} _____ Ft. lamberts _____ (Circle correct units)

Monitor Description	Center of Image Display	Top Left Corner	Top Right Corner	Bottom Right Corner	Bottom Left Corner
Console					

Luminance Uniformity:
Average of values obtained in four corners of screen: _____ Cd m^{-2}
Percent difference: _____ %

$$\% \text{ difference} = 200 * (L_{max} - L_{min}) / (L_{max} + L_{min})$$

7. Evaluation of Site's Technologist QC Program

1. Set up and positioning accuracy: (weekly)
2. Center frequency: (weekly)
3. Transmitter attenuation or gain: (weekly)
4. Geometric accuracy measurements: (weekly)
5. Spatial resolution measurements: (weekly)
6. Low-contrast detectability: (weekly)
7. Film quality control: (weekly)
8. Visual checklist: (weekly)

SPECIFIC COMMENTS:
_____
_____
_____
_____

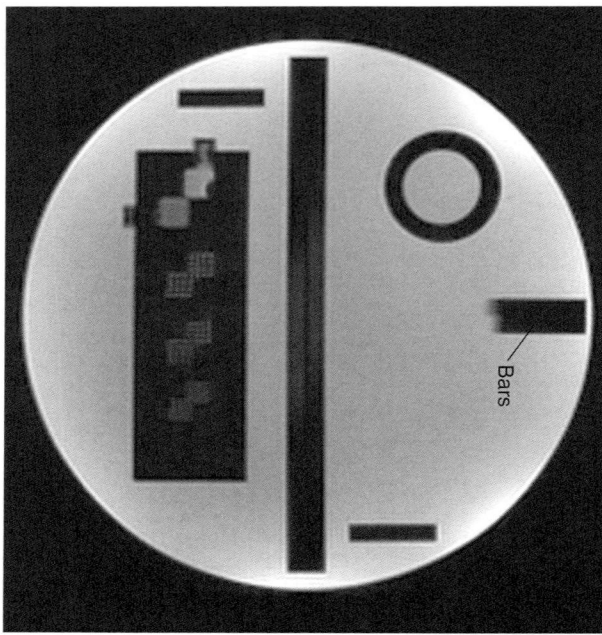

FIGURE 13-9 Slice 1 of American College of Radiology T1 series with pair of dark vertical bars from the 45° crossed wedges indicated. (*Courtesy St. Luke's Health System.*)

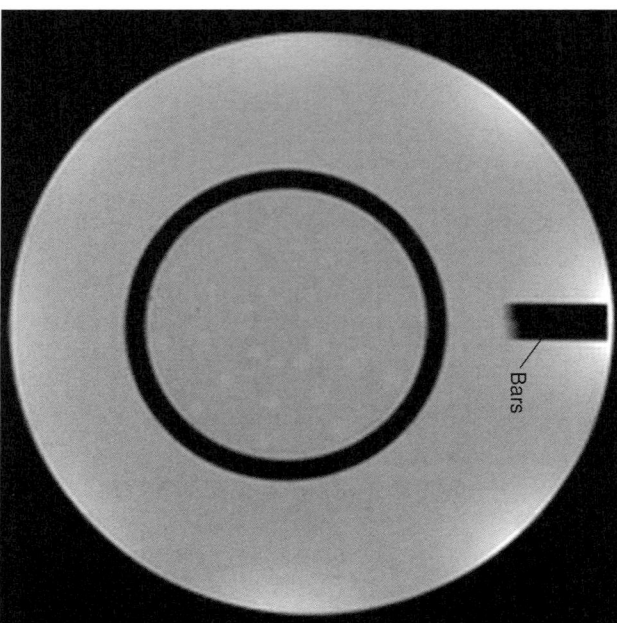

FIGURE 13-10 Slice 2 of American College of Radiology T1 series with pair of dark vertical bars from the 45° crossed wedges indicated. (*Courtesy St. Luke's Health System.*)

FIGURE 13-11 Magnified portion of slice 1 showing measurement for slice position error. The arrows indicate the difference in bar length. (*Courtesy St. Luke's Health System.*)

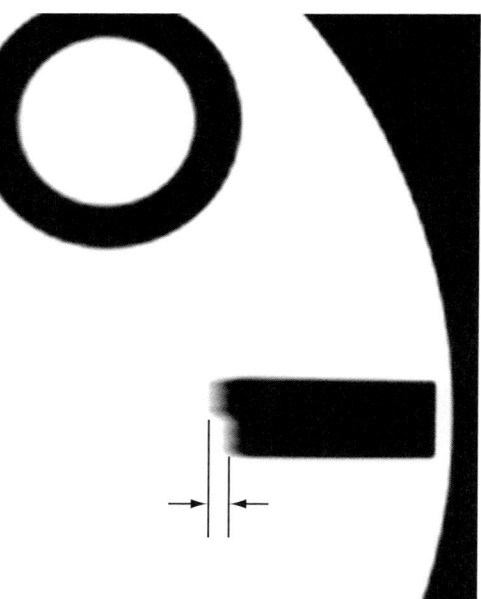

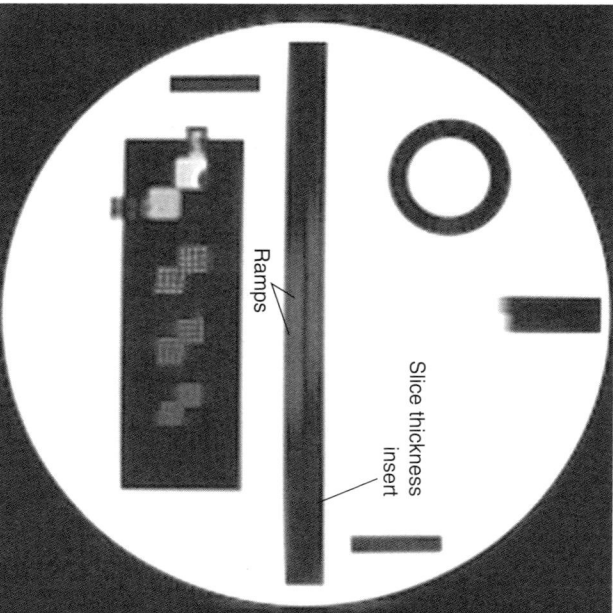

FIGURE 13-12 Slice 1 from American College of Radiology T2 series demonstrating the slice thickness insert and signal ramps. (*Courtesy St. Luke's Health System.*)

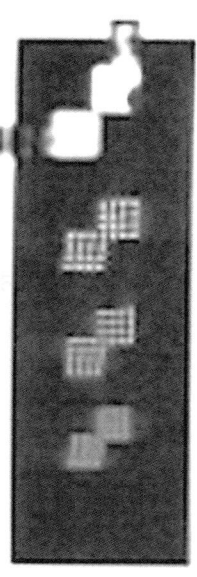

FIGURE 13-13 Magnified portion of slice 1 showing placement for rectangular regions of interest to measure average signal in the ramps. (*Courtesy St. Luke's Health System.*)

RF Coils (Fig. 13-15)

The performance of the RF coils used to generate MR images is critical to the overall performance of the MR system as a whole. Currently, the ACR requires three different measurements for volume coils and one measurement for surface coils. The QC tests required for volume coils provide measurements of image uniformity, SNR, and percent signal ghosting (PSG). The QC test used for surface coils measures only the maximum SNR.

CHAPTER 14

Ultrasound Equipment Quality Assurance

James A. Zagzebski*, James M. Kofler, Jr.*

KEY TERMS

Axial resolution
Depth of visualization
Horizontal distance measurement
Lateral resolution

Phantom
Scan image uniformity
Sensitivity
Slice thickness

String test
Vertical distance measurement

OBJECTIVES

At the completion of this chapter, the reader will be able to do the following:

- Discuss the importance of quality assurance for ultrasound equipment
- Describe the various phantoms used in ultrasound quality assurance
- Identify the basic quality control tests for ultrasound
- Explain the importance of documentation of quality assurance testing
- Describe the basic quality control testing for Doppler color flow equipment

OUTLINE

Components of an Ultrasound Quality Assurance Program
Quality Assurance and Preventive Maintenance
Tissue-Mimicking Phantoms
Tissue Properties Represented in Phantoms
Typical Quality Assurance Phantom Design
Cautions about Phantom Desiccation
Basic Quality Control Tests
Visual Inspection
Transducer Choice
System Sensitivity

Photography and Gray-Scale Hard Copy
Monitor Setup and Recording Devices
Routine Quality Assurance of Image Recording
Scan Image Uniformity
Distance Measurement Accuracy
Vertical Distance Measurements
Horizontal Distance Measurements
Other Important Instrument Quality Assurance Tasks
Documentation

Spatial Resolution Tests
Axial Resolution
Lateral Resolution
Cautions about Resolution Tests with Discrete Targets
Other Test Objects and Phantoms
Anechoic Voids
Objects of Various Echogenicity
Spherical Object Phantom
Doppler Testing
String Test Objects
Doppler Flow Phantoms
Electronic Probe Tests

---

*The author and publisher wish to acknowledge the previous edition's contributor.

COMPONENTS OF AN ULTRASOUND QUALITY ASSURANCE PROGRAM

In an imaging facility, quality assurance is a process carried out to ensure that equipment is operating consistently at its expected level of performance. During routine ultrasound imaging, each sonographer is vigilant for equipment changes that can lead to suboptimal imaging and might require service. Thus, in some ways, ultrasound equipment quality assurance is carried out every day, even when it is not identified as a process itself.

Quality assurance steps to be discussed here go beyond judgments of scanner performance that are made during routine ultrasound imaging. They involve prospective actions to identify problem situations, even before obvious equipment malfunctions occur. Quality assurance testing provides confidence that image data such as distance measurements and area estimations are accurate and that the image is of the best possible quality from the imaging instrument.

Quality Assurance and Preventive Maintenance

Various approaches are used by ultrasound facilities when setting up a quality assurance program for their scanners. Sometimes these programs include both preventive maintenance procedures performed by trained equipment service personnel and in-house testing of scanners with phantoms and test objects. Some facilities rely on only one of these measures. For preventive maintenance, emphasis is usually given to invasive electronic testing of system components such as voltage measurements at test points inside the scanner. Sometimes, preventive maintenance also involves an assessment of the imaging capability by scanning a phantom.

In-house scanner quality assurance programs usually involve imaging phantoms or test objects and assessing the results. In-house tests may be performed by sonographers, physicians, medical physicists, clinical engineers, or equipment maintenance personnel. Detailed recommendations from professional organizations and experts in ultrasound on establishing an in-house quality assurance program are available elsewhere (ACR Ultrasound Accreditation Program, 2012; Goodsitt et al., 1998; Zagzebski, 2000).

Tissue-Mimicking Phantoms

In-house scanner quality assurance tests most often are performed with tissue-mimicking phantoms. In medical ultrasound, a **phantom** is a device that mimics soft tissues in its ultrasound transmission characteristics. Phantoms represent 'constant patients,' and images can be taken at different times for close comparison. Image penetration capabilities, for example, are readily evaluated for changes over time when images of a phantom are available for comparison. Phantoms also have targets in known positions, so images can be compared closely with the region that is scanned. Examples include simulated cysts, echogenic structures, and thin 'line targets.'

Tissue Properties Represented in Phantoms

Tissue characteristics mimicked in commercially available phantoms are the speed of sound (speed of sound in phantom material is the same as that of human soft tissue, 1540 m/s); ultrasonic attenuation; and, to some degree, echogenicity (i.e., the ultrasonic scattering level). Phantoms cannot exactly replicate the acoustic properties of soft tissues. This is partially because of the complexity and variability of tissues. Instead, phantom manufacturers construct these objects to have acoustic properties that represent the average properties of many different tissues. Sometimes the term *tissue-equivalent* is used when phantoms are described; however, this term should not be interpreted literally because most phantom materials are not acoustically equivalent to any specific tissue.

Typical Quality Assurance Phantom Design

An example of a general purpose ultrasound quality assurance phantom is shown in Fig. 14-1. Such phantoms are examined with scanner settings that are similar to those used when patients are being scanned. The phantom images have gray-scale characteristics that are analogous to characteristics of organs, although the actual structures are not anatomically represented.

Fig. 14-1B shows the internal structure of this phantom. The tissue-mimicking material within the phantom consists of a water-based gelatin in which microscopic particles are mixed uniformly throughout the volume (Burlew et al., 1980; Madsen et al., 1978). The speed of sound in this material is about 1540 m/sec, the same speed assumed in the calibration of ultrasound instruments. The ultrasonic attenuation coefficient versus frequency is one of two values: either 0.5 or 0.7 dB/cm per megahertz (Box 14-1). Some users prefer the lower attenuating material because they find it easier to image objects in the phantom. However, standards groups recommend the higher attenuation because it challenges machines more thoroughly (Zagzebski, 2000).

Attenuation in the gel-graphite material in the phantom is proportional to the ultrasound frequency and mimics the behavior in tissues (Lu et al., 1999; Madsen et al., 1978; Maklad et al., 1984). Other types of materials have been used in phantoms, but only water-based gels laced with powder have both speed of sound and attenuation with tissue-like properties (Madsen et al., 1978; Zagzebski, 2000).

Small scatterers are distributed throughout the tissue-mimicking material; therefore, the phantoms appear echogenic when scanned with ultrasound imaging equipment (see Fig. 14-1C). Many phantoms have simulated

CHAPTER 14 Ultrasound Equipment Quality Assurance

evaluating the distance measurement accuracy of a scanner. Tests of the accuracy of distance measurements rely on the manufacturer of the phantom to have filled the device with a material with a sound propagation speed of 1540 m/sec or at least close enough to this speed that no appreciable errors are introduced in calibrations. These phantoms also rely on the manufacturer having defined the reflector positions accurately. With the correct speed of sound (1540 m/sec) and precisely known distances between point-like reflectors, it is easy to check the accuracy of distance measurements with calipers, as described later.

Phantoms often contain a column of reflectors, each separated by 1 or 2 cm, for vertical measurement accuracy tests. One or more horizontal rows of reflectors are used for assessing horizontal measurement accuracy. Additional sets of reflectors may be found for assessing the axial resolution and the lateral resolution of scanners.

Cautions about Phantom Desiccation

When a phantom made of water-based gels is used, loss of water (desiccation) may become a problem as the phantom ages. If this occurs, the speed of sound in the

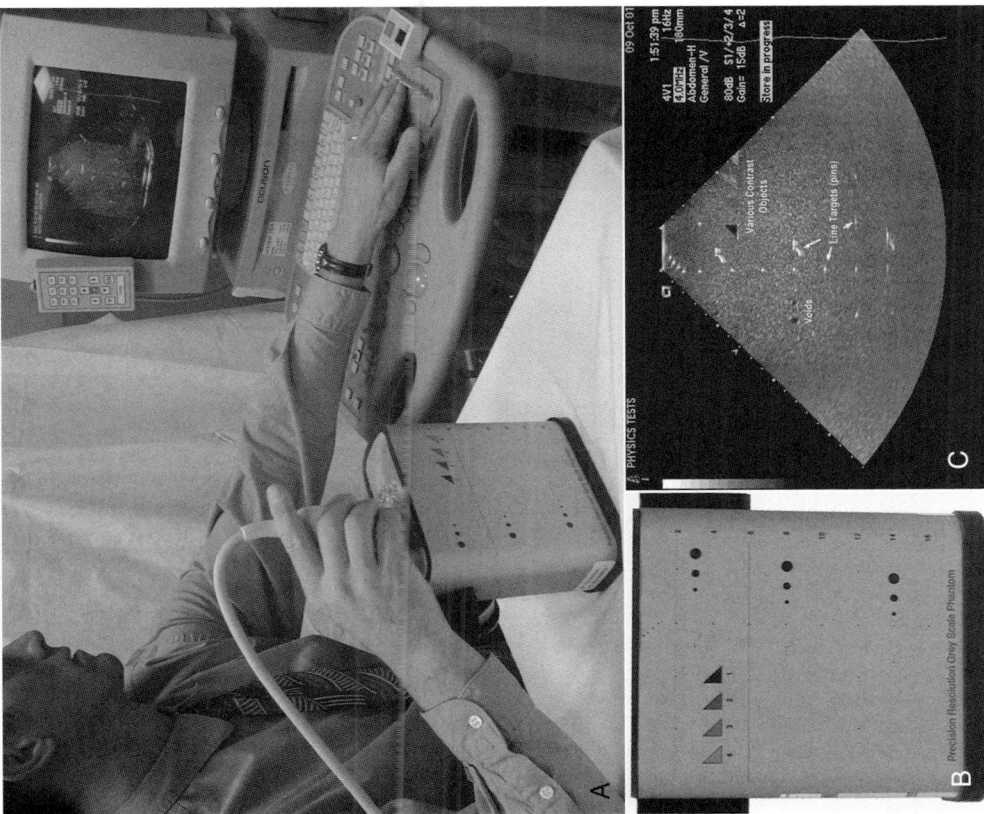

FIGURE 14-1 Example of a general-purpose quality assurance phantom. **A**, Phantom being imaged with an ultrasound scanner. **B**, Close-up of phantom, with diagram of interior contents. **C**, B-mode image of the phantom.

BOX 14-1 Tissue Attenuation Coefficients

Attenuation coefficients are normally specified in decibels per centimeter. To include the dependence of attenuation on frequency, phantom manufacturers divide the attenuation coefficient by the frequency at which the measurement is done. This yields units of decibels per centimeter per megahertz. Strictly speaking, this approach should be used only when attenuation is directly proportional to the frequency, as we often assume for tissues. The value of 0.7 dB/cm per megahertz is representative of the attenuation coefficient in difficult-to-penetrate fatty liver. The depth that structures can be visualized within tissue-mimicking material having this amount of attenuation more closely correlates with clinical penetration.

From Lu ZF, Lee FT, Zagzebski JA: Ultrasonic backscatter and attenuation in diffuse liver disease, *Ultrasound Med Biol* 25:1047, 1999.

'cysts,' which are low-attenuating, nonechogenic cylinders. These should appear echo free on B-mode images and should exhibit distal echo enhancement. Some tissue phantoms provide additional image contrast by having simulated masses or test objects of varying echogenicity. Such objects are evident in Fig. 14-1C.

Most quality assurance phantoms also contain discrete reflectors such as nylon-line targets to be used mainly for

BASIC QUALITY CONTROL TESTS

A recommended set of instrument quality control tests includes checks for the consistency of instrument sensitivity; evaluation of image uniformity; assessment of gray-scale photography or image workstation brightness levels; and, where necessary, checks of both vertical and horizontal distance measurement accuracy (ACR Ultrasound Accreditation Program, 2001; Goodsitt et al., 1998; Zagzebski, 2000). This group of tests can be performed by a sonographer in 10–15 min, which includes the time for recording the results on a worksheet or in a notebook.

Visual Inspection

The visual inspection is used to evaluate the physical condition of the scanner's mechanical components, along with a few quick scan tests. This should be performed monthly or according to the user manual provided by the manufacturer. A checklist for documentation of the visual inspection is found on the enclosed CD-ROM. Some of the items to check during the visual inspection are described as follows:

Transducers: Cables, housings, and transmitting surfaces should be checked for cracks, separations, delamination, and discolorations. Any bent or loose prongs on the plug should be fixed. Also verify that the transducers are cleaned after each use.

Power cord: The cable and plug should be checked for any fraying, cracks, discoloration, and damage.

Control panel: Check for dirty or broken switches and knobs as well as any burnt-out indicator lights.

Video monitor: The video display monitor should be clean and free of scratches. The brightness and contrast controls should be set at proper levels.

Wheels and wheel locks: All wheels should be checked to ensure that they rotate freely and that the unit is easy to maneuver. The wheels also should be seated securely, and wheel locks should be checked to ensure they lock securely.

Dust filters: Dust filters should be inspected and free of lint and clumps of dirt. Otherwise, overheating of the internal electronic components can occur and shorten the life span of the unit.

Scanner housing: The unit should be inspected for dents or other 'cosmetic' damage, which could indicate events that might have caused damage to the internal components.

Transducer Choice

Results of some test procedures depend on which transducer/frequency combination is used with the instrument. On systems in which several transducers are available, tests should be done with two transducers (ACR Ultrasound Accreditation Program, 2012). Choose the most common transducer used in most examinations; additionally, it is preferable to test another transducer that has a different frequency range and a different scan format. For example, with a general purpose scanner, a low-frequency (2–5 MHz) curvilinear or phased array, and an intermediate-frequency (5–8 MHz) or even a high-frequency linear array are appropriate. This transducer combination should be used for all subsequent test procedures. All necessary transducer assembly identification information should be checked including the frequency, size, and serial number so that future tests will be conducted with the same probe. If several identical scanners are available,

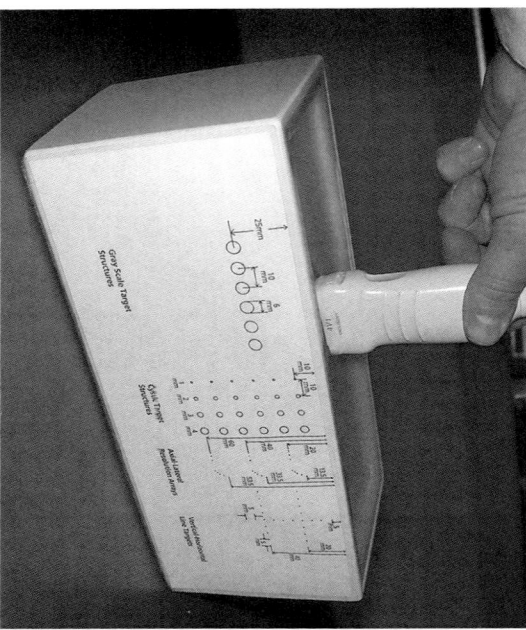

FIGURE 14-2 A phantom with rubber-based, tissue-mimicking small parts. Although the acoustic properties are not as precise as the water-based phantoms, less care is required during manufacturing and with on-site storage to minimize changes over time.

phantom may have changed. A scanning surface that has become concave is an indication of severe desiccation. Occasionally, water losses become so problematic that air entering the phantom window leads to the inability to image the phantom effectively. Users should follow the instructions given by the phantom manufacturer to avoid significant desiccation. For example, some manufacturers recommend storage in a humid, airtight container, and this practice should be adhered to if so stated.

Desiccation is not a problem with rubber-based phantom materials (Fig. 14-2) produced by some manufacturers. Storing these phantoms with the tissue-mimicking material directly exposed to the environment can be an advantage compared with water-based gels. The main disadvantages of rubber materials are that their speed of sound is lower than 1540 m/sec (≈1450 m/sec in some rubber-based phantoms) and that their attenuation is not proportional to the ultrasound frequency (Zagzebski, 2000). Therefore, they may not be as effective as water-based gel phantoms when imaging over a large frequency range.

CHAPTER 14 Ultrasound Equipment Quality Assurance

the same transducer/scanner pairs should be used for all subsequent testing.

System Sensitivity

The **sensitivity** of an instrument refers to the weakest echo signal level that can be detected and displayed clearly enough to be discernible on an image. Most scanners have controls that vary the receiver amplification (gain) and the transmit level (e.g., output or power). These are used to adjust the sensitivity during clinical examinations. The *maximum sensitivity* of the instrument occurs when these controls are at maximum practical settings. Often the maximum sensitivity is limited by electrical noise that appears on the display when the receiver gain is at maximum levels. The noise may be generated externally, for example, by electronic communication networks or by computer terminals. More commonly, the noise arises from within the instrument itself, such as in the first preamplification stage of the receiver amplifier.

Concerns during quality assurance tests are usually centered on whether notable variations in sensitivity have occurred since the last quality assurance test. Such variations might result from a variety of causes such as damaged transducers, damaged transducer cables, or electronic drift in the pulser-receiver components of the scanner. Questions related to the sensitivity of a scanner sometimes occur during clinical imaging; a quick scan of the quality assurance phantom and comparison with results of the most recent quality assurance test help determine whether there is cause for concern.

A commonly used technique for detecting variations in maximum sensitivity is the measure of the maximum **depth of visualization** for signals from scattered echoes in the tissue-mimicking phantom (ACR Ultrasound Accreditation Program, 2012; AIUM standard methods for measuring performance of ultrasound pulse-echo equipment, 1990; Carson and Goodsitt, 1995; Goodsitt et al., 1998; Zagzebski, 2000). The technique includes the following:

1. Adjust the output power transmit levels and receiver sensitivity controls so that echo signals are obtained from as deep as possible into the phantom. Now the output power control is positioned for maximum output, and the receiver gain is adjusted for the highest values without excessive noise on the display. (Experience helps in establishing these control settings; they should be recorded in the quality control worksheet, which is described later.)
2. Scan the phantom and estimate the maximum depth of visualization of texture echo signals (Fig. 14-3).
3. File a digital or hard-copy image of the phantom.

In the examples in Fig. 14-3, the maximum depth of visualization is 16.8 cm at 4 MHz. With a 2-MHz mode, the maximum depth of visualization is at least as deep as the length of the phantom, so it cannot be measured with

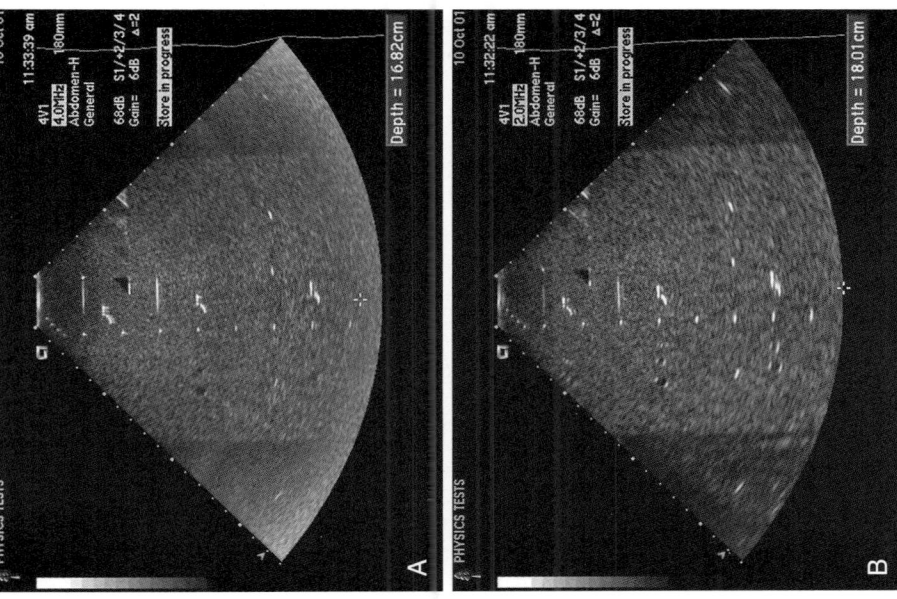

FIGURE 14-3 Images obtained for the maximum depth of the visualization quality assurance test with a multifrequency array transducer. The phantom has an attenuation coefficient of 0.7 dB/cm per megahertz. **A,** At 4 MHz, the maximum depth of visualization is 16.8 cm. **B,** At 2 MHz, the maximum depth of visualization cannot be determined with this phantom because visualization remains excellent all the way to the bottom of the phantom.

this phantom. The lower frequency results in a lower attenuation and therefore greater maximum depth of visualization.

For the test results to be interpreted, a comparison is made with maximum visualization results from a previous test, perhaps 6 months earlier. Results should agree within 1 cm. Normal trial-to-trial variations in scanning and interpretation prohibit closer calls than this. However, with digital or hard-copy images and records of maximum depth of visualization tests, ascertaining whether a scanner/transducer combination has drifted significantly over time in echo detection capabilities should be possible.

In addition to this measurement being made with the standard transducer, occasionally performing the test with different transducers is useful. For example, the test can be performed with all of the transducers that are available for each instrument when quality control tests are first established and semiannually thereafter. This method helps pinpoint the source of any decrease in the maximum sensitivity. If the maximum depth of visualization decreases on all of the transducers tested on a specific scanner, the problem is most likely associated with the scanner and not the transducer assemblies.

Photography and Gray-Scale Hard Copy

Perhaps the most frequent source of ultrasound instrument variability over time is related to image photography. Too often, drift in the imaging instrument, in the hard-copy cameras, or in film processing reduces image quality to the point that significant amounts of detail related to echo signal amplitude variations are lost on hard-copy B-mode images. However, if image viewing monitors and recording devices are set up properly and if sufficient attention is given to photography during routine quality control, these problems can be reduced. The advent of laser printers with automatic (or semiautomatic) calibration has greatly reduced much of the variability of producing a hard-copy image. However, even laser printers have problems.

Monitor Setup and Recording Devices. Most instruments provide both an image display monitor, which is viewed during scan buildup, and an image recording device. As a general rule, the display monitor should be set up properly first, and then adjustments should be made, if necessary, to the laser printers or other hard-copy recording devices to produce an acceptable gray scale on hard-copy images. The establishment of proper settings is expected only during the installation of a scanner, major upgrades, or detection of image problems. Changes made to the display settings are not automatically reflected in the printed image. Changing the display settings requires adjustment of the hard-copy device to properly match the printed image to the displayed image; therefore, image display settings should not be shifted routinely. Many facilities go so far as to remove the control knobs on image monitors once the contrast and brightness are adjusted to an acceptable level; thus, the temptation to change settings casually is removed.

An effective method for setting up both viewing and hard-copy devices has been described by Gray (1985).

It is recommended that adjustments be done with an image that contains a clinically representative sampling of gray shades.

1. First, attend to the display monitor viewed during scanning. With the contrast settings of the monitor initially set at minimum settings, adjust the brightness to a level that just allows television raster lines to be discernible.
2. After the adjustment, increase the monitor contrast until just before the text on the display begins to become distorted (the text, which is typically displayed at a maximum brightness, begins to smear to the left and right if the contrast is too high). Verify that the settings are adequate with a clinical image.

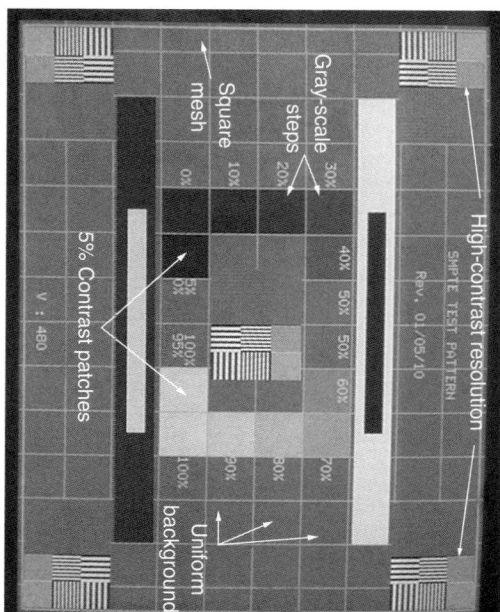

FIGURE 14-4 A test pattern of the Society of Motion Picture and Television Engineers (SMPTE). The pattern contains a gray-scale range in increments of 10% video level. There are also 5% contrast patches at the 0% (black) and 100% (white) levels, a mesh pattern to check for spatial distortions, and several resolution patterns.

After the viewing monitor is properly adjusted, make provisions to prevent casual changes in settings by department personnel.

3. Adjust the image recording device to obtain the same gray shades that appear on the display monitor. This adjustment may require several repetitions, varying the contrast and the overall brightness, until satisfactory results are obtained. Many manufacturers provide gray-scale test patterns such as the one by the Society of Motion Picture and Television Engineers (SMPTE) (Fig. 14-4) that can be displayed on the scanner. These patterns are useful for matching the hard-copy image to the display image. If such a pattern is unavailable, a small gray-scale bar is usually presented on the real-time image.

Routine Quality Assurance of Image Recording. Routine checks should be performed on the quality of gray-scale photography or other hard-copy recording media. Detailed analysis performed in some installations includes film sensitometry and film-emulsion batch crossovers. These processes are well established and documented in Chapter 3, and are not explained in detail. Images of a tissue-mimicking phantom, along with the gray-bar pattern that appears on the edge of most image displays, can be used for routinely assessing photography settings. In photography and processing, all brightness variations in the viewing monitor image should be successfully recorded on the hard-copy image.

A quick check of gray-scale recording can be done as follows:

1. On an image of a tissue-mimicking phantom (or of a patient), check to see whether weak echo signal dots appearing on the viewing monitor are successfully recorded on film.

2. Determine whether the entire gray bar is visible and whether all gray levels are distinguishable. For example, for a scanner with a gray bar including 15 levels of gray, along with the background, the hard-copy image should portray distinctions among all of the different levels. Continuous gray bars are more of a visual challenge when display bars are compared with printed gray levels. In this case, focus attention on the light and dark ends of the patterns and compare the differences in the extent of white and black areas on the bars. The suggested action level is any optical density that is greater than or equal to 0.2 optical density units from the baseline.

3. The entire length of the gray-bar pattern displayed on the viewing monitor should be visible on the final image (see Fig. 14-3B). For multiple images on a single sheet of film or paper, all images should have the same background brightness and should display the gray-bar pattern in the same manner. These images can be verified from clinical images taken on the same day the quality assurance tests are taken or from the quality assurance films themselves.

4. Some laser printers offer features for setting other characteristics of the printed image such as border width and background density. These settings should be decided, usually by trial and error, by all of those involved in reading the images. Once a conclusion has been reached, the settings should be installed in all printing devices used for ultrasound and documented for future reference.

Many imaging facilities now use digital images archived on computer systems and image workstations, rather than film recording. Workstation displays require periodic evaluation to ensure optimum performance. The displays should be cleaned periodically and before any quality assurance testing. Ideally, a lint-free cloth should be used for wiping the surface of the display. Cleaning solution should be applied to the cloth and not sprayed directly on the display. Some displays, especially flat-panel displays, may require specific cleaning products because of antiglare or other special coatings on the screen surface, so check the manufacturer's cleaning instructions before applying any chemical product to the display. Storing a cloth and cleaner solution next to the workstation display is a convenient practice to promote a dust-free, clean display screen.

The SMPTE pattern (see Fig. 14-4) is useful for the routine quality assurance of displays. The large squares on the SMPTE pattern are used to note any distortions caused by the display; they should appear as an array of perfect squares over the entire screen. Degradation of monitor resolution can be noted by viewing the high-contrast resolution patterns and the text on the SMPTE pattern. These should appear well-defined, not blurry or smeared. The 95% density patch within the 100% video (*white*) and the 5% density patch within the 0% video (*black*) square should be visible. The gray background of the SMPTE pattern should be uniformly gray across the entire display. The following characteristics should be noted when performing display quality assurance (Groth et al., 2001):

- *Monitor cleanliness.* The display screen should be free of dust or other markings (e.g., pen markings, fingerprints).
- *Spatial distortion.* The display should be serviced if the squares on the SMPTE pattern are distorted at the corners or if their aspect ratios (width/height) are not correct (e.g., a square shape that appears to be rectangular). Some displays provide controls that allow the user to correct minor spatial distortions.
- *Monitor resolution (edge definition).* Any high-contrast boundary such as white text on a dark background should be well-defined.
- *Gray-scale uniformity.* The intensity on the display should be consistent over the entire screen. This requires a test pattern that contains a constant gray level over the entire screen or at least at all four sides and in the center. Moving a small uniform image from one side of the screen to the other is typically an ineffective alternative to a single large image.
- *Low-contrast visibility.* The 5% difference in video level (on black and on white) of the SMPTE pattern should be noticeable on the display. Room lighting should be minimal when viewing low-contrast objects. Alternatively, the entire gray-bar pattern seen on the scanner monitor should be visualized on the workstation monitor.
- *Display artifacts.* The display should not contain streaks, lines, or dark/light patches. If a test pattern of uniform brightness is unavailable, the brightest pattern available should be used. In this case, the observer must 'look through' the test objects at the background of the image. A few nonfunctioning (dropped) pixels, which appear as small black dots, may be tolerable. However, a group of dropped pixels or several dropped pixels scattered over the screen warrants replacement of the display.

Scan Image Uniformity

Ultrasound phantoms typically contain a background material that is distributed throughout the phantom. However, with most phantoms it is impossible to acquire a view that does not contain any test objects. In these cases, **scan image uniformity** can be assessed by focusing attention solely on the background material of the phantom. Ideally, when a region within a phantom is scanned and the machine's gain settings are adjusted properly, the resultant image has a uniform brightness throughout (Fig. 14-5A). Nonuniformities caused by the ultrasound imager can occur because of the following situations:

- Bad elements in a linear or curved array or loose connections in beam former board plug-ins can lead to

FIGURE 14-5 Image uniformity tests. **A,** Good uniformity. **B,** Results with a transducer that should be repaired or replaced. Note the vertical streaks that are evidence of element dropout for this linear array transducer.

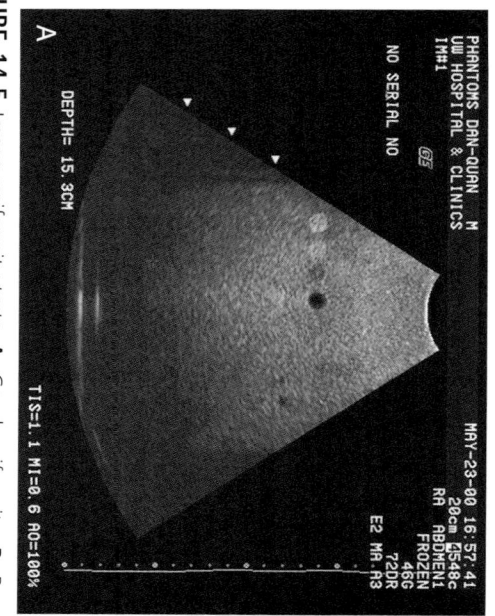
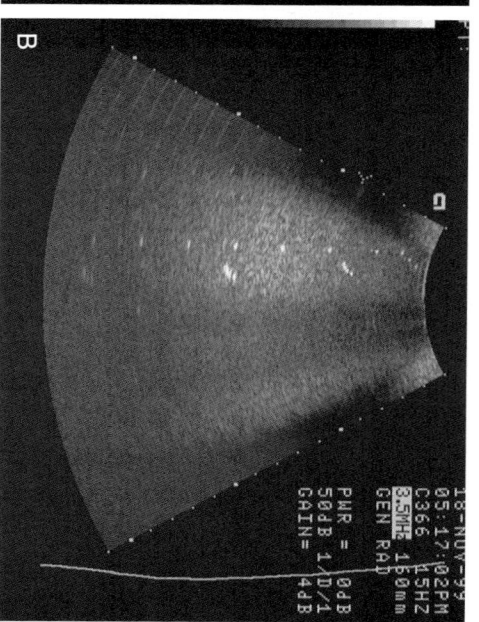

vertically oriented nonuniformities (Fig. 14-5B). (Boards can be loosened if the scanner is wheeled over bumps or if it is transported by a van to other hospitals or clinics.)
- Inadequate side-to-side image compensation in the machine can lead to variations in brightness from one side of the image to another.
- Inadequate blending of pixel data between transmit and receive focal zones can lead to horizontal or curved streaks parallel to the transducer surface. Quality assurance testing is an ideal time to assess whether such faults are noticeable. An image is taken of a uniform region in the quality assurance phantom, and the image is inspected for these problems.

A uniformity image is useful in the detection of subtle artifacts that may not be readily evident on the clinical images. Care should be taken to inspect the image thoroughly for any vertical or radially oriented streaks, any dark or light patches, or any gray-scale gradients in the axial or lateral directions. Occasionally a swirling pattern with the background texture may be noticed. However, this pattern is typically a result of the phantom manufacturing process, which can be verified by comparison with uniformity images from other transducers. The suggested action level would be nonuniformity greater than or equal to 4 dB or any consistent measurable change from the baseline.

Distance Measurement Accuracy

Instruments used for measuring structure dimensions, organ sizes, and areas can be tested periodically for accuracy of distance indicators. However, many individuals think that routine distance measurement accuracy checks are not useful because digital measurement systems on scanners exhibit satisfactory stability over time (ACR Ultrasound Accreditation Program, 2012; Goodsitt et al., 1998).

Distance indicators usually include 1-cm-deep markers on M-mode and B-mode scanning displays and electronic calipers on B-mode scanning systems. Calipers on workstations that are part of computer archiving systems also should be checked for accuracy. The principal distance measurement tests are separated into two parts: one part is for measurements along the sound beam axis, which is referred to as the *vertical distance measurement test*, or the *axial distance measurement test*, and the other part is for measurements taken perpendicular to the sound beam axis, which is called the *horizontal distance measurement test*. **Vertical Distance Measurements.** Vertical distance measurement accuracy also is called *depth calibration accuracy* in some texts.

1. To evaluate a scanner's vertical distance measurement accuracy, scan the phantom, ensuring that the vertical column of reflectors in the phantom is clearly imaged (Fig. 14-6).
2. Position the digital calipers to measure the distance between any two reflectors in this column.
   a. Correct caliper placement is from the top of the echo from the first reflector to the top of the echo from the second reflector or from any position on the first reflector to the corresponding position on the second reflector.
   b. When testing general purpose scanners, choose reflectors positioned at least 8–10 cm apart for this test. Most laboratories also measure a smaller spacing such as 4 cm. For small-parts scanners and probes, use a distance of 1 or 2 cm. In general, the largest separation allowed by the transducer/frequency combination and the target placement in the phantom is appropriate for the distance accuracy test.
3. Determine that the measured distance agrees with the actual distance given by the phantom manufacturer to within 1 mm or 1.5%, whichever is greater. If a larger discrepancy occurs, consult with the ultrasound scanner manufacturer for possible corrective measures.

CHAPTER 14 Ultrasound Equipment Quality Assurance

occasional attention. These include cleaning air filters on instruments that require this service (most do), checking for loose and frayed electrical cables, looking for loose handles or control arms on the scanner, checking the wheels and wheel locks, and performing recommended preventive maintenance of photography equipment, which may include dusting or cleaning of photographic monitors and maintenance chores on cameras.

DOCUMENTATION

An important aspect of a quality assurance program is keeping track of the test results. Most laboratories want to adopt a standardized worksheet on which to write the test results. The worksheet helps the user carry out the tests in a consistent manner by having enough information to assist recall of transducers, phantoms, and machine settings. It also includes blank spaces for recording the results. An example is shown in Box 14-2. Box 14-3 contains the American College of Radiology (ACR) Annual System Performance Evaluation Report—Ultrasound/Breast Ultrasound Equipment Evaluation Summary, to be completed by the medical physicist. Box 14-4 contains the ACR Evaluation of Site's Routine QC Program, to be completed by the technologist.

SPATIAL RESOLUTION TESTS

Some laboratories include spatial resolution in their quality assurance testing. Measurements of spatial resolution generally require more exacting techniques to achieve results that allow intercomparisons of scanners; therefore, many centers do not do such performance tests routinely but may do so only during equipment acceptance tests (Carson and Goodsitt, 1995). Common methods for determining axial resolution and lateral resolution are discussed in this section.

Axial Resolution

Axial resolution is a measure of how close two reflectors can be to one another along the axis of an ultrasound beam and still be resolved as separate reflectors. Axial resolution also is related to the crispness of the image of a reflector arranged perpendicularly to the ultrasound beam.

Axial resolution can be estimated by measuring the thickness of the image of a line target in the quality assurance phantom. Alternatively, some phantoms contain sets of reflectors for axial resolution testing. Fig. 14-8 shows both approaches. The axial separations between successive targets in this phantom are 2, 1, 0.5, and 0.25 mm. The targets are offset horizontally to minimize the effects of shallow targets shadowing the deeper ones. The pair most closely spaced yet clearly distinguishable in the axial direction indicates the axial resolution. This implies that to be considered resolved, the axial extent of

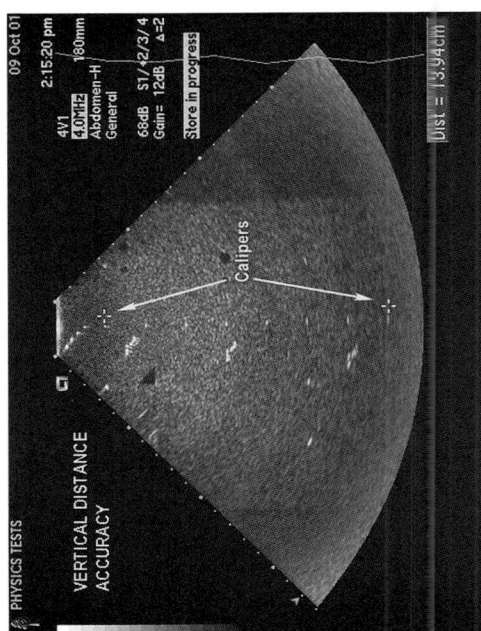

FIGURE 14-6 Vertical distance measurement check. The caliper reading (13.94 cm) is compared with the actual separation (14 cm) between pins positioned along a vertical column in the phantom. Shorter distances should be used when high-frequency transducers are evaluated.

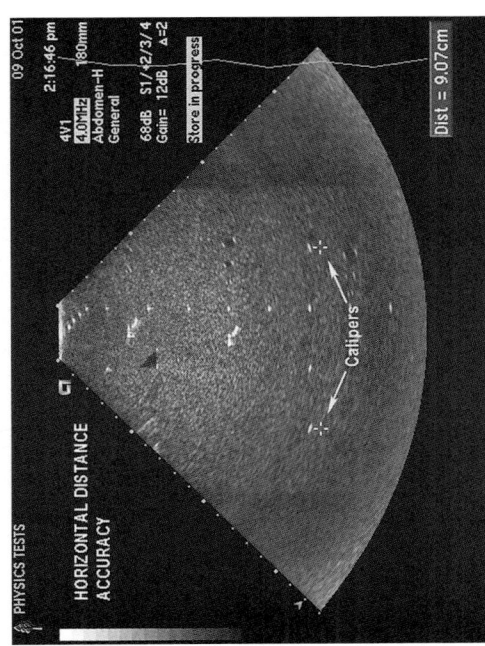

FIGURE 14-7 Horizontal distance measurement check. The caliper reading (90.7 mm) is for a measurement taken horizontally on the image and compared with the actual pin separation (90 mm).

Horizontal Distance Measurements. Horizontal measurement accuracy should be checked in a manner similar to vertical distance measurement. Measurements obtained in this direction (Fig. 14-7) are frequently less accurate because of beam width effects and scanner inaccuracies. Nevertheless, results should agree with the phantom manufacturer's distances to within 3 mm or 3%, whichever is greater. Correct caliper placement for this test is from the center of one reflector to the center of the second reflector. For the example in Fig. 14-7, measurement results are within 1 mm of the actual distance between the reflectors examined. This is well within the expected level of accuracy.

Other Important Instrument Quality Assurance Tasks

During routine performance testing, it is a good idea to perform other equipment-related chores that require

BOX 14-2 | Ultrasound Quality Control Results

Machine: Acuson 128   Room: E3 315
Transducer assembly: I.D.: V4   Serial no: 555-1212
Date: 9/09/97   Phantom: RMI 403 GS
Instrument settings:
  Power 0 dB   Dynamic range: 50 dB
  Pre 0/Persis 3/Post 0
  Gain: 12 dB   Transmit focus: 16 cm
  Image magnification: 18 cm

1. Depth measurement accuracy
   Electronic calipers
   Measured distance .... 98.8 mm
   Actual distance .... 100 mm
   Error .... 1.2 mm
2. Horizontal measurement accuracy
   Electronic calipers
   Measured distance .... 30.5 mm
   Actual distance .... 30 mm
   Error .... 0.5 mm
3. Depth of penetration (4 MHz)
   Measured distance .... 152 mm
   Baseline distance .... 150 mm
   Variation from baseline .... 2 mm
4. Image uniformity
   Significant   Excellent
   Nonuniformity   Uniformity
   1   2   3   ④   5
5. Photography
   Gray bars
   Number of gray bars visible 13
   Number of gray bars visible on baseline 15
   Variation 2
   Low-level echoes
   All echoes displayed on viewing monitor also seen on film:
   Yes X   No ___
   Contrast and brightness
   Level of agreement between contrast and brightness on viewing monitor and film:
   Poor   Excellent
   1   2   3   4   ⑤
6. Filters
   Clean _____   Dusty X _____

Lateral Resolution

Lateral resolution is a measure of how close two reflectors can be to one another, be perpendicular to the beam axis, and still be distinguished as separate reflectors on an image. One approach that is used for lateral resolution tests is to measure the width on the display of a point-like target such as a line target inside a phantom. For example, Fig. 14-9 shows such a measurement. The cursors indicate that the displayed width is 0.7 mm for this case. The displayed response width is related to the lateral resolution at the depth of the target. Through the imaging of targets at different depths, it is easy to see that the lateral resolution usually varies with depth for most transducers. Additionally, the lateral resolution measurement is sensitive to any focal zone placement. The suggested action level is any change greater than 1 mm from the baseline value.

Cautions about Resolution Tests with Discrete Targets

The lateral and axial dimensions of the displayed image of a point-like target depend on the power and gain settings on the machine. Such dependency is one of the difficulties of adopting such tests in routine testing. Quantitative results for axial and lateral resolution have been obtained by measuring the dimensions of point-like targets when they are imaged at specified sensitivity levels above the threshold for their display (AIUM standard methods for measuring performance of ultrasound pulse-echo equipment, 1990; Carson and Goodsitt, 1995). The procedure is as follows:

1. Obtain an image with the sensitivity of the scanner set so that the target is barely visible on the display.
2. Next, obtain a second image, with the scanner sensitivity increased 20 dB above the setting for display threshold.
3. Set the calipers to measure the lateral resolution at this scanner setting. Additional information is available elsewhere (Goodsitt et al., 1998; Zagzebski, 2000).

OTHER TEST OBJECTS AND PHANTOMS

Most general purpose phantoms contain additional objects for the evaluation of image performance. Although these tests are not considered essential to a routine quality assurance program, they may be useful for testing or optimizing specific imaging configurations. These tests are subjective; therefore, the comparison of results with those acquired previously is essential.

Anechoic Voids

Many phantom designs include cylindrical anechoic voids (Fig. 14-10). These voids appear as dark, circular one-pin depiction does not overlap with that of the next one below, even though the two pins may be distinguishable because of their lateral separation. Often, as in this phantom, the target pair separations are not finely spaced enough to allow a good measure of axial resolution; that is, the 0.25-mm pair in this example is not clearly resolved, whereas the 1-mm pair certainly is and the 0.5 mm is almost resolved. The vertical thickness of a single target (0.6 mm in this case) is sometimes used (Burlew et al., 1980) to obtain more detailed indication of the axial resolution (Method 2 in Fig. 14-8). The suggested action level is 1 mm (or 2 mm if transducer frequency is <4 MHz) or any consistent measurable change from the baseline value.

CHAPTER 14 Ultrasound Equipment Quality Assurance 311

BOX 14-3 | Annual System Performance Evaluation Report: Ultrasound/Breast Ultrasound Equipment Evaluation Summary

Annual System Performance Evaluation Report
Ultrasound/Breast Ultrasound Equipment Evaluation Summary

Site: _____ Report Date: _____

Facility UAP #: _____

Facility BUAP #: _____ Survey Date: _____

System Manufacturer: _____ Model: _____

System SN: _____

Building/Room #: _____ System ID: _____

Medical Physicist (or designee): _____

Signature: _____

Equipment Evaluation Tests

Test	Pass/Fail	Comments
1. Physical and Mechanical Inspection		
2. Image Uniformity and Artifact Survey		
3. Geometric Accuracy		
4. System Sensitivity		
5. Scanner Electronic Image Display Performance		
6. Primary Interpretation Display Performance*		
7. Contrast Resolution (Optional)		
8. Spatial Resolution (Optional)		

* If located at the facility where ultrasound is performed

Medical Physicist's (or designee's) Recommendations for Quality Improvement:

You must send ACR the entire, most recent Annual System Performance Evaluation report. It must include: • _Equipment Evaluation Summary form, signed by the medical physicist (or designee)_ • _Evaluation of Site's Routine QC Program form, AND_ • _All data pages from the report (not just the summary forms)_

CHAPTER 14   Ultrasound Equipment Quality Assurance

BOX 14-4   Evaluation of Site's Routine Quality Control Program

Evaluation of Site's Routine QC Program

| Facility UAP #: | | Facility BUAP #: | | Survey Date: | |

Test	Minimum Frequency	Pass/Fail	Comments
1. Physical and Mechanical Inspection	semiannually		
2. Image Uniformity and Artifact Survey	semiannually		
3. Geometric Accuracy (mechanically scanned transducers only)	semiannually		
4. Scanner Electronic Image Display Performance	semiannually		
5. Primary Interpretation Display Performance*,**	semiannually		

* If located at the facility where ultrasound is performed
** Semiannually, or as judged appropriate based on the specific display technology, or prior QC testing data

Specific Comments:

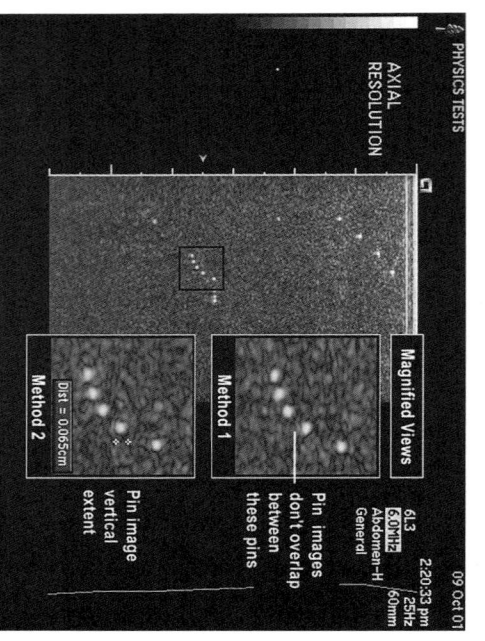

FIGURE 14-8 Axial resolution measurement. The thickness of the pin target is 0.65 mm. In the axial resolution target set (vertical separation 2, 1, 0.5, and 0.25 mm), the 1-mm pair is separated a sufficient distance vertically so that there is no vertical overlap of the images of these two targets, whereas the 0.5-mm pair overlaps if the two targets are on a vertical line. The axial resolution is just over 0.5 mm, in agreement with the estimate made from the thickness of the single target image.

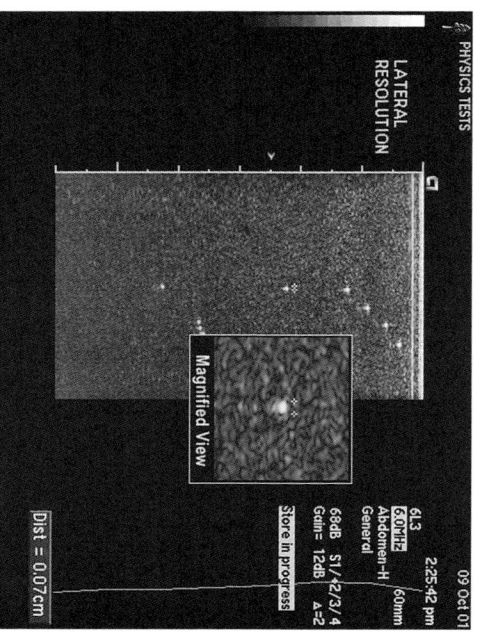

FIGURE 14-9 Lateral resolution measurement. The horizontal size of the pin target is 0.7 mm.

CHAPTER 14 Ultrasound Equipment Quality Assurance

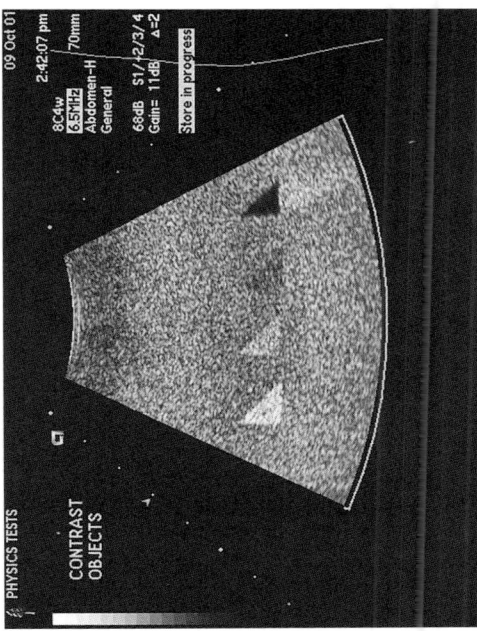

FIGURE 14-10 B-mode image of a phantom containing three anechoic cylinders of different sizes (6-, 4-, and 2-mm diameter) acquired with a 4-MHz linear transducer. Some echoes are evident within the voids, and the edges are well-defined. The smallest void is easily detectable.

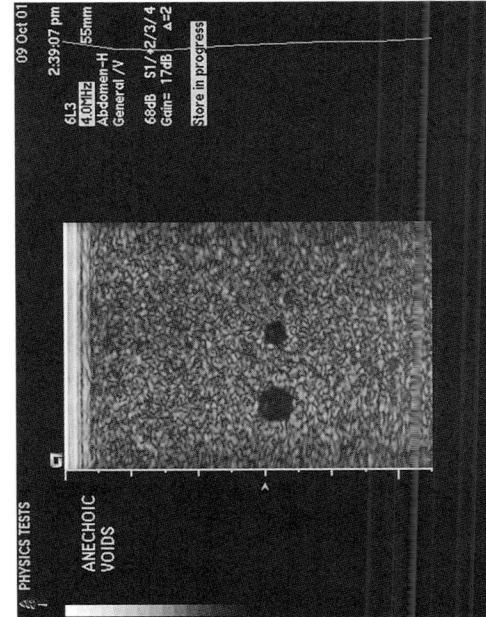

FIGURE 14-11 Image of a phantom containing four triangular-shaped objects of different contrast values acquired with a 6.5-MHz curvilinear transducer. The higher contrast objects (the outer two) are clearly visualized. The second object from the right is barely visible. The corners of the two inner objects are poorly defined.

objects on an ultrasound image and can yield a wide range of information about the performance of a scanner. The void depictions can be inspected for spatial distortions; the voids should not be elliptical. The edges of the voids should be relatively sharp, and the interior of the voids should be echo free. If voids of different sizes are available, the smallest visualized void can be noted.

Objects of Various Echogenicity

Many phantoms also include a set of objects with different inherent contrasts (Fig. 14-11). These objects can be visually assessed as a means of comparing one scan configuration with another or the performance of a specific scan configuration over time. For example, these objects may be useful to demonstrate the effect of changing the log compression. However, there must be caution when the impressions obtained by the set of various contrast objects are extrapolated into the clinical environment because the entire clinical range of inherent object contrasts may not be completely represented by the test objects. As with the anechoic voids, the perimeter of the objects can be inspected for edge definition.

Spherical Object Phantom

Another phantom becoming increasingly popular for spatial resolution tests is one that has simulated focal lesions embedded within echogenic tissue-mimicking material (AIUM standard methods for measuring performance of ultrasound pulse-echo equipment, 1990; Madsen et al., 1991). Different simulated lesion sizes and different object contrast levels (e.g., relative echogenicity) have been tried (Madsen et al., 1991). An example is shown in Fig. 14-12, in which the phantom imaged contained 4-mm-diameter, low-echo masses. The

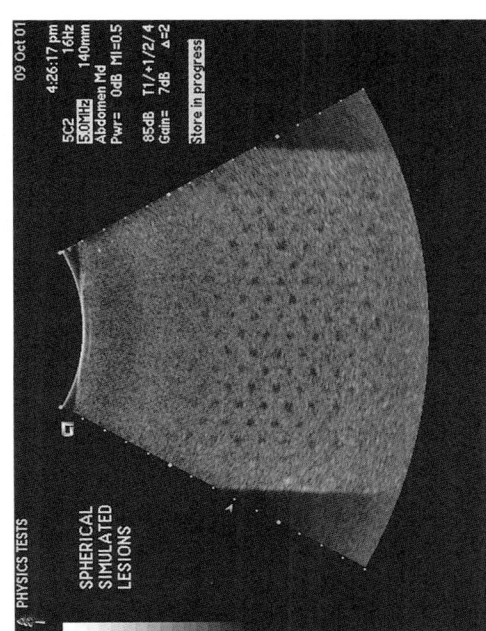

FIGURE 14-12 B-mode image of a phantom containing 4-mm low-scattering spheres that mimic cysts. The spheres are centered in a regular array within a plane, and the scanning plane is carefully aligned to coincide with the plane containing the spheres. They can be visualized from depths of 5.0–12.0 cm with this transducer.

centers of the masses are coplanar and distributed in a well-defined matrix.

A test of the ultrasound imaging system is used to determine the 'imaging zone' for detection of masses of a given size and object contrast (Madsen et al., 1991). The 5-MHz phased array used for Fig. 14-12 can successfully detect the masses over a 5- to 12-cm depth range. The **slice thickness** (Goodsitt et al., 1998) is too large for this transducer to pick up these structures at more shallow depths.

A particularly useful aspect of spherical mass phantoms is that they present realistic imaging tasks that readily demonstrate resolution capabilities in terms of resolution. For three-dimensional spherical targets, the resolution is a combined, effective resolution composed of axial, lateral, and slice thicknesses. If two-dimensional cylindrical objects are used as phantoms, only two dimensions, usually axial and lateral, are involved in their visualization. Because slice thickness is usually the worst measure of spatial resolution with array transducers, cylindrical objects can be misleading in terms of translating minimum sizes resolved into resolution of actual focal masses. The spherical lesion phantom is superior in this regard.

DOPPLER TESTING

Limited evaluations of Doppler and color flow equipment also can be made in the clinic. A number of devices including string test objects, flow velocity test objects, and flow phantoms are available to clinical users for carrying out tests of Doppler equipment (Hoskins et al., 1994; Performance criteria and measurements for Doppler ultrasound devices, 1993; Zagzebski, 1995).

String Test Objects

String test objects consist of a thin string wound around a pulley and motor-drive mechanism. The string is echogenic, so it produces echoes that are detected by an ultrasound instrument. The drive moves the string at precise velocities, either continuously or after a programmed waveform. This provides a way to evaluate the velocity measurement accuracy of Doppler devices. String test objects also may be used to evaluate the lateral and axial resolution in Doppler mode and can be used to determine the accuracy of gate registration on duplex Doppler systems (Hoskins et al., 1994).

The advantage of the string test object is that it provides a small target moving at a precisely known velocity. The disadvantages are that the echogenic characteristics of the string are not the same as those of blood and that actual blood flow, with its characteristic distribution of velocities across the vessel, is not mimicked.

Doppler Flow Phantoms

Doppler flow phantoms (Figs. 14-13 and 14-14) consist of one or more hollow tube coursing through a block of tissue-mimicking material. A blood-mimicking fluid is pumped through the tube(s) to simulate blood flowing through vessels in the body. Usually the blood-mimicking fluid is a solution of water and glycerol that has small plastic particles suspended in it. The blood-mimicking material should provide the same echogenicity as whole human blood at the ultrasound frequencies of the machine; reasonable representative blood-mimicking materials are now available for use in these phantoms. If the tissue-mimicking material in the body of the phantom has a representative amount of beam attenuation, the depth-dependent echogenicity of the fluid within the

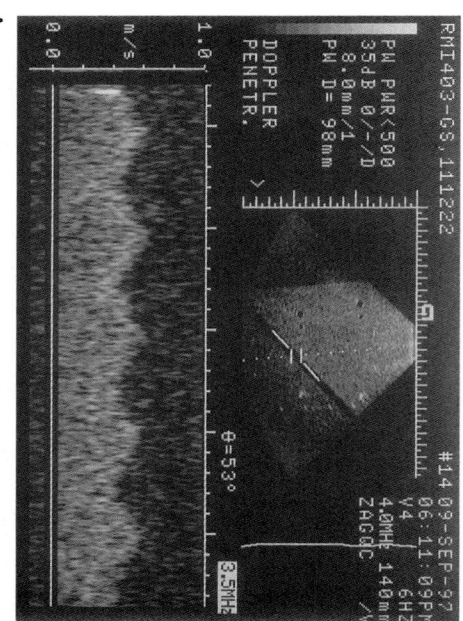

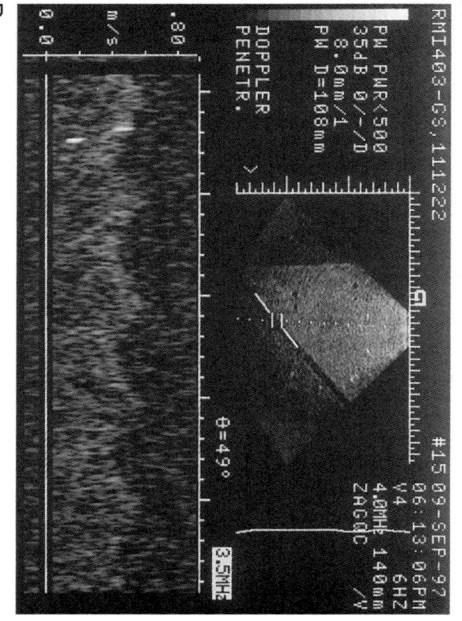

FIGURE 14-13 B-mode and spectral Doppler display of a flow phantom for evaluating Doppler penetration. **A**, A strong Doppler signal and a good signal-to-noise ratio is obtained when the sample volume is at a depth of 9.8 cm. **B**, The Doppler signal is just detectable above the electronic noise when the sample volume is at a depth of 10.8 cm. The maximum depth of detection of the Doppler signal in this case is 10.8 cm.

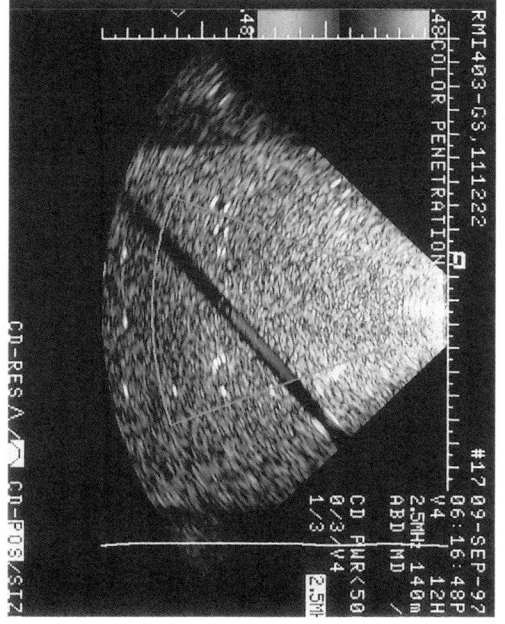

FIGURE 14-14 An example of a color flow image of a Doppler flow phantom used to determine the maximum penetration in color.

CHAPTER 14 Ultrasound Equipment Quality Assurance

phantom is representative of signal levels from actual vessels in vivo.

Doppler flow phantoms are used for the following types of tests of Doppler and flow imaging equipment (Hoskins et al., 1994; Zagzebski, 1995):

- *Maximum detection depth.* The maximum depth at which flow waveforms can be detected in the phantom has been used to assess whether the Doppler sensitivity has varied from one quality assurance test to another.[1] This is shown in Fig. 14-13. Penetration in this case is 10.8 cm.
- *Alignment.* The phantom can be used to evaluate whether the pulsed Doppler sample volume is aligned with the volume indicated on the B-mode image.
- *Volume flow accuracy.* Some Doppler flow phantoms have precise volume flow measuring equipment. A flow phantom can thus be used in assessments of the accuracy of flow measuring algorithms on Doppler devices.
- *Velocity accuracy.* If the velocity of the fluid within the phantoms can be determined accurately, then this can be used to evaluate velocity displays on Doppler and color flow machines.
- *Color flow penetration* (see Fig. 14-14). System sensitivity settings are at their maximum levels without excessive electronic noise. The maximum depth at which color data can be recorded in the flow phantom is noted. Any changes over time such as greater than 1 cm indicate a change in the sensitivity of the instrument.

[1] This measurement may be useful for consistency checks, which are an essential part of quality assurance, in attempting to verify that equipment is operating at least as well as when it was delivered or last upgraded. As an absolute measure of Doppler sensitivity, it is controversial because many factors are involved in the concept of Doppler sensitivity (Performance criteria and measurements for Doppler ultrasound devices, 1993).

- *Alignment of color flow image with B-mode image* (image congruency test). This test checks whether the color flow image and B-mode image are aligned so that they agree spatially. Color images of vessels should be completely contained within the B-mode image of the vessel. Sometimes bleeding out occurs, and this can be corrected by equipment service personnel.

ELECTRONIC PROBE TESTS

A frequent cause of nonuniformity on B-mode images is nonfunctioning elements in ultrasound transducer arrays. We previously saw that nonfunctioning elements in a transducer array often result in dark 'shadow-type' regions emanating from the transducer as seen on a B-mode image.

Quantitative tools for assessing transducer integrity now are becoming available. One of these is a mode on a scanning machine for testing transducers. Although not available generally, such modes would greatly facilitate routine quality assurance in the clinic and would allow operators to do tests quickly and routinely. Beta versions of the transducer test mode separately address each element in the transducer and channel in the machine. The test mode excites the element with the system pulser and measure the resultant ring-down signal. Criteria are then applied to the signal to judge whether the element is operating normally or is faulty. In this way, a profile of the array functionality can be obtained. Although such modes are not yet available on scanners, manufacturers are encouraged to provide this information to enable more convenient assessment of transducer integrity than can be done at the present time.

An alternative, more sensitive means to evaluate transducer function is to use an electronic probe tester. Special purpose transducer testers, such as the Aperio by Sonora (Longmont, CO, USA; Fig. 14-15) are available.

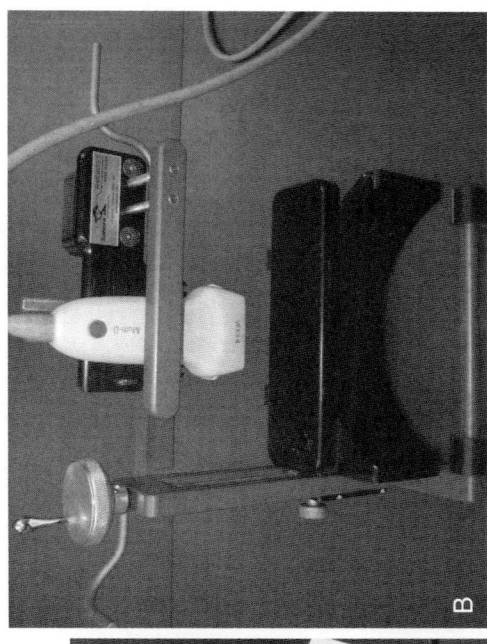

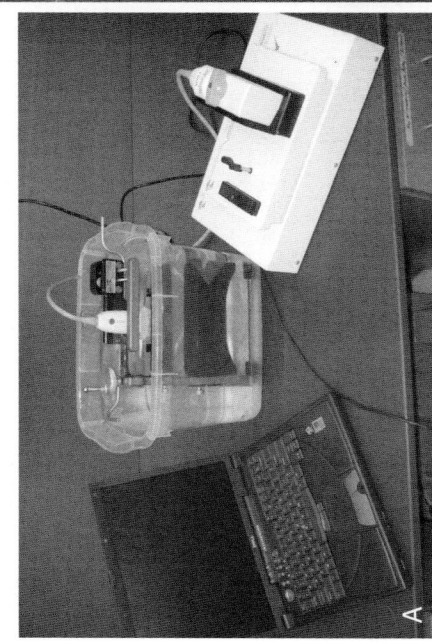

FIGURE 14-15 **A**, Arrangement for testing transducers using an electronic probe tester. The transducer is connected to the tester through its port. The tester may have various special ports to adapt to different manufacturer's transducer connectors. The face of the probe is immersed in water and directed toward a smooth reflector. A computer controls the tester and produces printouts of test reports. **B**, Typical arrangement for testing a linear array transducer. Positioners on the holder enable users to orient the transducer so that beams are perpendicular to the smooth reflecting surface. The mount is immersed in a water bath so that the path from transducer to the reflector is water.

CHAPTER 14 Ultrasound Equipment Quality Assurance

Analogous to the probe testing mode just described, the function of the probe tester is to evaluate each element in an array transducer, testing its transmission and echo detection capability and its acoustic and electrical properties.

The transducer to be tested is immersed in water and oriented to transmit waves toward a specular interface (Fig. 14-15). Users select a planar interface for testing linear arrays (Fig. 14-15B) and phased arrays, while a concave shaped interface is selected for testing curvilinear arrays. Transducer data provided by the probe tester includes manufacturer guide placement of the transducer, and a screen that displays the echo amplitude and exact distance between selected elements and the reflector aids users to achieve the correct transducer orientation. When alignment is satisfactory, users switch the software into test mode. In this mode, each element is isolated, a short electrical pulse is applied to it, and the resultant echo from the interface is detected and analyzed. Information including the amplitude of the signal produced by the element, the frequency content of this echo, and the electrical capacitance is provided.

Graphs that depict the amplitude of the signal from each array element (Fig. 14-16) are used to evaluate the condition of the transducer. The top record in this figure shows this transducer has eight elements that are compromised in some way, as seen by the relative amplitudes of their signals. The electrical capacitance test in the lower figure helps engineers pinpoint whether the problem is likely caused by electrical malfunctions or by mechanical problems, such as delaminations of the matching layers that exist between the transducer and the medium. This transducer was operating poorly enough to warrant replacement following the test. Advantages of the probe tester include the following:

1. This is a more sensitive test than use of images of uniform phantoms for establishing whether a transducer is functioning well or not.
2. Users can readily establish objective pass-fail criteria for a transducer. For example, the test manufacturer suggests that if there are three or more nonfunctioning elements in a typical 128-element transducer, the probe should be replaced.
3. Often the data provided by the electronic probe tester enable users to determine the cause of any dead elements and consider whether repair is possible. An auxiliary test of the electrical capacitance of transducer elements helps pinpoint whether a dead or weak element is a result of a disconnect in the electrical path between the probe cover and the transducer housing or whether the flaw is caused by delaminations between the element and the lens material or matching layers.

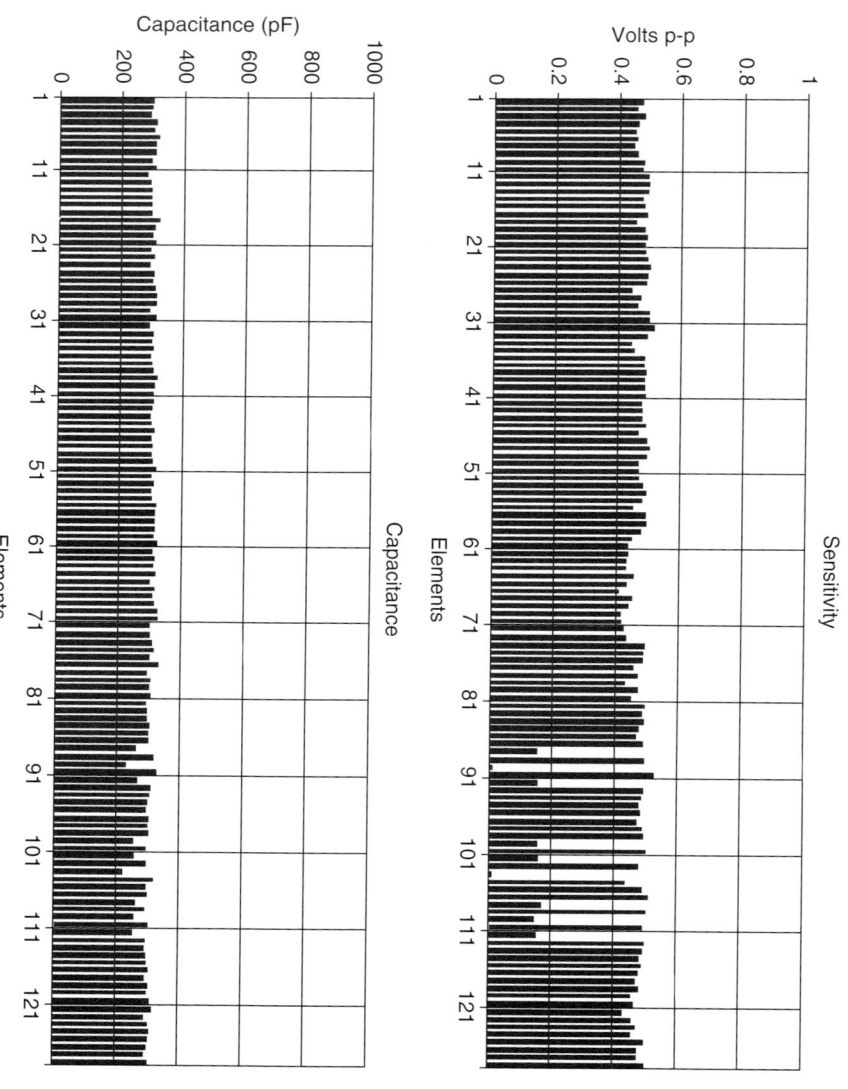

FIGURE 14-16 Typical probe test result for a transducer with eight dead elements. 'Volts p-p' in the top record indicates the relative amplitude of the echo signal detected by each element from the specular reflector. For eight of the elements, the signal clearly is much weaker than for the other elements. The lower record displays the electrical capacitance of each element and its electric lead.

CHAPTER 14 Ultrasound Equipment Quality Assurance

Disadvantages of the system include the following:

1. The system is costly. Besides the basic test unit and target fixture, individual transducer adapters are needed for different manufacturer's transducers.
2. Not all transducers are testable. The pin connection of transducer connectors are not standardized in the probe industry, requiring extensive testing by the electronic probe tester manufacturer to provide 'probe definition files' that apply to each transducer.
3. New transducers such as multidimensional and two-dimensional arrays are less likely to have probe definition files available because of the complicated nature these transducers must operate.

In spite of these shortcomings, many large imaging centers where dozens of transducers are available and must be evaluated in a quality assurance testing environment find electronic probe testers essential to their routine ultrasound quality management program.

Refer to the Evolve Website at https://evolve.elsevier.com for Student Experiment 14.1: Ultrasound System Visual Inspection.

REVIEW QUESTIONS

1. Which term best describes routine tests done to determine that an ultrasound scanner is operating at its expected level of performance?
   a. Equipment acceptance tests
   b. General equipment maintenance
   c. Quality assurance
   d. Instrument upgrades

2. Which one of the following statements is true about quality assurance tests of ultrasound scanners?
   a. They require expertise of a hospital engineer or physicist.
   b. Quality assurance for each scanner takes approximately 2 hours per week.
   c. Good record-keeping is an essential component.
   d. Quantitative results generally are not necessary.

3. In-house quality assurance programs usually involve all but which of the following?
   a. Tests with phantoms
   b. Inspection and cleaning of air filters
   c. Records and worksheets with test results
   d. Voltage measurements at specified points

4. Material making up the body of a typical quality assurance phantom is 'tissuelike' in terms of its _____ properties.
   a. Attenuation and perfusion
   b. Sound speed and attenuation
   c. Sound speed and reflector location
   d. Echogenicity and reflector location

5. To be used for tests of geometric accuracy, the _____ and _____ in a phantom must be precisely specified.
   a. Echogenicity; reflector location
   b. Sound speed; reflector location
   c. Attenuation; reflector location
   d. Echogenicity; attenuation

6. What is the percentage error in the caliper readout if the actual distance between two reflectors in a phantom is 4 cm but the digital caliper readout indicates it is 3.8 cm?
   a. Less than 1%
   b. 1.5%
   c. 5%
   d. 10%

7. Which of the following tests does not need to be performed routinely as part of a quality assurance program?
   a. Uniformity
   b. Distance accuracy
   c. Axial resolution
   d. Maximum depth of visualization

8. What is a string phantom useful for measuring?
   a. The maximum depth of Doppler signal detection
   b. Velocity accuracy on a spectral Doppler display
   c. Axial resolution in B-mode
   d. Vertical distance measurement accuracy

9. What are Doppler flow phantoms useful for determining?
   a. The maximum depth of Doppler signal detection
   b. The vertical distance measurement accuracy
   c. The acoustic output during color flow imaging
   d. The horizontal distance measurement accuracy

10. For echo signals to be produced that are of a similar magnitude as blood in the body, what two factors in a Doppler phantom must be comparable to human tissues?
    a. Phantom material attenuation and mimicking material blood echogenicity
    b. Phantom material density and mimicking material blood attenuation
    c. Mimicking material blood viscosity and attenuation
    d. Mimicking material blood velocity and acceleration

REFERENCES

ACR Ultrasound Accreditation Program: *ACR Ultrasound Accreditation Program 2012*, Reston, VA, 2012, American College of Radiology.

AIUM standard methods for measuring performance of ultrasound pulse-echo equipment: *AIUM standard methods for measuring performance of ultrasound pulse-echo equipment 1990*, Laurel, 1990, American Institute of Ultrasound in Medicine. MD committee report.

Burlew M, et al.: A new ultrasound tissue-equivalent material with a high melting point and extended speed of sound range, *Radiology* 134:517, 1980.

Carson P, Goodsitt MM: Acceptance testing of pulse-echo ultrasound equipment. In Goldman L, Fowlkes B, editors: *Medical CT and ultrasound: current technology and applications*, Madison, WIS, 1995, Advanced Medical Publishers.

Goodsitt M, et al.: Real-time B-mode ultrasound quality control test procedures, Report of AAPM ultrasound task group no 1 *Med Phys* 25:1385–1406, 1998.

Gray J: Test pattern for video display and hard copy cameras, *Radiology* 154:519, 1985.

Groth D, et al.: Cathode ray tube quality control and acceptance program: initial results for clinical PACS displays, *Radiographics* 21:719, 2001.

Hoskins PR, Sheriff SB, Evans JA: *Testing of Doppler ultrasound equipment*, York, UK, 1994, The Institute of Physical Sciences in Medicine. Rep no 70.

Lu ZF, Lee FT, Zagzebski JA: Ultrasonic backscatter and attenuation in diffuse liver disease, *Ultrasound Med Biol* 25:1047, 1999.

Madsen L, et al.: Tissue mimicking material for ultrasound phantoms, *Med Phys* 5:391, 1978.

Madsen L, et al.: Ultrasound lesion detectability phantoms, *Med Phys* 18:1771, 1991.

Maklad N, Ophir J, Balara V: Attenuation of ultrasound in normal and diffuse liver disease in vivo, *Ultrason Imaging* 6:117, 1984.

Moore GW, et al.: The need for evidence-based quality assurance in the modern ultrasound clinical laboratory, *Ultrasound* 13:158–162, 2005.

Performance criteria and measurements for Doppler ultrasound devices: *Performance criteria and measurements for Doppler ultrasound devices 1993*, Laurel, 1993, American Institute of Ultrasound in Medicine. MD committee report.

Thijssen JM, et al.: Objective performance testing and quality assurance of medical ultrasound equipment, *Ultrasound Med Biol* 33:460–471, 2007.

Zagzebski J: Acceptance tests for Doppler ultrasound equipment. In Goldman L, Fowlkes B, editors: *Medical CT and ultrasound: current technology and applications*, Madison, WIS, 1995, Advanced Medical Publishers.

Zagzebski J: US quality assurance with phantoms. In Goldman L, Fowlkes B, editors: *Categorical course in diagnostic radiology physics: CT and US cross-sectional imaging*, Oak Brook, Ill, 2000, Radiological Society of North America.

CHAPTER 15

Quality Assurance in Nuclear Medicine

*Joanne M. Metler**

KEY TERMS

American College of Radiology
Bioassay
Center of rotation
Chemical impurity
Chi-square test
Chromatography
Collimator
Count rate
Counts per minute
Disintegrations per minute
Dose calibrator
Energy resolution
Field uniformity
Gamma camera
Gas-filled detector
Geiger–Müller meters
Hydrolyzed reduced technetium
Molybdenum-99
Multichannel analyzer
Nuclear Regulatory Commission
Occupational Safety and Health Administration
Optically stimulated luminescent dosimeter
Photomultiplier tubes
Photon
Photopeak
Pixel size
Positron emission tomography
Pulse height analyzer
Radionuclide impurity
Scintillation crystal
Scintillation detectors
Sensitivity
Single-photon emission computed tomography
Spatial linearity
Spatial resolution
Spectrum
Standardized uptake value (SUV)
Technetium-99m
Technetium-99m pertechnetate
The Joint Commission
Thermoluminescent dosimeter
Uniformity correction flood

OBJECTIVES

At the completion of this chapter the reader will be able to do the following:

- Describe the principles of radiation detection and measurement
- Describe the scintillation crystal
- Describe the basic principles of the gamma camera
- Describe the scintillation camera performance characteristics of image linearity, image uniformity, intrinsic spatial resolution, detection efficiency, and counting rate problems
- Describe the design and performance characteristics of commonly used collimators
- Describe planar camera quality control testing methods of calibration, gamma energy spectrum, window determination, daily floods (intrinsic and extrinsic), weekly resolution (intrinsic and extrinsic), counting efficiency and sensitivity, and multiwindow spatial registration
- Describe gamma camera single-photon emission computed tomography (SPECT) systems
- Describe SPECT quality control (i.e., flood uniformity, center of rotation, attenuation correction, and pixel size)
- Describe positron emission tomography and its quality control
- Describe nuclear medicine nonimaging equipment and related quality control procedures (i.e., gas-filled detectors such as dose calibrators, survey meters, Geiger–Müller meters, and scintillation detectors such as the multichannel analyzer and thyroid probe)
- Describe quality control procedures in a radiopharmacy and radionuclide generator quality control evaluation of contaminant such as molybdenum, aluminum, and hydrolyzed reduced technetium

---

*The author and publisher wish to acknowledge the previous edition's contributor.

15

Quality Assurance in Nuclear Medicine

OUTLINE

The Scintillation Gamma Camera
Quality Control Procedures for Imaging Equipment
  Energy Resolution and Photopeaking
  Counting Rate Limits
  Field Uniformity
  Spatial Resolution and Spatial Linearity
  Sensitivity
  Multiple-Window Spatial Registration
Quality Assurance of Spect Cameras
  Uniformity Correction Flood
  Center of Rotation
  Pixel Size

SPECT Quality Control during and after Patient Procedures
Positron Emission Tomography
Positron Emission Tomography/Computed Tomography Systems
Quality Control of Nonimaging Equipment
  Gas-Filled Detectors
    Ion-Detecting Radiation Detectors
    Geiger–Müller Meters
    Dose Calibrator
  Nonimaging Scintillation Detectors
Quality Assurance in the Radiopharmacy

Sealed Radioactive Source
Molybdenum-99/Technetium-99
Radionuclide Generator
Radiopharmaceuticals
Radiation Protection of Nuclear Medicine Personnel
  Personnel Monitoring
  Area Monitors
  Radioactivity Signposting
  Package Shipment, Receipt, and Opening
  Infection and Radiation Exposure Control
Radiopharmaceutical Administration

Nuclear medicine technology is a scientific and clinical discipline involving the diagnostic, therapeutic, and investigative use of radionuclides. The nuclear medicine professional performs a variety of responsibilities in a typical day, including formulating, dispensing, and administering radiopharmaceuticals; performing in vivo and in vitro laboratory procedures; acquiring, processing, and analyzing patient studies on a computer; performing all daily equipment testing; preparing the patient for the studies; operating the imaging and nonimaging equipment; and maintaining a radiation safety program. Because of the variety of responsibilities in the nuclear medicine department, **The Joint Commission** (TJC) has recognized the necessity for an established quality assurance program in nuclear medicine. TJC states that "There shall be quality control policies and procedures governing nuclear medicine activities that assure diagnostic and therapeutic reliability and safety of the patients and personnel" (Accreditation manual for hospitals, 1993). The **American College of Radiology** (ACR) also offers accreditation of nuclear medicine departments and mandates that certain quality assurance procedures be performed. This chapter discusses the many quality assurance procedures routinely performed in nuclear medicine. In the summer of 2008, Congress passed the Medicare Improvements for Patients and Providers Act of 2008, which mandates that any nonhospital institution performing advanced diagnostic services (such as nuclear medicine) must be accredited by a Centers for Medicare & Medicaid Services (CMS) designated accrediting organization to receive federal funding (Medicare reimbursement). As of the writing of this edition, CMS has approved three national accreditation organizations: ACR, the Intersocietal Accreditation Commission, and TJC. This rule affects providers of magnetic resonance imaging, computed tomography (CT), **positron emission tomography** (PET), and nuclear medicine imaging services for Medicare beneficiaries on an outpatient basis. The accreditation applies only to the suppliers of the images and

not to the physician's interpretation of the image. The Consumer Assurance of Radiologic Excellence bill (discussed in Chapter 1) if passed, would make similar requirements for hospital-based facilities. Therefore, accreditation programs are becoming mandatory for nuclear medicine departments to succeed.

THE SCINTILLATION GAMMA CAMERA

The scintillation **gamma camera** was first developed by Hal Anger in 1958 and has undergone many changes in design and electrical sophistication since its inception. However, the basic components of the gamma camera remain the same (Fig. 15-1) (Anger, 1958). The camera

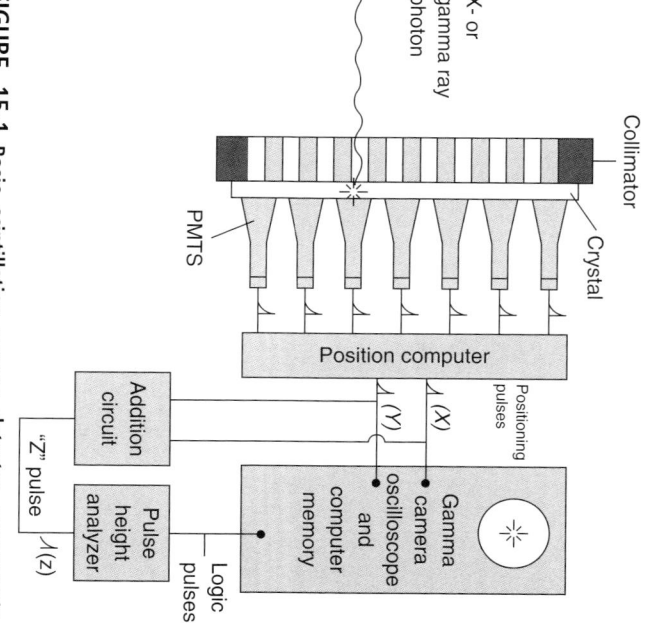

FIGURE 15-1 Basic scintillation camera detector components. PMTS, photomultiplier tubes. *From Thrall and Ziessman (1995).*

CHAPTER 15 Quality Assurance in Nuclear Medicine

consists of a circular or rectangular detector mounted on a gantry, which allows flexible manipulation around a patient, and electronic processing and display components. In addition, the camera system is interfaced to a computer to control study acquisition, analysis, and display. The detector head contains a thallium-activated sodium iodide (NaI(T1)) crystal, **photomultiplier tubes** (PMTs), preamplifiers, a position energy circuit, a pulse height analyzer, and a display mechanism.

Because radiation is a random process, gamma rays are not easy to control. The energy of the ionizing gamma radiation is too high to be deflected like visible light. However, the gamma **photon** can be directed through holes in a **collimator** while it blocks tangential or scattered photons. For a resolving image to be obtained, the collimator must be placed on the face of the detector head; this placement allows the desirable gamma photons to pass through to the NaI(T1) crystal. A collimator is a lead-filtering device that consists of holes through which a gamma photon can pass. These holes are separated by lead septa (Fig. 15-2). The photons that are not absorbed or scattered by the lead septa pass straight through to the NaI(T1) crystal and subsequently create an image of the isotope distribution from the patient. With high-energy photons, thicker lead septa are required to prevent scatter from degrading the image.

Collimators are available from several manufacturers. The collimator chosen for a patient study depends on the isotope energy and resolution required for the specific diagnostic procedure. Collimators commonly used in nuclear medicine include low-, medium-, and high-energy parallel hole; high-resolution parallel hole; high-sensitivity parallel hole; general all-purpose parallel hole; pinhole; and converging and diverging collimators (Early and Sodee, 1995). Because collimators are made specifically to operate within a gamma photon's energy range, a nuclear medicine department must have collimators suitable for several types of applications. The most common type used for diagnostic studies is the parallel-hole collimator. The parallel-hole collimator is preferred because it directs photons from a patient onto the scintillation crystal without varying the image. Once the photon passes through the collimator, it reaches the NaI(T1) **scintillation crystal** and is converted to light. The number of light photons produced is directly proportional to the energy of the gamma photon. Typically, 30 photons are produced per kiloelectron volt (keV) of energy (Murray and Ell, 1994). The NaI(T1) crystals vary in diameter, shape, and thickness. Changing the parameters of the crystal affects sensitivity or resolution (i.e., if sensitivity is increased by the use of a thicker crystal, then the resolution is compromised and vice versa). The NaI(T1) crystal is hygroscopic and extremely sensitive to sudden temperature changes. The environment of the gamma camera must remain stable, and precautions must be taken to prevent moisture from entering the NaI(T1) crystal and sudden temperature shifts (Early and Sodee, 1995). In addition, an accidental impact may cause the crystal to crack.

The scintillation, or light, photon interacts with the PMT. The light generated in the NaI(T1) crystal is then converted to electrical signals. The electrons produced are amplified and accelerated a million-fold in the PMT system. After conversion to an electrical pulse, a position circuit produces X and Y position signals, which are directly related to the location of the photon interaction on the NaI(T1) crystal. Because of the high potential of

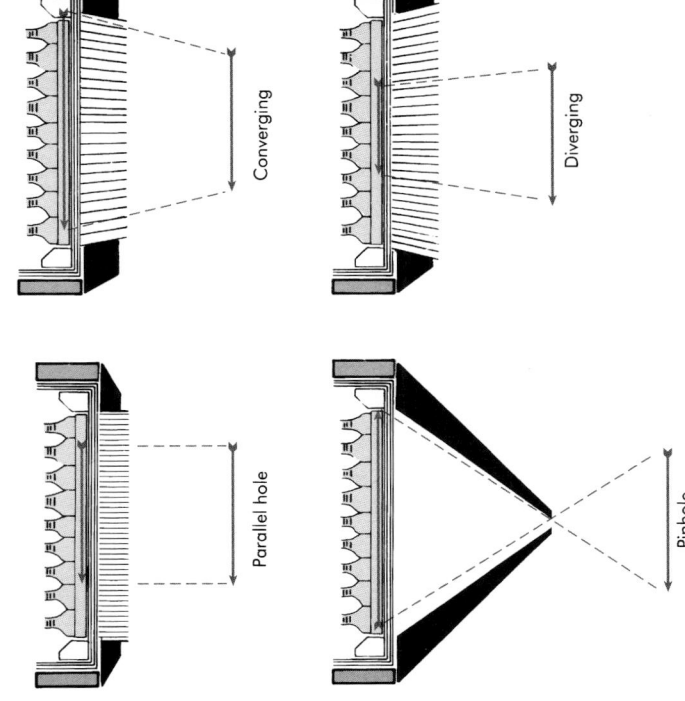

FIGURE 15-2 Four common types of collimators used on gamma cameras. *From Bernier et al. (1997).*

ionizing radiation interacting with matter, not all of the gamma photons detected by the NaI(Tl) crystal are the original primary gamma photons of interest. The interactions with matter from the patient and through the camera system can cause scatter radiation. Too much scatter radiation can cause degradation in the resolution of the final image. It is therefore possible to electronically exclude undesirable photons by only accepting the gamma ray photons above a certain energy.

The discrimination and selection of the gamma photon are performed with a **pulse height analyzer** (PHA). The PHA can be preset to accept only specific energy signals from the detector. The gamma photon energy required is specified by creating an energy "window" in the PHA. The energy window designates lower and upper limits of the gamma photon energy of interest. The model and age of equipment determine how a window is set; three different methods can be used. A threshold window may be set with a window reading above it; the reading is usually expressed in a percentage of total kiloelectron volts of the gamma energy in question. A midline energy may be set at the energy of the gamma ray or at the maximum count position of the voltage or gain adjustment. The percent window is then applied above and below this midpoint or peak. Finally, some instruments allow setting window thresholds at any position, including overlapping energies and multiple discrete windows for multiple isotope studies. Multiple windows also may be set up for those radionuclides that emit more than one gamma ray (e.g., thallium-201, indium-111, gallium-67). The signal is then sent to a display controller to produce a numeric display and an image. The display can occur simultaneously on a cathode-ray tube, a scalar, a film, and a computer screen. Many camera systems can display an analog or a digital image, or both. An analog camera allows the image to be displayed directly onto film in a cassette with or without the use of a computer. The analog camera also may be interfaced to a computer that simultaneously collects the image in the computer and displays it digitally. Finally, a digital camera digitizes the output of each PMT to create a digital image.

Various gamma camera configurations are available. The gamma camera detector may have a small or large field of imaging capability. The detector also may be circular or rectangular. In addition, the gamma camera system may hold one, two, or three detectors. These configurations are better known as single-, dual-, or triple-head cameras. In addition, some gamma cameras are fixed, whereas others are mobile. The scintillation gamma camera system is a complex mechanism accompanied by a variety of components that are crucial to producing a reliable and factual clinical image. The quality of the nuclear medicine image is determined by a variety of parameters. These parameters must be perpetually evaluated to guarantee that the image the physician is interpreting is accurate and truly diagnostic of the patient's pathologic condition.

According to the National Electrical Manufacturers Association (NEMA), 12 acceptance test standards are performed at the factory on all gamma cameras (Murphy, 1987; National Electrical Manufacturers Association, 1980, 1986). Box 15-1 lists the tests that are performed. The quality control measures taken at the factory ensure the good working condition of the new system. However, once the gamma cameras are in the nuclear medicine department, it is impractical and sometimes impossible for all of the NEMA standard acceptance tests to be performed (Sorenson and Phelps, 1987). However, the quality control procedures listed in Table 15-1 are required by TJC (Accreditation manual for hospitals, 1993) and regulatory agencies and are to be performed routinely (Rao et al., 1986). The quality control procedures performed on all imaging equipment ensure that the patient's diagnostic study is safe and accurate.

QUALITY CONTROL PROCEDURES FOR IMAGING EQUIPMENT

Energy Resolution and Photopeaking

Before any quality control or patient procedure, the correct energy setting for the radionuclide being used must be selected and the primary gamma ray energy,

BOX 15-1 NEMA Acceptance Tests for Scintillation Cameras (SPECT)

Intrinsic Spatial Resolution
Intrinsic Energy Resolution
Intrinsic Field Uniformity
Intrinsic Count Rate Performance
Intrinsic Spatial Linearity
Multiple Spatial Registration
Sensitivity
Angular Variation of Spatial Position
Angular Variation of Flood Field Uniformity and Sensitivity
Reconstructed System Spatial Resolution
Spatial Resolution with and without Scatter
System Count Rate Performance with Scatter

From NEMA (1986). NEMA, National Electrical Manufacturers Association; SPECT, single-photon emission computerized tomography; Intrinsic Spatial Resolution.

TABLE 15-1 Gamma Camera Quality Control

Quality Control Procedure	Frequency
Peaking	Daily and before each new radionuclide used
Counting rate limits	Daily
Field uniformity	Daily, after repair
Spatial resolution	Weekly, after repair
Spatial linearity	Weekly, after repair
Sensitivity	Quarterly

CHAPTER 15 Quality Assurance in Nuclear Medicine

or **photopeak**, centered around an energy window. The quality control is performed daily, either manually or automatically, depending on the manufacturer's specifications. The PHA is centered about the photopeak(s) of the radionuclide of interest, usually with a 5–10% window. This is generally referred to as "peaking" the camera. It is accomplished by adjusting the baseline window setting of the PHA around the specific energy of the gamma ray. For example, **technetium-99m** (^{99m}Tc) is used daily in a nuclear medicine department. The primary gamma ray of ^{99m}Tc has an energy of 140 keV. The window generally used for imaging is 20% around 140 keV; therefore, reserving a 20% window "tells" the PHA to accept only gamma photons with energies from 126 to 154 keV and to center the photopeak at 140 keV. The camera must be peaked before any radionuclide is used.

Because radioactive decay is random, each step in converting the radiation to an electrical current is subject to random error. The **spectrum** (curve) of the radionuclide of interest is not a straight line representing complete absorption of the gamma ray, but a Gaussian distribution resulting from random error, Compton scattering, or material attenuation (Fig. 15-3). The light photons emitted by the NaI(Tl) crystal are given off in all directions with random probability. The **energy resolution** can then be expressed as the spread, or width, of the spectrum divided by the center photopeak. The spread of the spectrum or the full width at half maximum (FWHM) measurement is the energy range of the widest width of the spectrum, which is halfway down from the photopeak (Fig. 15-4). The energy resolution is calculated as follows:

$$\text{Percent energy resolution} = \frac{\text{FWHM at half maximum}}{\text{Photopeak center}} \times 100$$

The narrower the curve, the better is the energy resolution of the detector. A good energy resolution is between 8% and 12%, which enables the camera system to better discern gamma rays with close energies. A reliable energy resolution is significant because it represents the system's ability to accurately depict two separate events in space, time, or energy. The ability of a system to detect separate radiation events becomes clinically relevant, especially when used for in vitro or in vivo counting, which potentially leads to a patient's clinical diagnosis. Performing a test of energy resolution also verifies that scatter rejection is sufficient to provide optimal contrast in clinical studies.

Counting Rate Limits

The sensitivity (counting ability) of a gamma camera generally decreases with increased amounts of activity. If the activity is too high, the detector is "paralyzed" and cannot count. The system's inability to count is referred to as *dead time*. Dead time describes the duration the detector requires to process the ionizing events as they occur in the NaI(Tl) crystal. The manufacturer's specification of the **count rate** limit per second states that the observed count rate through a 20% window should not exceed 20% of the counts lost as a result of dead time (Greer et al., 1985). The electronic circuitry of most contemporary gamma cameras reaches counting limits of 120,000–150,000 counts per second before experiencing a 20% loss because of dead time (Henkin et al., 1996). Before any quality control procedure is performed, the count rate of the radioactive point or flood source must be determined to ensure that the counts per second do not exceed the manufacturer's specifications. Once the count rate is determined to be within the counting rate limits for that gamma camera, only then can the quality

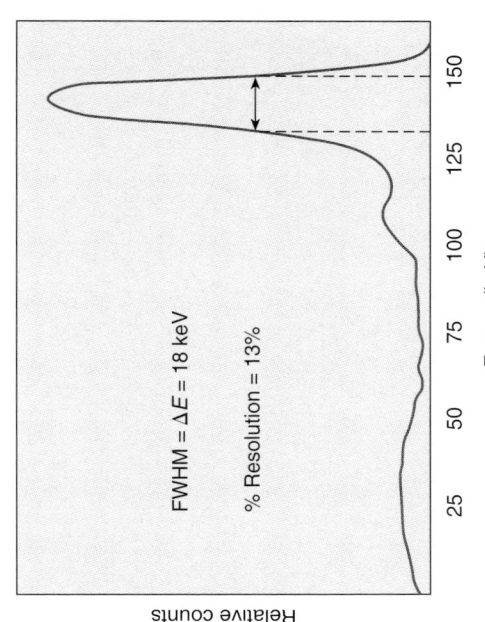

FIGURE 15-3 Energy spectrum of the radionuclide technetium-99m (^{99m}Tc). kcts, kilocounts; keV, kiloelectron volt.

Energy resolution = % 11.544
Y T1/2 (UP) = keV 131.96
Y T1/2 (DWN) = keV 148.12
^{99m}Tc Peak is at : 140.67 keV

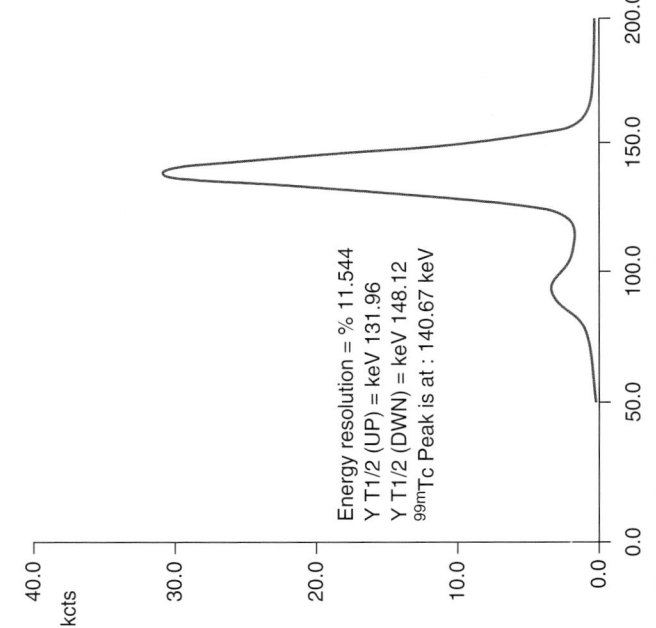

FIGURE 15-4 Energy spectrum of technetium-99m (^{99m}Tc). The full width at half maximum (FWHM) is 18 kiloelectron volts (keV). The energy resolution is 13%. ΔE, Change in energy. *From Thrall and Ziessman (1995).*

FWHM = ΔE = 18 keV
% Resolution = 13%

images and loss of counts (Henkin et al., 1996). If the counts-per-second rate is too high and it is necessary to decrease the count rate, the radioactive source is repositioned at an increased distance, or the amount of radioactivity in the source is decreased.

Field Uniformity

Field uniformity refers to the gamma camera's ability to detect a uniform source of radiation and responds exactly the same at any location within the imaging field. The uniform response of the gamma camera results in an image with an even distribution of radioactivity (Fig. 15-5). The uniformity of the gamma camera depends on the uniform response of the NaI(Tl) crystal and the PMTs. The response of each PMT must match that of all the other PMTs. In addition, the counting window must be centered around the photopeak. Mispositioning the photopeak may alter the field uniformity (Fig. 15-6). Nonuniformity also may arise because of, for example, the use of the incorrect photopeak for a specific radionuclide, a malfunctioning PMT, a cracked NaI(Tl) crystal, or total system malfunction (Fig. 15-7). Because the uniformity of the camera determines the accuracy of a patient's image and, ultimately, the diagnosis, it is imperative that the field uniformity or flood be performed daily. This quality control procedure must be performed before any patient studies.

The measurement of the daily field uniformity can be performed intrinsically or extrinsically. Intrinsic uniformity is the measurement of the uniformity of the gamma camera detector with no collimator in place. The procedure is generally performed with a point source of radioactivity placed at a distance equivalent to four to five diameters of the detector's field of imaging (Scintillation Camera Acceptance Testing and Performance Evaluation, 1980). Caution should be taken that the counts-per-second rate does not exceed that particular system's limits. The intrinsic uniformity determines the integrity of the NaI(Tl) crystal and its electronic components. The phenomenon known as *edge packing* can show up as a bright rim of activity around the perimeter of the flood. To prevent edge packing, most manufacturers provide a lead-shielded ring that masks the effect when attached to the edge of the camera head. These tests also monitor a scintillation unit for electronic problems and crystal deterioration (hydration).

Extrinsic uniformity testing is also the measurement of the camera's field uniformity; however, it is performed with the collimator (which is used for imaging) in place. A uniform flood source of radioactivity is placed directly on the collimated camera (Fig. 15-8). The two commonly used extrinsic radioactive sources are (1) an acrylic plastic (Plexiglas) container filled with water and generally 1–10 mCi of ^{99m}Tc and (2) a solid-sealed 10 mCi cobalt-57 sheet (Steves, 1992). The ^{99m}Tc liquid-filled acrylic plastic (Plexiglas) source does have

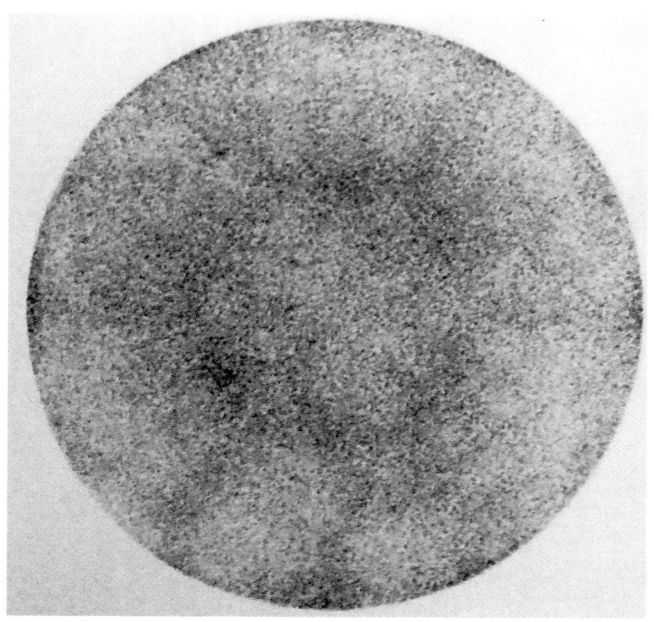

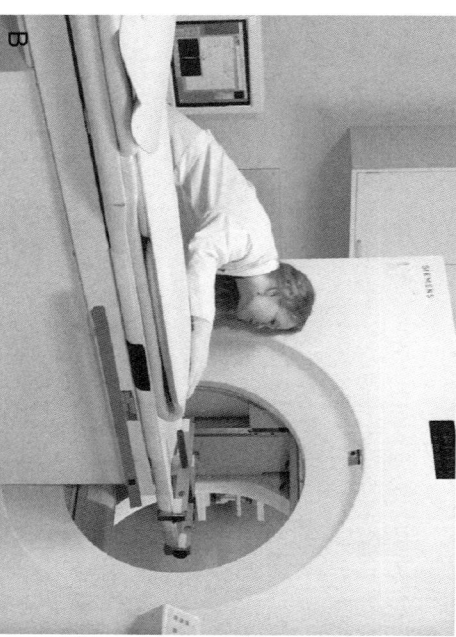

FIGURE 15-5 **A**, Field uniformity flood and resolution pattern. **B**, Nuclear medicine technologist preparing to obtain a field flood uniformity on a dual-head camera system. **B**, *Courtesy Northwest Community Hospital, Arlington Heights, IL.*

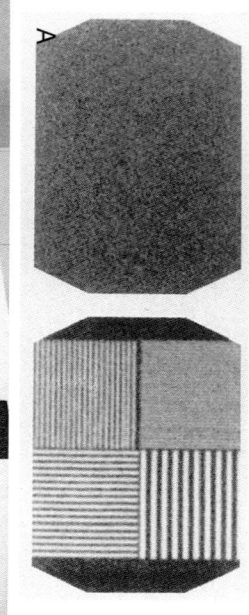

FIGURE 15-6 Mispositioned photopeak resulting in a nonuniform flood.

control testing continue. The procedures to determine count rate are simple: The radioactive source is placed at the appropriate location necessary for quality control, and the time/count scalar continuously displays the counts per second. Count rates that exceed the gamma camera's design limits can result in degradation of the

CHAPTER 15 Quality Assurance in Nuclear Medicine

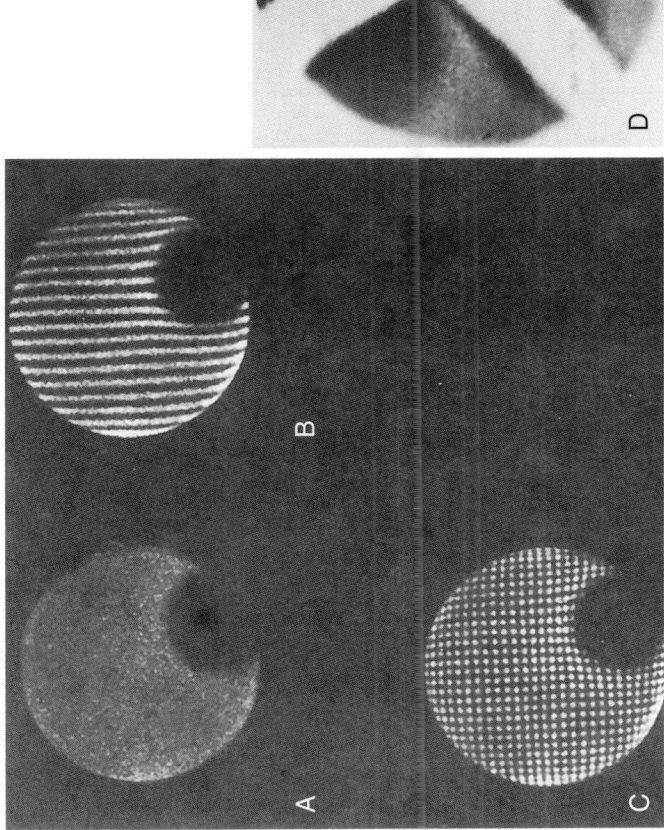

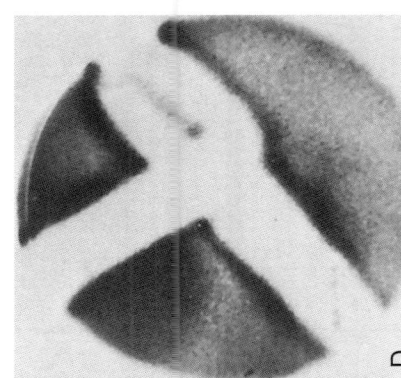

FIGURE 15-7 **A**, Example of a nonfunctioning photomultiplier tube (PMT) seen in the flood field; **B**, the orthogonal hole resolution pattern; and **C**, the parallel-line equal space (PLES) phantom. **D**, Examples of nonuniform flood fields caused by a cracked crystal. **A**, from Rollo FD: Nuclear medicine physics, instrumentation, and agents, St Louis, 1997, Mosby; **B**, from Early and Sodee (1995).

and equipment; thus, the technologist's risk of radiation exposure is increased. The extrinsic uniformity, in addition to evaluating the NaI(Tl) crystal and electrical components, allows visualization of a defect or damage to the collimator. Annual inspection of collimators with extrinsic field uniformity testing is recommended and should become a routine part of any quality assurance program. A defect in a collimator will visualize in an image as photopenic areas (Fig. 15-9).

A flood field image of 1–3 million is generally acquired whether the intrinsic or extrinsic method is used. However, it is recommended that the quality control for each gamma camera should be carefully evaluated according to the manufacturer's specifications and the department's needs. The quality control test used should remain consistent. The consistency allows visual inspection of any nonuniformity of the camera system to be easily monitored. The uniformity flood must be performed daily on every piece of imaging equipment. Visual inspection of the flood and comparison with that of the previous days reveal any subtle changes in uniformity that are not always apparent by looking at one image. Any areas of nonuniformity of the detector must be noted and repaired before clinical use. In addition to the performance of daily floods, the TJC quality assurance program recommends that every piece of equipment also has a preventive maintenance program performed biannually (Accreditation manual for hospitals, 1993).

Gamma cameras of the late 1970s until the present have been developed to correct some of the nonuniformities seen in older images. A microprocessor built into the gamma camera generates a correction factor for each

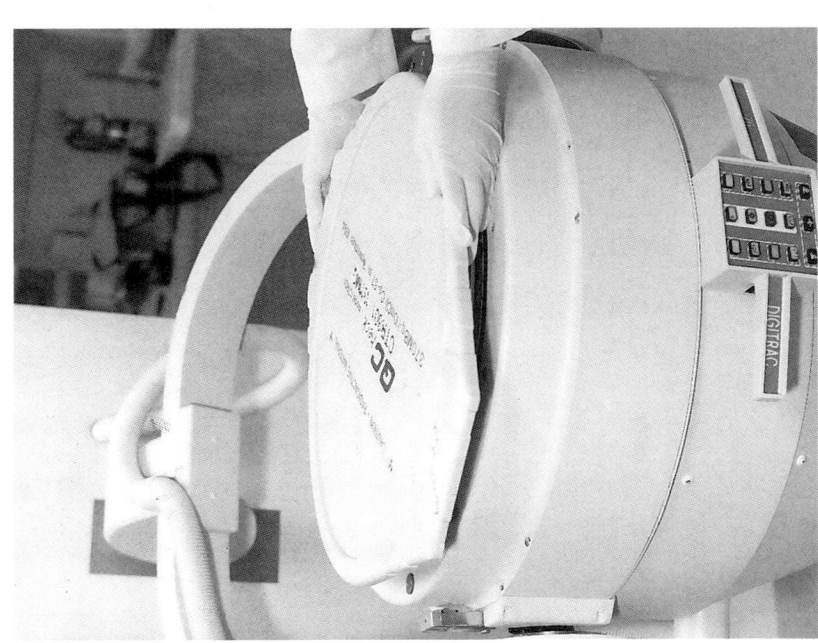

FIGURE 15-8 Extrinsic flood uniformity with a cobalt-57 (^{57}Co) sheet source.

some disadvantages. It must be manually filled with technetium and thoroughly mixed to secure even distribution of the radionuclide. The procedure increases the risk of radioactive contamination to the technologist

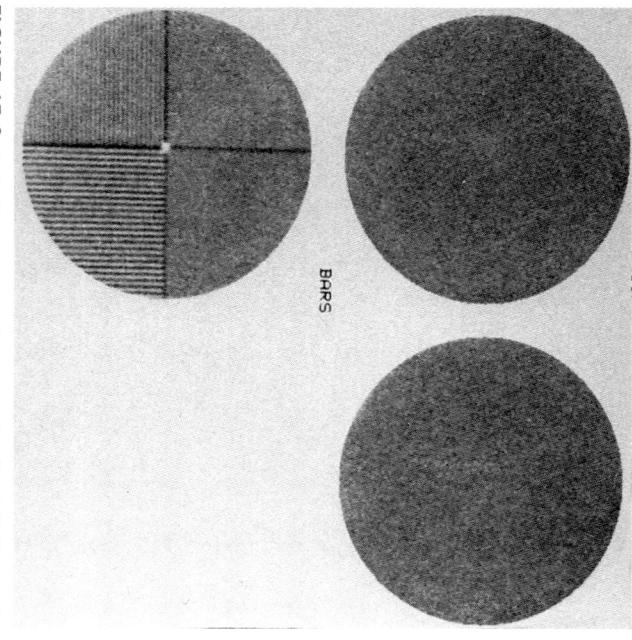

FIGURE 15-9 Note the photopenic area in the flood field and the resolution bar pattern. These are due to collimator damage.

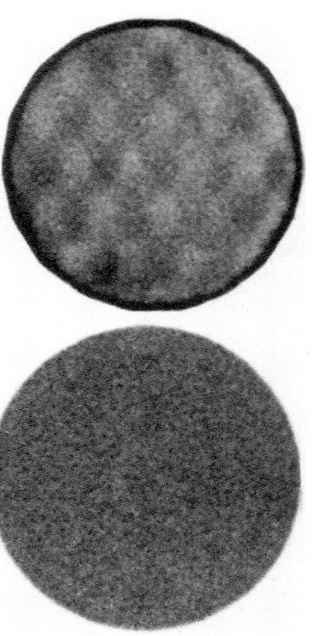

FIGURE 15-10 An uncorrected and a microprocessor-corrected uniformity flood.

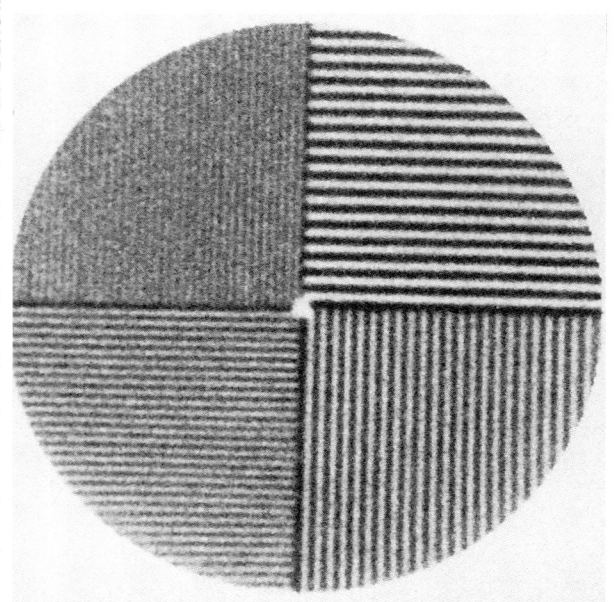

FIGURE 15-11 Spatial resolution with a four-quadrant bar pattern. Four images are obtained 90 degrees apart.

pixel of the matrix, according to the variation in counts of different pixels (Saha, 1993). Fig. 15-10 demonstrates the difference between an uncorrected and corrected uniformity flood. Subsequently, when patient images are generated, the correction factors are applied to each pixel; thus, nonuniformity is reduced (Saha, 1993).

Spatial Resolution and Spatial Linearity

Spatial resolution is the gamma camera's ability to reproduce small details of a radioactive distribution (Greer et al., 1985). The smaller the details that a camera can reproduce, the better the spatial resolution is for that system. The spatial resolution quality control procedure is required to be performed a minimum of once a week on every imaging system. The quality control determines the camera's ability to detect and image fine differences of a radioactive distribution that exist in closely spaced areas. In essence, the gamma camera detects the small abnormalities of different radioactive concentrations that may subsequently be seen on patient images. For the exact spatial resolution of a gamma camera system to be determined, one of the following resolution test pattern transmission sources must be used: four-quadrant bar phantom with varying size bars, parallel-line equal space (PLES) bar pattern with constant bar and spacing sizes, or an orthogonal hole phantom with varying sizes of holes (Bernier et al., 1997; Eisner, 1985).

The manufacturer of every gamma camera system determines the intrinsic spatial resolution specific for the gamma camera. This is important when choosing the type and size of a transmission resolution pattern. For example, if the manufacturer specifications say that gamma camera 1 has an intrinsic spatial resolution of 3 mm, then the four-quadrant bar phantom used must have bars between 2 and 5 mm. The resolution pattern is placed on the collimator or camera for an intrinsic resolution quality control test and on the collimator for an extrinsic resolution quality control test. The resolution pattern is placed in the center of the field of view (FOV) in such a way that the center of the pattern is directly over the center of the detector. A ^{99m}Tc or cobalt-57 (^{57}Co) sheet source is then placed on the resolution pattern so that the radioactivity is transmitted through the resolution pattern. It is recommended that when the four-quadrant bar pattern is used, four images should be obtained at 90° between positions (Bernier et al., 1997; Henkin et al., 1996). This allows verification of the spatial resolution in the X and Y positions and allows the bars barely resolved to be evaluated in each quadrant of the FOV (Fig. 15-11).

The PLES bar resolution pattern is sometimes preferable to the four-quadrant pattern. A PLES pattern is preferable for testing spatial resolution because it is specifically designed to minimize the number of images that are actually required to evaluate resolution (Henkin et al., 1996).

determines the accuracy of the dose calibrator's response to measure a wide range of activities. The dose calibrator should be able to measure a full range of activities from microcuries to millicuries. *Two methods are readily used and accepted by the NRC.* The first linearity test requires assaying a decaying source of ^{99m}Tc sequentially over 3–5 days. The readings are compared with the actual decay of ^{99m}Tc at the same time intervals. The second method involves the use of precalibrated lead sleeves that are placed sequentially over the same source. The advantage of using the lead sleeves is that the procedure only takes about 5 minutes and results in a much lower level of radiation exposure to the technologist. The linearity test is performed at installation, at 3-month intervals, and after any repair. *The observed values in either method must be within 10% of the actual calculated activities.*‡

Nonimaging Scintillation Detectors

Along with the scintillation gamma camera systems mentioned previously, there are also nonimaging systems found in nuclear medicine that use the NaI(Tl) crystal and detect radiation with the same basic principle of scintillation. The **scintillation detectors** used in nuclear medicine have many functions. The single-channel or **multichannel analyzers** (well counters) are scintillation detectors that are used to count blood and urine samples obtained from in vitro procedures such as red cell mass and plasma volume determinations and Schilling tests. In addition to in vitro patient studies, well counters are used to count the quality control **chromatography** strips required to evaluate radionuclides and radiopharmaceuticals (Zimmer, 1991). The advantage of the multichannel over the single-channel analyzer is that samples with multiple radioisotopes presenting low to high energy can be analyzed simultaneously. In addition, because the spectrum display is directly proportional to the radionuclide energy, it is possible to determine the unknown radiation that might be present in some contamination. It is also possible to see at a glance the whole spectrum and proper peaking over the energy of interest. This is important when performing NRC-required, daily, area-wipe surveys to locate, identify, and quantitate any contamination. The quality control procedures required for a scintillation detector are listed in Table 15-3.

Calibration is performed to determine and preset the correct operating voltage that is necessary for the detector to place the gamma energy peak in the center of the spectrum window. This results in achieving the highest and most accurate count rate. Generally, a long-lived radionuclide such as ^{137}Cs, with a gamma photon energy of 662 keV, is used. The voltage is adjusted so that the pulse height of 662 keV is at the center of the spectrum and the window is spaced equally above and below 662 keV.

TABLE 15-3 Scintillation Detector Quality Control

Quality Control Procedure	Frequency
Energy calibration	Daily
Peaking	Daily and before each new radionuclide used
Background	Daily and before each new radionuclide used
Constancy	Daily
Instrument calibration	Annually, after repair
Energy resolution	Annually, after repair
Efficiency	Annually, after repair
Chi-square test (reproducibility)	Quarterly, weekly recommended

Because the scintillation detectors count a variety of radionuclides (e.g., ^{99m}Tc, iodine-123, iodine-125, iodine-131, ^{57}Co), the detector must be photopeaked before each new radionuclide is counted. Once this is accomplished, the detector's high voltage is adjusted properly for that specific radionuclide. When environmental samples are counted for contamination, windows are set wide to capture the gamma rays of all radionuclides that may be potentially released as contaminants. Matching the photopeaks on the spectrum to specific energies allows identification of the radionuclide in the sample.

A background measurement with no radionuclide present is taken to ensure that no contaminating radioactivity will affect the true counts. The background is taken for the same period that the sample is counted. The background counts must be subtracted from each sample's gross counts to obtain the true, or net, counts (i.e., net counts = gross counts − background counts). A new background count must be taken for each radionuclide and for each separate procedure to obtain accurate clinical data.

A constancy test is performed daily to verify the stability of the detector. A long-lived source such as ^{137}Cs is counted, and the counts per minute per microcurie are determined and compared with the counts per minute per microcurie at the time of calibration. A change of more than 10% indicates that repair is necessary (Graham et al., 1996).

An annual calibration is performed to regulate the gain and high-voltage settings in such a way that dial settings of the channels read directly to the energy kiloelectron volt of the radionuclide. A ^{137}Cs source is used in the detector, and the energy peak is set on 662 keV with a 5% window. The voltage and gain are adjusted until the center, or photopeak, is exactly centered on 662 keV.

The energy resolution can be thought of as the ability of the scintillation detector to accurately discern two different energies as separate. Energy resolution quality control is discussed in the section on quality control of imaging equipment. To review, the energy resolution can then be expressed as the spread or width of the spectrum divided by the center photopeak. The spread of the spectrum or the FWHM is the energy range of the widest

The energy resolution of most scintillation systems that use ^{137}Cs is between 8% and 12% (Bernier et al., 1997).

The efficiency of a counting detector is measuring the sensitivity of the detector. It is expressed as the observed count rate divided by the disintegration rate of a radioactive sample (Sorenson and Phelps, 1987).

$$\text{Percent energy resolution} = \frac{\text{FWHM at half maximum}}{\text{Photopeak center}} \times 100$$

$$\text{Percent efficiency} = \frac{\text{Counts per minute}}{\text{Disintegrations per minute}}$$

This concept is important because counts per minute must be converted into **disintegrations per minute** (dpm) for the technologist to know whether regulatory requirements are being met for keeping environmental contamination within specific contamination limits for both fixed and removable contamination. For the same sample activity and geometry, every instrument registers a different count per minute on the basis of several detector design factors; therefore, an efficiency factor must be determined for each instrument used to count in counts per minute and convert to disintegrations per minute.

Radioactive decay of an atom is a random process, so when a radioactive source is said to undergo a number of disintegrations per second, the value represents only the average. Because the number of disintegrations per unit time varies, it can be expected that the counts obtained also vary. The variation to be expected when counting the same sample is due to random error. A statistical test called the **chi-square test** is used to evaluate the reliability of the detector. The results of the chi-square test indicate whether the error that exists in counting is due to randomness. If the error is due to some other problem such as a technical or mechanical error, the detector must be serviced before clinical use. The chi-square quality control test is easy to perform. A radioactive sample is counted 10 times for 1 minute each time. The sample must be placed at a distance from the detector that results in a minimum of 10,000 counts. The 10,000 counts are necessary to obtain good statistical data within 1% SD. The data are then used to determine the chi-square value:

$$\text{Chi-square} = \frac{\text{Sum}(x_i - \text{mean})^2}{\text{Mean}}$$

where x_i = individual count rates

The result is then located on the table of chi-square values to determine the probability that the discrepancy between the observed and expected frequency is due to random error. Most scintillation detectors are computer driven and maintain the statistical programs that automatically calculate the chi-square values.

Another NaI(Tl) scintillation detector used in nuclear medicine is the thyroid uptake probe. The thyroid probe is used clinically to determine the function of the patient's thyroid. A percent uptake of an ingested radioisotope of iodine is calculated. The thyroid uptake probe is a multichannel analyzer with a flat-face crystal and PMT encased in an open-field collimator that faces the patient's thyroid during the procedure. The collimator is generally 20–30 cm long, which is the length required to obtain the proper counting geometry of the patient's thyroid. All of the quality control procedures required for a scintillation detector are performed on the thyroid probe. However, because distance and geometry are crucial in measuring a patient's iodine uptake, a thyroid phantom is used in all daily quality control procedures (Fig. 15-18). The thyroid phantom has been designed to mimic the location of a thyroid in a patient. The phantom ensures that the quality control procedures are accurate and can be related to the patient study.

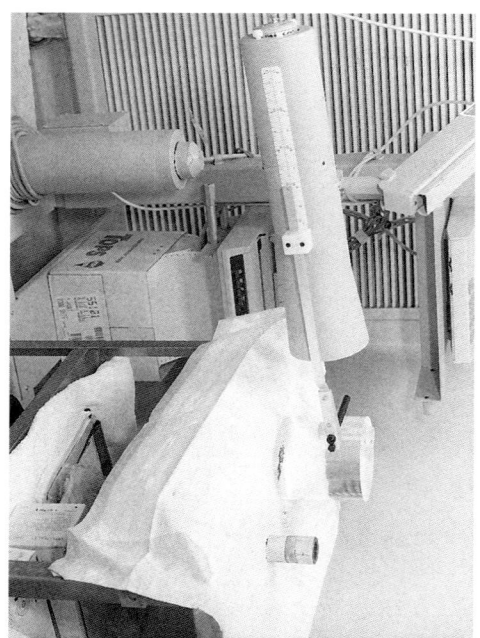

FIGURE 15-18 Thyroid probe quality control with a neck phantom.

QUALITY ASSURANCE IN THE RADIOPHARMACY

Sealed Radioactive Source

The sealed sources used in the previously mentioned calibrations and for calibration of other nonimaging and imaging equipment must be tested for any leakage of radioactive material. The NRC requires that all photon-emitting sealed sources containing 100 μCi or more be tested for leakage biannually (USNRC Regulatory Guide, 1977). Any sealed sources with more than 0.005 μCi of removable activity per test must immediately be removed, properly stored, and reported to the NRC (USNRC Title 10, 2013). In addition, the NRC requires that all sealed sources be inventoried and surveyed quarterly for radiation exposure.

Molybdenum-99/Technetium-99 Radionuclide Generator

The radionuclide generator system, a long-lived parent yielding to a shorter-lived daughter, allows the production of useful radionuclides for clinical use. The combination of half-lives of the radionuclides in the generator system makes the shipping of radionuclides from a commercial nuclear pharmacy to a hospital more cost-effective; deliveries are required once a week rather than daily. Most of the radiopharmaceuticals prepared by the nuclear medicine technologist are labeled with ^{99m}Tc. The most commonly used generator system in hospitals and clinics is the **molybdenum-99/technetium-99m** ($^{99}Mo/^{99m}Tc$) system. The $^{99}Mo/^{99m}Tc$ generator is an alumina ion-exchange column onto which ^{99}Mo, the parent, has a high affinity. Subsequently, ^{99m}Tc has a lower affinity to the column; therefore, the separation of ^{99m}Tc from the parent, ^{99}Mo, is simple. When saline solution is pulled through the alumina column by means of an evacuated collection vial, the daughter, ^{99m}Tc, is removed, or eluted, from the column. The technetium eluted is in the radiochemical form $^{99m}TcO_4^-$ (**technetium-99m pertechnetate**), and the ^{99m}Tc is in the valence state of +7. Quality control procedures are essential on the technetium eluent each time the generator is eluted, to ensure that the eluent does not contain any contaminants or impurities including **radionuclide impurity** of ^{99}Mo, molybdate, **chemical impurity** of Al^{+3}, alumina, or radiochemical impurity of **hydrolyzed reduced technetium** (HR-Tc).

A common contaminant found in the generator eluent is the parent, ^{99}Mo. The appearance of ^{99}Mo in the eluent is called *moly breakthrough*. If any ^{99}Mo is injected into a patient, the liver absorbs the ^{99}Mo and receives unnecessary radiation.

Testing for moly breakthrough is simple to perform. A lead container, which absorbs the ^{99m}Tc 140-keV energy but allows the passage of the higher-energy 740 and 780 keV ^{99}Mo photons, is used. The generator eluent vial is placed in the moly lead shield and assayed in the dose calibrator. The amount of ^{99}Mo contamination is calculated by dividing the total amount of ^{99}Mo assayed by the total amount of ^{99m}Tc. *The NRC allowable limit is 0.15 µCi of ^{99}Mo activity per 1 mCi of ^{99m}Tc activity at the time of injection of the administered dose* (USNRC Title 10, 2013). *This is critical because the concentration of $^{99}Mo/^{99m}Tc$ may creep up and exceed limits several hours after elution.*

The chemical impurity that can be present in the generator eluent is alumina, Al^{+3}, which comes from the ion-exchange column. The U.S. Pharmacopoeia (USP) has established that the Al^{+3} concentration limits not exceed 10 µg of Al^{+3} per milliliter eluent. Aurin tricarboxylic acid is used for colorimetric spot testing (Thrall and Ziessman, 1995). The color reaction for a standard alumina sample is compared with the generator eluate. The comparison is qualitative and made by visual inspection.

Excessive levels of aluminum can interfere with normal distribution of some radiopharmaceuticals.

In addition, the radiochemical impurity that may exist in the eluent solution is HR-Tc. Technetium that is eluted is expected to have a valence state of +7, which is the desired chemical form for most kit preparations. If the ^{99m}Tc is present in other forms, then the distribution of the final radiopharmaceutical product in a patient is altered. Unbound, or free, $^{99m}TcO_4^-$ accumulates in the stomach, thyroid gland, and salivary gland. ^{99m}Tc-colloidal uptake occurs in the reticuloendothelial system, especially the liver. The USP standard for the generator eluent is that 95% or more of the technetium activity be in the +7 valence state (Klingensmith et al., 1995).

Radiopharmaceuticals

Because radiopharmaceuticals are intended for diagnostic and therapeutic patient procedures, quality control procedures are crucial in ensuring the safety and effectiveness of these preparations (Zimmer, 1991). When a nuclear medicine department uses unit doses provided by a commercial nuclear pharmacy, the preparations undergo extensive quality control procedures by the manufacturer or the commercial nuclear pharmacy. However, many radiopharmaceutical preparations are prepared with lyophilized radiopharmaceutical preparation kits and short-lived radionuclides such as ^{99m}Tc. As a result, the absolute responsibility for the quality assurance of the radiopharmaceuticals lies with the radiopharmacist or the nuclear medicine technologist preparing the kits.

Whether the radiopharmaceuticals are prepared by commercial manufacturers or at the hospital nuclear pharmacy, they must be subjected to physiochemical and biologic testing including physical state examination and osmolality, pH, chemical, radionuclidic and radiochemical purity, sterility, and pyrogenicity testing (Zimmer, 1991).

Sterility represents the absence of metabolic products such as endotoxins in the final product. Sterility testing uses USP standard media such as thioglycollate and soybean casein digest media to determine the presence of bacteria and fungi in the radiopharmaceutical solution (Thrall and Ziessman, 1995). Because many radiopharmaceuticals are prepared just before patient administration, the sterility test must be performed retrospectively. Pyrogens or microorganism metabolites that may exist in the radiopharmaceutical solution can cause a fever if injected into a patient. The pyrogen test uses the USP limulus amebocyte lysate test to detect the presence of pyrogens.

The radiochemical and radionuclidic purity of a radiopharmaceutical may be assessed by many different methods including paper chromatography, thin layer chromatography, high-performance liquid chromatography, and gel electrophoresis (Robbins, 1984; Zimmer, 1991; Zimmer and Pavel, 1977; Zimmer and Spies, 1991). Because of the characteristics of short-lived radionuclides used in the preparation of radiopharmaceuticals, time is critical. Miniaturized chromatography procedures are used to evaluate the radiochemical purity of radiopharmaceuticals because they are rapid and easy to use (Webber et al., 1983; Zimmer and Pavel, 1977). The miniaturized chromatography system developed by Zimmer (Zimmer and Spies, 1991) uses a support medium such as thin-layer chromatography and a developing solvent to routinely evaluate radiopharmaceutical preparations subsequent to patient administration (Taukulis et al., 1979).

The chromatography procedures involve spotting the radiopharmaceutical being tested on the origin line of the respective paper strips and eluting the strips in the designated solvent system (Fig. 15-19). After solvent migration to the solvent front line, the strips are removed, cut at the cut line, and counted for activity with appropriate counting systems such as the dose calibrator or the well counter (Fig. 15-20). The labeling efficiency or the fraction of total radioactivity incorporated into the radiolabeled material is calculated by subtracting the sum of the fraction of the impurities of free technetium and HR-Tc from 100%.

Percent labeling efficiency = 100 − (Sum of all impurities).

The percent labeling efficacy for most radiopharmaceuticals should be more than 98% (TJC Accreditation Manual, 2013).

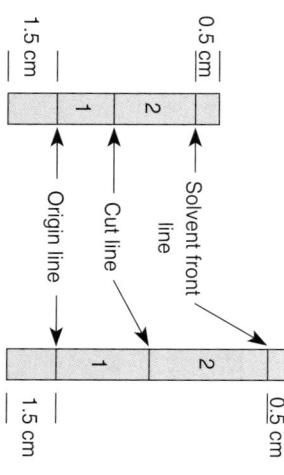

FIGURE 15-19 Eluting chromatography strips.

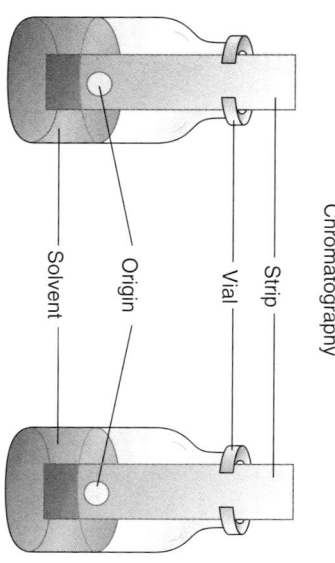

FIGURE 15-20 Typical chromatography strips.

Radiation Protection of Nuclear Medicine Personnel

Through mutual cooperation, several regulatory agencies control the radiation exposure of radiation workers in the United States. The Department of Transportation, the Environmental Protection Agency (EPA), OSHA, individual state nuclear safety agencies, and the U.S. Nuclear Regulatory Commission Council on Radiation Protection and Measurements determined and provided the radiation dose exposure recommendations used for establishing the regulations and statutes of the NRC (Bernier et al., 1997). Table 15-4 lists the current acceptable radiation dose limits for occupational radiation workers (USNRC Title 10, 2013).

To ensure that the occupational radiation worker maintains an exposure far below the federal limits, the radiology communities adhere to the philosophy that the radiation dose exposure be "as low as reasonably achievable," or ALARA (Bernier et al., 1997). The NRC states that the ALARA concept should maintain radiation doses to personnel working in radiation areas of a medical institution to less than 10% of the federal limits of occupational exposure (Bernier et al., 1997).

Personnel Monitoring. All radiation workers in the medical institution who may run the risk of exposure to ionizing radiation during routine duties must be provided with and wear a film badge dosimeter, **thermoluminescent dosimeter (TLD)**, or **optically stimulated luminescent dosimeter (OSL)** personnel monitoring device. The detector must be worn on the body part likely to receive the highest radiation exposure. It is recommended that the detector be worn between the shoulders and the waist. Nuclear medicine technologists or others who handle radionuclides or radiopharmaceuticals also must wear a ring or wrist radiation monitor (usually a TLD) so that radiation exposure of fingers and extremities can be estimated. A female technologist who has a declared pregnancy should be issued a second monitoring device to be worn at the waist area to determine any fetal dose. The average period that a radiation worker routinely wears the personnel monitoring device

TABLE 15-4 Nuclear Regulatory Commission Dose Equivalent Limits per Year

Anatomic Category	Dose Equivalent Limit/Year
Whole body, head, trunk, blood-forming organs, gonads, and lens of the eyes	50 rem (500 mSv)
Hands, forearms, feet, and ankles	5 rem (50 mSv)
Skin of whole body	30 rem (300 mSv)
Fetus of radiation worker	0.5 rem (5 mSv)*

mSv, Millisievert; rem, roentgen equivalent, man.
*Dose equivalent for entire gestation period.

CHAPTER 15 Quality Assurance in Nuclear Medicine

is recommended not to exceed 1 month for film badge dosimeters and OSLs and 3 months for TLDs. In addition, it is the responsibility of the radiation safety officer to review at least quarterly the results of personnel radiation monitoring and investigate and document any radiation dose exposure exceeding action Level II (30% of the federal limit; Regulatory Guide 8.7, 1992).

In addition to personnel monitoring, any individual handling certain amounts of radioiodine (10 CFR 35 315(a)(8)) must have a bioassay performed. The **bioassay** is performed to determine whether any iodine activity in the thyroid is due to ingestion or inhalation. The assay is performed with the thyroid uptake probe. The bioassay must be performed between 6 and 72 hours after handling for any individual dispensing, preparing, or administering a therapeutic dose of sodium iodide-131. Individuals who handle less than 30 mCi of iodine are required to undergo a bioassay each calendar quarter if it is volatile. The NRC recommends that corrective action be taken if the ^{131}I thyroid activity of the radiation worker exceeds 40 nCi.

Area Monitors. In addition to monitoring radiation exposure with personal dosimeters, individuals working in areas with radioactive materials also must monitor themselves before meals and before going home. The individuals can use a portable survey instrument such as a survey meter to determine any contamination to the body or clothing. In addition, each radiation work area must be surveyed daily to ensure that only background levels of radiation are present. If an area exceeds background radiation, it must be decontaminated. Because the survey meter is the best instrument to detect radiation but not quantitate or identify radionuclide contaminant, a daily wipe test also is required in any radiation areas. The wipe test is a survey designed to detect any removable radiation contamination by wiping the area to be evaluated with a cotton swab or some other absorbent paper such as filter paper. The wipe sample is analyzed in a scintillation detector such as a well counter or multichannel analyzer to determine the extent of the radionuclidic contamination. Although the NRC only requires a detector sensitive enough to detect any contamination of 2000 dpm, it recommends that if the wipe sample results are more than or equal to 200 dpm/100 cm^2, *the specific area must be decontaminated and checked again* (USNRC Regulatory Guide, 1977).

The NRC mandates that areas where radioactive gaseous materials are used such as the nuclear pharmacy, as well as rooms where xenon-133 lung ventilation studies are performed, have negative airflow pressure with respect to surrounding areas (USNRC Title 10, 2013). With this pressure, airborne activity that might be generated within the room can be removed through the exhaust system. The negative airflow pressure does not permit xenon-133 to passively diffuse into any surrounding areas. The exhaust must be a dedicated system

and provide enough ventilation to dilute and remove radioactive concentrations that may be released into the room (USNRC Regulatory Guide, 1977). The exhaust also must release at a distance away from the public such as the roof top and meet EPA regulations for effluents released. Quality control procedures must be performed to demonstrate that the airflow at the perimeters of these rooms is toward the room (Regulatory Guide 8.25, 1992). The airflow must be checked a minimum of every 6 months to demonstrate proper and unchanged ventilation.

Radioactivity Signposting. *Specific signs are required by the NRC* (Bernier et al, 1997; Early and Sodee, 1995; USNRC Regulatory Guide, 1977). They must be posted near the entrance to any room where radioactive material may be used or stored. This is done to inform anyone entering the area of the potential hazard of radiation exposure. Each sign must bear the three-bladed international warning symbol for ionizing radiation (Fig. 15-21). The three-bladed symbol can be either magenta, purple, or black on a yellow background. Four different signs are used depending on the amount of potential exposure, as listed in Table 15-5.

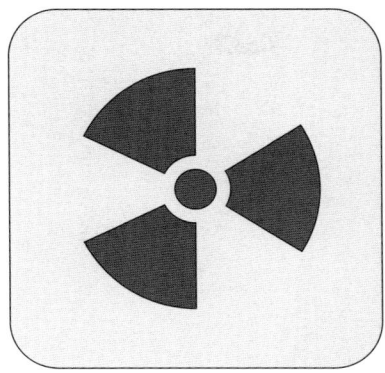

FIGURE 15-21 The three-bladed international warning symbol for ionizing radiation.

TABLE 15-5 Radiation Signs

Type of Sign	Radiation Exposure Potential
Caution, radioactive materials	Areas in which radioactive material is stored or used in amounts not exceeding 5 mrem in 1 h
Caution, radiation area	Areas in which an exposure could result in excess of 100 mrem in any 1 h
Caution, high radiation area	Areas in which an exposure could be >5 mrem in 1 h or >100 mrem in 5 consecutive days
Caution, airborne radioactivity area	Areas in which the airborne radioactivity level may exceed the restricted limit or may exceed 25% of the restricted area limit when averaged over 1 week

mrem, Millirem.

Package Shipment, Receipt, and Opening.

NRC Regulation Part 20 recommends that all radioactive materials be monitored on receipt or within 3 hours if received during normal working hours or within 18 hours if received after normal working hours (USNRC Title 10, 2013). A good quality assurance program recommends that any radioactive package be handled with disposable gloves, visually inspected, verified for contents, and checked for breakage or leaks. The radiation safety officer is to be notified of any irregularities. The package must then be monitored with a survey meter at the surface of the package and at 3 ft from the package. In addition, a wipe survey of the exterior surface is performed to determine any removable contamination present. *Any value in excess of 0.01 µCi/100 cm² of surface area tested is a reportable level and must be decontaminated.* In addition, exposure levels exceeding 200 mR/h on the surface or 100 mR/h at 3 ft from the package require notification of the radiation safety officer (USNRC Title 10, 2013). *These must be documented daily on receiving forms.*

Infection and Radiation Exposure Control.

Protective shielding in a variety of forms must be used when working with radioactive material. Several protective measures must be followed to minimize radiation contamination and exposure. Some examples of shielding protection materials are lead bricks, disposable gloves, leaded glass, shielded bench tops, syringe shields, vial dose, lead-shielded containers to transport radioactive materials outside of the nuclear medicine department, and shielded waste receptacles. Use of the gloves and shielding are considered mandatory for the nuclear medicine worker. The department/institution must have a plan in place in case of a spill of radiopharmaceuticals, and training of non-nuclear medicine personnel must be provided and documented.

In addition, OSHA requires that all personnel who work with needles and blood products minimize their chance of exposure to the human immunodeficiency virus and the hepatitis virus by practicing standard precautions. When working with patient procedures that include needles and patient blood products, personnel are now required to wear disposable gloves. The standard precaution guidelines assert the prevention of recapping of needles at all costs. The used syringe must be placed in an approved infectious control needle and syringe receptacle, or sharps container (Fig. 15-22). Because nuclear medicine deals with radioactive needles and syringes, the sharps container also must be properly shielded, be decayed, and have stored a minimum of 10 half-lives before disposal to the biohazard department.

Radiopharmaceutical Administration

After preparation and quality control testing, the radiopharmaceutical is ready to be dispensed and administered

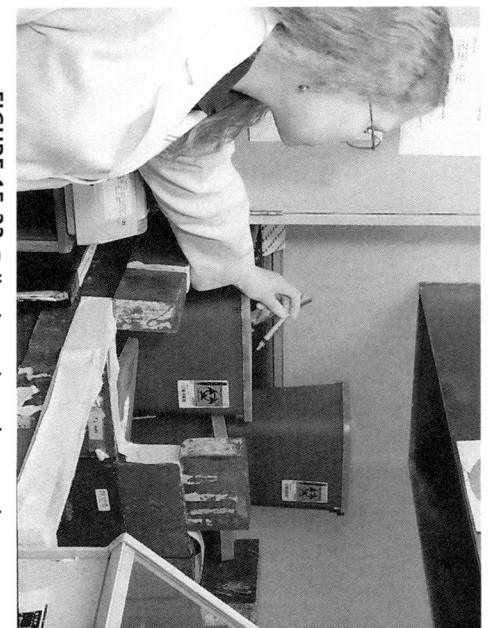

FIGURE 15-22 Following universal precautions.

to a patient. Quality assurance does not stop here. The individual who is dispensing and injecting the radiopharmaceutical should again verify the requisition, the identity of the radiopharmaceutical, the activity, and the patient. The following information must be visually inspected and verified on each request before the nuclear medicine procedure is initiated:

- Patient's name
- Hospital identification number and room number
- Requesting physician's name
- Patient history, condition, and preliminary diagnosis
- Examination agreement with the physician's orders and possible diagnosis of the patient
- Correct radiopharmaceutical for the examination
- Contraindications that can interfere with the radiopharmaceutical biodistribution
- Patient's physical limitations
- Allergies or potential drug interactions
- Potential nuclear medicine radiopharmaceutical interference with other diagnostic or therapeutic procedures
- Patient concerns

After the information has been checked and it is determined that the examination is correct, the person who is administering the radiopharmaceutical must continue to practice good quality assurance. The radiopharmaceutical, the activity, and the volume to be administered must be verified. Before administration, the patient's name and hospital identification number must be verified on the patient's wristband. Finally, if an outpatient is being treated, he or she must be identified through name, birth date, and social security number. If misadministration occurs, the radiation safety officer must be notified immediately. The radiation safety officer determines what NRC classification of misadministration has occurred and immediately takes appropriate action (USNRC Title 10, 2013) including notification of ordering physician, medical director, patient, and NRC or agreement state. An

CHAPTER 15 Quality Assurance in Nuclear Medicine

investigation must be conducted to determine all factors contributing to the misadministration and a plan made of corrective action including training to prevent future occurrences.

REVIEW QUESTIONS

1. The scintillation detector is based on the principle that certain crystals _____ after deposition of energy by some ionizing radiation.
   a. Vibrate
   b. Refract
   c. Emit light
   d. Trap

2. The crystal that is used in most planar and SPECT gamma cameras is the _____ crystal.
   a. Cesium iodide (CsI(T1))
   b. Cesium fluoride (CsF)
   c. Lithium iodide LiI(Eu)
   d. NaI(T1)

3. _____ testing involves performing a quality control performance evaluation of the camera system without the collimator.
   a. Extrinsic
   b. Intrinsic
   c. Phantom
   d. Dead time

4. What are the two most important quality control procedures that must be performed on a scintillation gamma camera?
   a. Intensity; persistence
   b. Counting efficiency; sensitivity
   c. Flood field uniformity; spatial resolution
   d. Linearity; geometry

5. A dose calibrator is an example of an ionization chamber. The following quality control procedures are mandated by the NRC except for which of the following?
   a. Geometry
   b. Chi-square
   c. Linearity
   d. Accuracy
   e. Constancy

6. Which of the following values is the allowable (NRC) limit of molybdenum in the generator eluent of ^{99m}Tc pertechnetate?
   a. 0.0015 μCi/mCi
   b. 0.015 μCi/mCi
   c. 0.15 μCi/mCi
   d. 1.5 μCi/mCi
   e. 1.5 mCi/μCi

7. _____ is the gamma camera's ability to see detail in any image.
   a. Spatial linearity
   b. Spatial resolution
   c. Relative position
   d. Energy resolution

8. In addition to the routine quality assurance procedures required for planar gamma cameras, the SPECT systems require evaluation of its tomographic performances, as well as reconstruction algorithms. Uncorrected center-of-rotation errors greater than 1/2 pixel can produce significant loss of spatial resolution. The quality control procedure COR aligns the COR projected onto the computer matrix with the center of the _____ used for reconstruction.
   a. Camera
   b. Patient
   c. Computer matrix
   d. Camera gantry

9. Evaluating the equipment used in a SPECT system is important, as is evaluating each patient study for artifacts or errors. The sinogram of a selected tomographic slice is a summed image of all the projection data. It is useful in detecting _____, which can degrade the quality of the SPECT study.
   a. Patient motion
   b. Dead time
   c. Correct acquisition time
   d. Incorrect radionuclide energy

10. Impurities found in radiopharmaceutical preparations are placed in all of the following categories except which of the following?
    a. Chemical impurities
    b. Nuclidic impurities
    c. Radionuclide impurities
    d. Radiochemical impurities

REFERENCES

Accreditation manual for hospitals: *Accreditation manual for hospitals*, vol. 1. Oakbrook Terrace, IL, 1993, Joint Commission on Accreditation of Healthcare Organizations: Standards.

Anger HO: Scintillation camera, *Rev Sci Instrum* 29:27, 1958.

Bernier DB, Christian PE, Langan JM, et al.: *Nuclear medicine: technology and techniques*, ed 4, St Louis, 1997, Mosby.

Cherry S: *Physics in Nuclear Medicine*, ed 4, St. Louis, 2012, Mosby.

Christian P, Waterman-Rich K: *Nuclear medicine and PET/CT*, ed 7, St. Louis, 2013, Mosby.

Early PJ, Sodee BD: *Principles and practices of nuclear medicine*, ed 2, St Louis, 1995, Mosby.

Eisner R: Principles of instrumentation in SPECT, *J Nucl Med Technol* 13:23, 1985.

English RJ: *SPECT single-photon emission computerized tomography: a primer*, ed 3, Reston, VA, 1995, The Society of Nuclear Medicine.

Esser PD, Sorenson JA, Westerman BR: *Emission computed tomography*, New York, 1983, The Society of Nuclear Medicine.

Graham SL, Kirchner PT, Siegel BA: *Nuclear medicine: self study program II: instrumentation*, Reston, VA, 1996, The Society of Nuclear Medicine.

Greer K: Quality control in SPECT, *J Nucl Med Technol* 13:76, 1985.

Henkin RE, et al.: *Nuclear medicine*, vol. 1. St Louis, 1996, Mosby.

Karp JS, et al.: Performance standards in positron emission tomography, *J Nucl Med* 2:2342, 1991.

Klingensmith III WC, Eshima D, Goddard J: *Nuclear medicine procedure manual: 1995-1996*, Englewood, CO, 1995, Wick.

Murphy PH: Acceptance testing and quality control of gamma cameras including SPECT, *J Nucl Med* 28:1221, 1987.

Murray IPC, Ell PJ: *Nuclear medicine in clinical diagnosis and treatment*, vol. 1. Edinburgh, 1994, Churchill Livingstone.

National Electrical Manufacturers Association: NEMA standards for performance measurements of scintillation cameras, Washington, DC, 1986, The Association. Pub No NU1-1986.

National Electrical Manufacturers Association: *NEMA standards for performance measurement of positron emission tomographs*, Washington, DC, 2001, Publication 2-2001.

National Electrical Manufacturers Association: *Performance measurements of scintillation camera*, Washington, DC, 1980, The Association.

Rao DV, Early PJ, Chu RY, et al.: *Radiation control and quality assurance surveys: nuclear medicine—a suggested protocol*, American College of Medical Physicists, 1986, Rep No 3.

Regulatory Guide 8.25: Air sampling in the workplace, Washington, DC, 1992, US Nuclear Regulatory Commission.

Regulatory Guide 8.7: Instructions for recording and reporting occupational radiation exposure data, Washington, DC, 1992, US Nuclear Regulatory Commission.

Robbins PJ: *Chromatography of technetium-99m radiopharmaceuticals: a practical guide*, New York, 1984, The Society of Nuclear Medicine.

Saha GP: *Physics and radiobiology of nuclear medicine*, New York, 1993, Springer-Verlag.

Scintillation camera acceptance Scintillation camera acceptance testing and performance evaluation, Chicago, 1980, American Association of Physicists in Medicine. Rep 6.

Sorenson JA, Phelps ME: *Physics in nuclear medicine*, ed 2, Philadelphia, 1987, WB Saunders.

Steves AM: *Review of nuclear medicine technology*, New York, 1992, The Society of Nuclear Medicine.

Strasinger SK, Di Lorenzo MA: *Phlebotomy workbook for the multiskilled healthcare professional*, Philadelphia, 1996, FA Davis.

Taukulis RA, et al.: Technical parameters associated with miniaturized chromatography systems, *J Nucl Med Technol* 7:19, 1979.

Thrall JH, Ziessman HA: *Nuclear medicine: the requisites*, St Louis, 1995, Mosby.

The Joint Commission: *Accreditation Manual 2013*. Oak Brook, IL 2013. The Joint Commission.

USNRC Regulatory Guide: 8.18: Information relevant to insuring that occupational radiation exposures at medical institutions will be as low as reasonably achievable, Washington, DC, 1977, US Nuclear Regulatory Commission.

USNRC Title 10: *Code of Federal Regulations, Part 20: standards for protection against radiation*, Washington, DC, 2013a, US Nuclear Regulatory Commission.

USNRC Title 10: *Code of Federal Regulations, Part 20: standards for protection against radiation*, Fed Reg 56(89):23390, 2013b.

USNRC Title 10: *Code of Federal Regulations, Part 20: standards for protection against radiation*, Fed Reg 56(98):23390, 2013c.

USNRC Title 10: *Code of Federal Regulations, Part 35: human uses of byproduct material*, Washington, DC, 2013d, US Nuclear Regulatory Commission.

Webber DJ, Zimmer AM, Spies SM: Common errors associated with miniaturized chromatography, *J Nucl Med Technol* 11:66, 1983.

Ziessman H, et al.: *Nuclear medicine*, ed 4, Philadelphia, 2013, Saunders.

Zimmer AM: *Miniaturized chromatography procedures for radiopharmaceuticals*, Chicago, 1991, Northwestern University Medical Center.

Zimmer AM, Pavel DG: Rapid miniaturized chromatographic quality control procedures for Tc-99m radiopharmaceuticals, *J Nucl Med* 18:1230, 1977.

Zimmer AM, Spies SM: Quality control procedure for newer radiopharmaceuticals, *J Nucl Med Technol* 19:210, 1991.

Index

Resolution (Continued)
monitor, 307
spatial, in tomographic imaging, 115, 115f
temporal, 134
Resolution chart
for focal spot size estimation, 104-105, 105f
for spatial resolution, 47-48, 47f
Resonance frequency, 285-287, 285b
Resource Conservation and Recovery Act (1987), 59-62, 83b
Resources Conservation/Hazardous Waste Act (1976), 83b
Respect and caring, 12
Responsibility, assigning, 11
Restrainer, in developer, 55
Reticulation marks, 182
Rhodium, as target material, 197
Risk, definition of, 28
Risk analysis, 28-29
Risk management, 20, 28-29
policies and procedures in, 29
risk analysis in, 28-29
Risk priority numbers (RPN), 17
Risk to others, to diagnostic imaging department, 29
Risks to employees and medical staff, to diagnostic imaging department, 28
Risks to patients, to diagnostic imaging department, 28
Road mapping, 153
Roentgen (R), 97
Roller subsystem, of film processor, 63
Root cause analysis (RCA), 10
Rotatable spoke test pattern, 134, 134f
Run chart or run-sequence plot, 25-26, 26f
Rusting, of steel wool cartridge, 84-85

S

Safelight, 38-39, 38f-39f
testing, 40, 40f
Safelight fog, 185
Safe Medical Devices Act (SMDA), 2, 4
Safety
in care environment, 12
chemical, 59-62
magnetic resonance imaging, 284-285
mechanical and electrical, 95
from radiation, 20, 29-33
Safety and loss prevention. see Risk management
Sample, 20
Saturation, 143-144
Scan image uniformity, 307-308, 308f
Scan lines, 189f
Scanner housing, visual inspection of, 304
Scatter, increased sensitivity to, 188
Scatter diagram, 25, 25f
Scatter plot, 25, 25f
Scattered radiation, 346
Scheduled maintenance, 72
Scientific management, 3
Scintillation crystal
in automatic exposure control systems, 110, 110f
in gamma camera, 321
Scintillation detectors, 335-336, 335t, 336f

Scintillation gamma camera, 320-322, 320f-321f
acceptance tests for, 322b
quality control of, 322-328, 322t
counting rate limits in, 323-324
energy resolution and photopeaking in, 322-323, 323f
field uniformity in, 324-326, 324f-326f
multiple-window spatial registration in, 327-328, 328f
sensitivity in, 327, 327f
spatial resolution and spatial linearity in, 326-327, 326f-327f
Scintillator digital radiography system, 146
Scrap exposed film, 88
Scratches, 186
Screen speed. see also Intensifying screens.
factors affecting, 44-45
intensifying, 44-45, 44t
older names for, 44t
optical density and, 344
quality control testing of, 45-46
uniformity of, in mammography, 204
S distortion, 123f, 124
Sealed radioactive source testing, 336
Secondary capture, 138-140, 139f-140f
Section level, tomographic, 114, 114f
Section thickness, tomographic, 114, 114t, 115f
Section uniformity, of tomographic system, 115-116
Self-managed teams (SMTs), 10
Sensitivity
diagnostic, 178, 191
for processor monitoring, 77, 77b, 79f
gamma camera, 327, 327f
ultrasound instrument, 305-306, 305f
Sensitometer
for processor monitoring, 73-74, 74f
for safelight testing, 40b
Sensitometric curve
for film contrast, 346-347, 346f
for processor monitoring, 77, 77b, 79f
Sensor, automatic exposure control, 110, 110f
Sentinel event indicator, 11
Sequestering agent
in developer, 55
in fixer, 58
Serious adverse event, 265b
Serious complaint, 264, 265b
Service recovery, 6
Setup and table positioning accuracy, in magnetic resonance imaging equipment, 285, 285b
Severity number, 16-17
Shading test in digital radiography, 149b, 150f
Shape distortion, 350
Sharpness, image, 348
Shewhart, Walter A., 15-16, 26
Shielding, 33, 340
of breast areas, 31
Short-scale or high radiographic contrast, 345
SID. see Source-to-image distance (SID)
Sigma, 17, 21

Signal-to-noise ratio (SNR)
consistency, in magnetic resonance imaging, 297-299, 297f-298f, 298b
contrast resolution and, 46-47
Silver
consumer of, 82
worldwide supply of, 83
Silver flake, 86, 86f
Silver recovery, 82-89
from film, 87-88
justification for, 83-84
monetary return for, 83
pollution laws and, 83-84, 83b
from processing chemicals, 84-87
chemical precipitation for, 87
direct sale of used fixer for, 86-87
electrolytic, 85-87, 85f-86f, 86b-87b
ion exchange or resin systems for, 87
metallic replacement for, 84-85, 84f, 85b
Single-energy X-ray absorptiometry, 174
Single-phase generator, 91-92, 91f
Single-photon absorptiometry, 173-174
Single-photon emission computed tomography cameras, 328-330, 329t
center of rotation in, 330
pixel size of, 330
quality control during/after procedures for, 330, 331f
uniformity correction flood in, 329, 329f
Single-photon emission computed tomography (SPECT), 328
Six Sigma, 17, 22
Size distortion, 350
Slice position accuracy, 293, 293b
Slice thickness
in computed tomography, 274-275, 275f, 275b
in magnetic resonance imaging, 293-296, 293b, 296f-297f
in ultrasound, 313
Slow scan, in digital fluoroscopy, 154
Smudge static, 186
SNR. see Signal-to-noise ratio (SNR)
Society of Motion Picture and Television Engineers (SMPTE) test pattern, 134
for electronic display devices, 158-159, 159f
for magnetic resonance imaging hard-copy images, 290
for multiformat camera, 163
for ultrasound images, 306-307, 306f
Sodium vapor lamp, 38-39, 39f
"Soft-copy" viewing, 156
Solarization, 41, 347, 347f
Solid-state detectors, 110
Solution concentration, 55, 71
Solvent
in developer, 55
in fixer, 58
Source-skin distance, for fluoroscopic unit, 132, 132b
Source-to-image distance (SID)
for mammography, 197
optical density and, 344
for radiographic unit, 108, 109f, 109b
recorded detail and, 348
size distortion and, 350

Index

Quality control film, 77, 77b, 78f
Quality control (QC), 7
  basic tenets of, 269
  history of, 3
  levels of testing in, 7
Quality improvement, 3. *see also* Continuous quality improvement.
Quality improvement team, 10
Quality management, 1–18
  components of, 20
  history of, 3–8
  process improvement in, 8–17
  tools and procedures for, 19–34
Quality management technologist duties, 27b
Quantitative computed tomography (QCT), 174–175
Quantitative ultrasound, 175
Quantum mottle, 184
  in computed tomography, 272
  contrast resolution and, 46–47
  in digital radiography, 187, 187f

R

Radiant flux, 42b
Radiation Control for Health and Safety Act, 3
Radiation exposure. *see also* Patient dose
  in computed radiography, 143–144
  control of, 340
  dose limits for, 339t
Radiation field, light field congruence with, 105–106
Radiation fog, 185
Radiation measurement, 96–97
Radiation output
  of mammographic equipment, 204–205
  in radiographic equipment, 98, 98b
Radiation protection
  patient, 30–32
  personnel, 32–33, 338–340, 338t–339t, 339f
  principles of, 33
  visitor, 32
Radiation quality, subject contrast and, 46–47
Radiation safety program, 20, 29–33
Radioactive source, sealed, 336
Radioactivity signposting, 339, 339f
Radiochemical, 334
Radiochemical impurity, 337
Radiofrequency coils, in magnetic resonance imaging, 296–298, 297f
Radiofrequency shielding effectiveness, 293b
Radiographic contrast, 345
Radiographic equipment
  ancillary, 90–119
  portable and mobile X-ray generators, 117–118
  control or operating console, 93–94
  conventional tomographic systems, 109–113
  automatic exposure control systems, 113–115
  high-voltage generator in, 94
  quality control program for, 94–109
  environmental inspection in, 95–96
  performance testing in, 96–109, 96f

Radiographic equipment (*Continued*)
  beam alignment in, 107, 107f
  beam quantity in, 98
  beam restriction system in, 105–107
  filtration check in, 98
  focal spot size in, 103–105
  kilovolt (peak) accuracy in, 98–100, 100f
  milliampere and exposure time linearity and reciprocity in, 103, 103b
  overload protection in, 108–109
  radiation measurement in, 96–97
  radiation output in, 98, 98b
  reproducibility of exposure in, 97–98
  source-to-image distance and tube angulation indicators in, 108, 109f, 109b
  timer accuracy in, 101–102, 102f
  voltage waveform in, 100–101, 100f
  X-ray tube heat sensors in, 109
  visual inspection in, 94–95
  X-ray generators, 91–93
  X-ray tube, tube accessories, and patient support assembly in, 94
Radiographic examinations
  ALARA program for, 30
  dose reduction for, 143, 144t
Radiographic images
  outcomes assessment of, 177–193
  artifact analysis in, 181–189
  diagnostic performance measurement in, 189–191
  repeat analysis in, 178–181, 178t, 179f–180f
Radiographic mottle, contrast solution and, 191, 192f
  quality of, 343
  in computed tomography, 271–274
  contrast in, 345–348
  distortion in, 350
  optical density and, 343–345
  recorded detail in, 348–350
  statistical phantom for, 191, 192f
Radiographic table, inspection of, 95
Radioiodine, 339
Radiological Society of North America (RSNA), 171
Radiology Information System (RIS), 171
Radionuclide, 334
Radionuclide generator, molybdenum-99/technetium-99, 337
Radionuclide impurity, 337
Radiopharmaceuticals, 334, 337–338, 338f
  administration of, 340–341
  positron-emitting, 330
Radiopharmacy, 336–341
  personnel protection in, 338–340, 338t–339t, 339f
  radionuclide generator in, 337
  radiopharmaceutical administration in, 340–341
  radiopharmaceuticals in, 334, 337–338, 338f
  sealed radioactive source in, 336
Rads, 97
Random errors, 21
Range, 21

Rare earth phosphors, 45
  emission color of, 45t, 46f
  line spectrum from, 46f
Rate meters, 97
Rebromination, 347
Receiver gain, in magnetic resonance imaging, 293b
Receiver operator characteristic (ROC) curve, 191, 192f
Reciprocity
  law failure, in automatic exposure control, 113
  milliampere and exposure time, 103, 103b
Recirculating electrolytic unit, 86
Recorded detail, 343, 348–350
  digital imaging and, 349–350
  factors affecting, 348
Record-keeping system, 28
Records
  of image, ultrasound routine quality assurance, 306–307
  in mammography, 263–265
  patient, 5, 12
Reducing agents, 54
Reflection, display, 160b–161b
Reflective layer, screen speed and, 45
Refresh rate, 156–157
Regeneration system, of film processor, 66
Region of interest (ROI), 272
Regulator in developer, 55
Reimbursement, 2, 6
Relative conversion factor, 133
Relative density difference (DD), 75b–76b
Relative operator characteristic curve, 191, 192f
Relative sensitivity test in computed radiography, 149b
Relative speed value, 44
Reliability, 21
Repeat analysis, 178–181
  advantages of, 178
  causal repeat rate in, 178–180
  for mammography, 235–237, 239f
  total repeat rate in, 180–181
  worksheets for, 179f–180f
Repeat examinations, 31
Replenishment rate, chemical activity and, 70–71
Replenishment system, of film processor, 66
Reporting requirements, mandatory, 4, 5t
Reproducibility
  of automatic exposure control, 112, 112b
  of exposure
    of fluoroscopic unit, 128b
    of X-ray generator, 97–98
  of radiographic equipment, 97, 97b
Resin systems, for silver recovery, 87
Resolution
  in computed radiography, 143
  in computed tomography, 271–272, 271b–272b, 273f
  in digital imaging, 349–350
  in digital mammography, 200
  of gamma camera, 326–327, 326f–328f
  of image receptor, 349
  of intensifying screen, 46–50

369

Index

Passboxes, 38
Patient artifacts, 183
Patient comfort, 27
Patient dose
 in cinefluorography vs. video recording, 168
 in computed radiography system, 143, 144t
 in computed tomography, 276, 276f, 276b, 277t
 in digital mammography, 201
 repeat analysis and, 178
Patient exposure, in tomography, 115–116, 116b
Patient motion, detection of, 330, 331f
Patient position, improper, 183
Patient Protection and Affordable Care Act, 6
Patient radiation protection, 30–32
Patient records
 data collection from, 12
 privacy standard for, 5
 security standard for, 5
Patient support assembly, 94
Patient surveys and questionnaires, 12
Patient thickness, fluoroscopic image brightness and, 123b
Patient-to-image intensifier, distance, 32
Penetrometer, 40f, 40b
Penumbra effect, 348
Percent signal ghosting, in magnetic resonance imaging, 297–298, 298b
Performance evaluation, 7
Performance measurement system, 14
Performance measures, identifying, 11
Performance testing, of fluoroscopic equipment, 128–134
Permissible exposure limits (PELs), for darkroom chemicals, 37
Perpendicularity, X-ray beam, 108, 108b
Personal protective equipment (PPE), 4, 59
Personnel monitoring in nuclear medicine, 338–339
Personnel performance, 27–28
Personnel protection from radiation, 32–33, 32t, 338–340, 338t–339t, 339f
PET. *see* Positron emission tomography (PET)
Pete, 87
pH, 54f, 55
 chemical activity and, 71
 developer solution, 55
 fixer solution, 87b
Phantom image artifact, 187, 188f
Phantoms
 cine-video, 169, 170f
 for computed tomography, 268, 268f–269f
 for digital radiography, 149f–150f, 149b
 for digital subtraction angiography, 155–156, 156f
 for dual-energy X-ray absorptiometry, 175f
 for fluoroscopy, 130
 for gamma camera, 326, 326f–327f
 homogenous, 111b, 112f
 for magnetic resonance imaging equipment, 284, 284f
 for mammography, 204, 204f, 235, 235f–237f, 235b
 statistical, 191, 192f
 thyroid, 336, 336f

Phantoms (*Continued*)
 for ultrasound
  anechoic voids in, 310–313, 313f
  desiccation of, cautions about, 303–304, 304f
  design of, 302–303, 303f
  Doppler flow, 314–315, 314f
  objects of various echogenicity, 313, 313f
  spherical object, 313–314, 313f
  tissue-mimicking, 302
  tissue properties represented in, 302
Phenidone, 54, 54f
Phosphor crystals, size of, screen speed and, 45
Phosphor materials
 photostimulable, 140
 recorded detail and, 349
 spectral matching for, 46, 46f
 thickness of layer of, 45, 45f
 type of, screen speed and, 44–45
Phosphorescence, 44
Photocathode, of image intensifiers, 121f, 122
Photoconductor digital radiography system, 146–147
Photodetectors, 110, 110f
Photoemission, 122
Photofluorography, 169–170
Photofluorospot camera, 126, 169
Photographic light meter, 41, 42f
Photography, in ultrasound, 306–307
Photometry, 42b–43b
Photomultiplier tubes (PMTs), 110, 110f
 in gamma camera, 320–321, 320f, 325f
Photon, 321
Photopeak
 of gamma camera, 322–323, 323f
 of scintillation detector, 335
Photostimulable phosphors, 140
Photostimulated luminescence, 140
Phototimer, 110
Picture Archiving and Communication System (PACS), 170, 171t
 cloud-based, 172t
 computed radiography and, 143
 for mammography, 201
 secondary capture for, 139
 test pattern for, 172f
Picture element, 138
"Piggybacking," of metallic replacement, 84f, 85b
Pi lines, 182, 182f
Pincushion distortion, 123, 123f
Pinhole camera, 103–104, 104f, 104b
Pixels, 138, 145–146, 145f
Pixel pitch, 156–157
Pixel size
 spatial resolution and, 349
 in SPECT camera, 330
Planetary rollers, 63, 63f
Plasma displays, 158
Plumbicon, 124
Pluridirectional tomography, 113, 114f, 116f
PMTs. *see* Photomultiplier tubes (PMTs)
Pocket dosimeters, 96, 97t
Point spread function, 48, 48f
Poisson distribution, 22
Pollution laws, 83–84, 83b
Population, 20

Portable X-ray generators, 117
Positive beam limitation systems, 106–107
Positive predictive value, 191
Positron emission tomography/computed tomography systems, 332–333
Positron emission tomography (PET), 330–333
Posteroanterior (PA) projection, 31
Postprocessing
 in computed radiography, 141
 in digital mammography, 200
Power assist, in fluoroscopic unit, 126
Power cord, visual inspection of, 304
Power ratings, 93
PPE. *see* Personal protective equipment (PPE)
Practice guidelines and parameters, 14
Precipitation, 87
Precision, 21
Prejudice, 21
Premix or ready-mix developer solution, 56
Preprocessing in computed radiography, 141
Preservative
 in developer, 54
 in fixer, 57
Pressure injectors, 173
Pressure marks, 185
Prevalence, 190–191
Preventive maintenance
 of processor, 72
 of ultrasound equipment, 302
Primary protective barrier, in fluoroscopic unit, 127
Printer errors, 189, 190f
Probability number, 17
Problem identification and analysis, 9–11
Problem-solving teams, 10–11
Process, 8
Process improvement, 8–17
Processing, optimum conditions for, 31
Processing area condition, 40–41, 41b
Processing artifacts, 181–183
Processing time
 developer, 70, 70f
 film processor, 67
Processor, quality control of, in mammography, 209–234
Progressive scan monitors, 125
Proportional counter, for radiation measurement, 97
Protective curtain, in fluoroscopic unit, 126–127
Psychrometer, 36–37, 36f
Pulsed interlaced scan mode, in digital fluoroscopy, 154
Pulsed progressive scan mode, in digital fluoroscopy, 154
Pulse height analyzer (PHA), 322
Pupin, Michael, 44

Q

Quality
 cost of, 3
 levels of, 2
Quality assessment, 7
Quality assurance (QA), 7
 agencies, organizations, and committees, 351
Quality circles, 10

Material Safety Data Sheet (MSDS), 59, 60f–62f
Matrix size, 349
Maximum density (D_{max}), 75b–76b
Maximum detection depth, in Doppler flow phantoms, 315
Maximum entrance exposure rate, for fluoroscopic unit, 130, 130f, 130b–131b
Maximum exposure time, for automatic exposure control, 111, 111b
Maximum gradient strength, in magnetic resonance imaging, 293b
Maximum sensitivity, 305
Mean, 21
Mean computed tomography number, 268
Measure in Cycle for Improving Performance, 14, 15f
Measurement error, 21
Median, 21
Medicaid, 4
Medical audit and outcomes analysis, for mammography, 263–264
Medical devices classification of, 30 reporting requirements for, 4
Medicare, 3–4
Medicare Improvements for Patients and Providers Act (MIPPA), 2, 4, 268–269, 320
Medicare Improvements for Patients and Providers Act of 2008, 283–300
Medium-frequency generators. see High-frequency generator
Metallic replacement, 84–85, 84f, 85b
Metol, 54
Mid-density point (MD), 75b–76b
Milliampere emission spectrum and, 196, 196f of fluoroscopic equipment, 31 of fluoroscopic equipment, linearity of, 129, 129b image brightness and, 123b optical density and, 344 of radiographic equipment for automatic exposure control, 111, 111b
Milliampere-second (mAs), of radiographic equipment, 30 linearity and reciprocity of, 103, 103b
Minification gain, 122
Minimum density (D_{min}), 75b–76b
Minimum exposure time, for automatic exposure control, 111
Mirror optics, 124
Miscellaneous equipment, inspection of, 95
Mixing procedure, developer, 56
Mobile X-ray generator, 117–118, 117t
Mode, 21
Modulation transfer function, 48–50, 49f, 49b
Moiré effect, 184, 185f
Moly breakthrough, 337
Molybdenum, as target material, 196f, 197
Molybdenum-99, 337
Molybdenum-99/technetium-99 radionuclide generator, 337
Molybdenum-rhodium-tungsten alloy, as target material, 197

Monitors cleanliness, 307 setup, for ultrasound, 306
Motion artifacts due to, 183, 330, 331f recorded detail and, 349
Multichannel analyzers, 335
Multifield image intensifier, 122, 123f
Multiformat cameras, 161–163 components of, 161–163 format patterns for, 165f quality control of, 163, 163b
Multiple-window spatial registration, of gamma camera, 327–328, 328f
Multivoting, 10

N
National Center for Devices and Radiological Health, 3
National Council on Radiation Protection (NCRP), 30
National Electrical Manufacturers Association (NEMA) standards DICOM-3, 170 focal spot and, 105, 105t, 203, 204t scintillation camera, 322, 322b
National Pollutant Discharge Elimination System (NPDES) permit, 59–62, 83b
National Radiology Data Registry (NRDR), 14
Negative predictive value, 191
New modality film, 39
Nightingale, Florence, 3
Nit, 43b
Noise in computed tomography, 273–274, 273f in digital radiography, 149b in fluoroscopy, 132–133, 133b optical density and, 344
Non-rare earth phosphors, 44–45, 46f
Noninvasive Evaluation of Radiation Output (NERO) system, 7, 96, 96f
Nonscheduled maintenance, 72–73
Normal distribution. see Gaussian distribution
Nuclear medicine, quality assurance in, 319–342 counting rate limits of, 323–324 energy resolution and photopeaking of, 322–323, 323f field uniformity of, 324–326, 324f–326f multiple-window spatial registration of, 327–328, 328f sensitivity of, 327, 327f spatial resolution and spatial linearity of, 326–327, 326f–327f nonimaging equipment for, 333–336 dose calibrator, 334–335, 334f gas-filled detectors in, 333–334 scintillation detectors in, 335–336, 335f, 336f positron emission tomography positron emission tomography/computed tomography systems in, 332–333 radiation protection for, 336–341 radiopharmacy in, 338–340, 338f–339f, 339f

Nuclear medicine, quality assurance in (Continued) radioactive source in, 337 radiopharmaceutical administration in, 340–341 radiopharmaceuticals in, 334, 337–338, 338f sealed radioactive source in, 336 scintillation gamma camera in, 320–322, 320f–321f, 322t, 322b SPECT camera for, 322b, 328, 329f, 329t, 331f center of rotation of, 330 pixel size of, 330 quality control during/after procedures for, 330, 331f uniformity correction flood of, 329, 329f
Nuclear Regulatory Commission (NRC), 30, 333, 338t
Nyquist frequency, 47–48, 147

O
Objective plane, 113
Object-to-image distance (OID) optical density and, 344 recorded detail and, 348 size distortion and, 350
Observation, in fluoroscopic unit, 127
Occupational Safety and Health Administration (OSHA), 333 hazard communication standards of, 59 infection control policy of, 4, 340, 340f permissible exposure limits, 37 radiation safety standards of, 30
Occupational Safety and Health Administration (OSHA) 2000 Log, 28
Optical density, 343–345 digital imaging and, 345 excessive, 183 factors influencing, 343–345 improper, 183 inherent, 345 insufficient, 183 measurement of, 74, 75
Optically stimulated luminescent dosimeter (OSL), 338–339
Orthicon, 124, 124f
Orthochromatic film, 39
OSHA. see Occupational Safety and Health Administration (OSHA)
Output, 9
Output phosphor, of image intensifier, 122, 125
Overhead lighting, in darkroom, 38
Overhead tube crane, inspection of, 95
Overload protection, 108–109
Oxidation/reduction reaction, 53

P
PACS. see Picture archiving and communication system (PACS)
Panchromatic film, 39
Pareto chart, 24–25, 25f
Park position interrupt, in fluoroscopic unit, 127
Part thickness consistency of exposure and, 111–112, 112b optical density and, 344

Index

J
Joint Commission. *see* The Joint Commission (TJC)
Juran, Joseph, 3

K
K-edge effect, 45
Kennedy-Kassebaum Act, 5
Kerma, 130
Key process variables, 9
Key quality characteristics, 9
Kilovolt (peak)
  of fluoroscopic equipment, 31
    accuracy of, 129b
    half-value layer values for, 179t
    image brightness and, 123b
  of mammographic equipment, 195
    accuracy and reproducibility of, 203
    emission spectrum and, 196, 196f
    optical density and, 343–344
  of radiographic equipment, 30, 91
    accuracy of, 98–100, 100f
    consistency of exposure with varying, for automatic exposure control, 111, 111b–112b
    screen speed and, 45, 46f, 46b
Kilowatt rating, 93

L
Lambert, 42b
Larmor frequency, 285, 285b
Laser, computed radiography, 349
Laser cameras, 163–166, 165f, 166b
  components of, 164–165, 164f
  quality control of, 166, 166b–167b
Laser film printer control chart, 277, 279f
Laser jitter test, 149b
Laser light accuracy, 271, 271f, 271b
Laser printers. *see* Dry laser printers
Laser scanning digitizer, 139, 139f
Last frame-hold feature, 153
Last-image-hold feature, 32
Latensification, 36
Latent image, 52
Lateral resolution, in ultrasound, 310, 312f
Law of Reciprocity, 113
Lazio, Rick, 3–4
Lead aperture, of tomographic test tool, 115f
Lead apparel, 32
Lead aprons, 33
  in fluoroscopic unit, 128
Leakage testing
  light, 39–41
  and processing area condition, 40–41, 41b
Lean process improvement, 17
LED safelight, 39
Leeds Test Object Kit, 150f
Legislation and government regulations affecting healthcare delivery, 2
  for quality management, 3–6, 5t
Lens coupling, 125, 125f
Level incrementation, tomographic, 114–115
Level of expectation, 12
Licensure and certification, 3–4
Light-absorbing dyes, screen speed and, 45, 45f

Light field-radiation field alignment (congruence), 105–106
Light fog, 185
Lights/meter function, in fluoroscopic unit, 127
Limiting resolution, 271b
Limiting spatial resolution, 47–48, 147
Linearity
  in computed radiography, 149b, 155–156
  in computed tomography, 275–276, 275f–276f, 276b
  milliampere, fluoroscopic, 129, 129b
  milliampere and exposure time, 103
  spatial
    of gamma camera, 327
    of magnetic resonance imaging, 287, 287f
Linear (rectilinear) tomography, 113, 113f
  lead aperture with, 116f
Line focus principle, 103, 104f
Line spread function, 48, 48f
Liquid crystal display (LCD)
  for fluoroscopy, 125
  quality control of, 158, 158f
Local area network (LAN), 171
Locational effect, 75b–76b
Long-scale or low radiographic contrast, 345
Look-up tables (LUTs)
  for computed radiography, 140f, 142
  for digital image contrast, 347–348, 348f
Loss control management. *see* Risk management
Loss potential, 29
Lossless compression, 172
Lossy compression, 172
Low-contrast resolution
  in computed tomography, 272, 272b, 273f
  of display device, 160b–161b
  of fluoroscopic unit, 132, 132b, 132f
  in magnetic resonance imaging, 289, 289b
Low-contrast visibility, 307
Low density (LD). *see* Minimum density (D_{min})
Luminance, 42b, 159
Luminescence, 44
Luminous flux, 42b

M
Magnetic field homogeneity, 290–293
Magnetic fringe field, 299
Magnetic resonance imaging equipment
  artifact analysis for, 289–290, 290f
  center frequency of, 285–287, 285b–286b
  detectability, 289, 289b
  evaluation form, 294b–295b
  geometric accuracy of, 287, 287f–289f, 287b–288b
  high-contrast resolution of, 287–289, 289f
  interslice RF interference, 298
  low-contrast resolution of, 289, 289b
  magnetic field homogeneity in, 290–293
  medical physicist/system engineer, 293b
  optional tests of, 299
  phantoms for, 284, 284f
  quality control for, 283–300

Magnetic resonance imaging equipment (Continued)
  hard copy images, 290, 290b–291b
  testing frequency, 284–285
  visual checklist, 292b
  radiofrequency (RF) coils of, 296–298, 297f
  setup and table positioning accuracy for, 285, 285b
  slice position accuracy of, 293, 293b
  slice thickness accuracy of, 293–296, 293b, 296f–297f
  soft-copy display devices for, 299
  transmit gain of, 287
  visual checklist, 292b
Magnification, 35f
  in fluoroscopy, 122, 123f
  in mammography, 199–201
Magnification mode, in fluoroscopy, 32
Main drive chain, 64
Main drive shaft, 64
Maintenance
  preventive, ultrasound, 302
  processor, 72–73, 72b–73b
  silver recovery unit, 87b
Mammographic quality standards, 194–266
Mammography, 195
  archiving images for, 88
  display devices for, 147
  equipment dedicated to, 195–201
    compression by, 197–198, 197b
    digital systems in, 199–201
    film processors in, 199
    grids in, 198
    image receptors in, 198–199, 198f
    magnification by, 199
    major repairs to, 205
    performance of, 263
    stereotactic localization by, 201
    X-ray generator, 195, 195f
    X-ray tube and window of, 195–197, 196f–197f
  quality assurance for, 201–265
    FDA inspection in, 263, 264b–265b
    legislation for, 201–202
    medical physicist responsibility in, 203
    for digital systems, 205–209, 210f–233f
    for film/screen systems, 203–205, 206f–208f
    radiologic technologist responsibility in, 209, 263t
    for digital systems, 241–263, 242f–262f
    for film/screen systems, 209–265, 234f–241f, 235b, 237b, 239b–240b
    radiologist responsibility in, 203, 263t
    repeat rates for, 180–181
    statistical phantom for, 191, 192f
Mammography Quality Standards Act (MQSA), 2, 4–5, 199, 201–202
Mammography Quality Standards Reauthorization Act (MQSRA), 2, 201–202
Manifest image, 52
Manual film processing, 53
Master rollers, 63

Index

Gaussian distribution, 22, 22f
Gear reduction mechanism, 64
Gears, drive subsystem, 64, 64f
Geiger-Müller counter, 97
Geiger-Müller (GM) meters, 334
Gelatin buildup, 181
Geometric accuracy, in magnetic resonance imaging, 287, 287f–289f, 287b–288b
Geometric distortion in display device, 159
Geometric factors, in recorded detail, 348–349
Geometric unsharpness. *see* Penumbra effect
Ghost intensity, 293b
Glass envelope, of image intensifiers, 121–122
Gloves
  in fluoroscopic unit, 128
  inspection of, 95
  for nuclear medicine, 340
  personal protective equipment standards, 59
  protective, 33
Gonadal shielding, 31
Gray level performance of computed tomography scanner display monitors, 281, 281b
Grays (Gy), 97
Gray-scale hard copy, in ultrasound, 306–307, 306f
Grayscale processing, 200
Gray-scale uniformity, 307
Green film, 88
Grid alignment
  in mammography, 198
  in tomographic system, 116
Grid uniformity
  in fluoroscopic system, 129b
  in tomographic system, 116, 116b
Group dynamics, 9–11
Guide shoe marks, 181–182, 182f

H

Half-value layer
  for fluoroscopic filtration, 129t
  minimum mammographic, 204, 204t
  for radiographic filtration, 98, 99f, 99t
Half-wave rectified generator, 91, 92f, 101
Halo artifacts, 189
Handling and storage artifacts, 184–186
Hard-copy viewing, 156
Hardener
  in developer, 55
  in fixer, 58
Hazard communication standards, 59
Healthcare delivery, changes in, 2
Health Information Technology for Economic and Clinical Health Act, 5, 5t
Health Insurance Portability and Accountability Act (HIPAA), 5, 171
Health Level 7 (HL7) standard, 171
Heat blur, 187

Heat sensors, X-ray tube
  for fluoroscopic unit, 129, 129b
  for radiographic unit, 109
Heel effect, 348–349
Hesitation marks, 182, 183f
High-contrast resolution, in fluoroscopy, 131–132, 131f
High-contrast spatial resolution in computed tomography, 271–272, 271b
High-density (HD). *see* Maximum density (D_{max})
High-frequency generator, 93, 93f
  for mammography, 195
High-pass filtering, 350
High transmission cellular (HTC) grid, 198
High-voltage generator, 94
HIPAA. *see* Health Insurance Portability and Accountability Act (HIPAA)
Histogram
  for computed radiography system, 141f
  in information analysis, 23–24, 25f
Histogram error, 187
Homogenous phantom, 111b, 112f
Horizontal distance measurement, in ultrasound, 308–309, 309f
Hospital Care Quality Information from the Consumer Perspective survey, 27
Hospital Corporation of America, 15–16
Hospital Information System (HIS), 171
Humidity, 36–37, 41
Hurter and Driffield curve, 73, 77, 346
Hydrolyzed reduced technetium, 337
Hydrometer, 55, 71, 71f
Hydroquinone, 54, 54f
Hypo in fixer, 57, 57b
Hyporetention, 53, 183, 184b
  in mammographic films, 237, 237b, 240f
  test kits for, 58, 58f

I

Illuminance, 42b
Illuminator bulb brightness, 107, 107b
Image archiving and management networks, 170–173, 172f, 173b
Image compression, 172
Image congruency test, 315
Image contrast, 153
Image duplicating units, 153
Image enhancement, in digital fluoroscopy, 153
Image intensifier tube digital fluoroscopy systems, 153, 153f
Image intensifiers
  artifacts of, 122–124, 123f
  components of, 121–122, 121f–122f
  image brightness and, 122, 123b
  multifield, 122, 123f
Image intensity uniformity, in magnetic resonance imaging, 297, 297b
Image inversion, 200
Image lag, in fluoroscopy, 132, 133b
Image monitoring systems, 124–126
Image reader device, in computed radiography, 140–141, 140f–141f, 349

Image receptors. *see also* Film/screen image receptors
  for computed radiography, 140
  flat-panel digital, 153
  for mammography, 198–199, 198f, 204
  in positive beam limitation system, 106–107
Image receptor system speed, 344, 346
Image receptor systems, high-speed, 30–31
Image recording devices, 306
  in ultrasound, 306–307
Image restoration, 153
Image uniformity
  in computed radiography, 155–156
  in computed tomography, 272–273, 272b, 273f
  in magnetic resonance imaging, 298b
  in ultrasound, 307–308, 308f
Imaging plate for computed radiology, 187, 187f, 349
Immersion time, developer activity and, 55, 57f
Improve in Cycle for Improving Performance, 14, 15f
Incident, 29
Incident light, 74f, 75
"Incident report," 29
Independent variables, 21
Indicator, 11
Indirect-conversion digital radiography system, 146
Infection control policy, 4
  in mammography, 264
  in nuclear medicine, 340, 340f
Information analysis, 20–26
  terminology used in, 23–26
  tools for, 23–26
Input, 9
Input phosphor, of image intensifiers, 121f–122f, 122
Integrating Healthcare Enterprise, 171
Intensification factor, 44
Intensifying screens
  cleaning of, 50b, 234–235
  condition of, 50, 50f
  resolution of, 46
  speed of, 44–45, 44t
  factors affecting, 44–45
  optical density and, 344
  quality control testing of, 45–46
Interlaced horizontal scanning, 125
Intermittent fluoroscopy, 32
Internal customers, 9
Interpolation, 156–157
Interslice RF interference, 298
Interventional procedures, fluoroscopic systems for, 134, 134b
Ion chambers
  in automatic exposure control system, 110
  for radiation measurement, 96, 96f
Ion-detecting radiation detectors, 333–334
Ion exchange, of silver recovery, 87
Ionization survey meter, 333
Ionomat, 110
Iron-impregnated foam cartridge, for silver recovery, 85
Ishikawa diagram, 23, 24f
Isodose curves, for computed tomography, 276, 276f

365

Index

E

Environmental Protection Agency (EPA), 59–62, 83
Equipment performance, in mammography, 263
Equipment quality control, 20
Erasure test in digital radiography, 149b, 150
Error, 21
Error correction tests, 7
Ethylenediamine tetraacetic acid (EDTA), 55
Exposure angle, tomographic, 114
Exposure artifacts, 183–184
Exposure latitude, film contrast and, 347, 347f
Exposure switch, in fluoroscopic unit, 127
Exposure time
 for automatic exposure control, 111, 111b
 milliampere linearity/reciprocity and, 103, 103b
 for multiformat camera image, 163
Extended processing, 199
External customers, 9
Eyeglasses, protective, 33
Eyewash station, 59

F

FADE model, 14, 15f
Fading, 140
Failure Mode and Effects Analysis (FMEA), 16
False negative (FN), 190–191
False positive (FP), 190–191
F-centers, 140
FDA. *see* Food and Drug Administration (FDA)
Federal pollution laws, 83–84, 83b
Fiber optics, 125, 125f
Field size
 consistency of exposure and, 112, 112b
 limiting, 31
 optical density and, 344
Field uniformity
 of gamma camera, 324–326, 324f–326f
 of SPECT camera, 329, 329f
Fill factor, 147
Film
 archival quality of, 58
 handling of, 36
 quality control, 77, 77b, 78f
 safelight for, 38
 silver recovery from, 82, 87–88
Film bin, 38, 38f
Film changers, 173
Film emulsion, contrast and, 346
Film gamma, 346
Film or inherent contrast, 346
Film processing, 52–68. *see also* Automatic film processors
 automatic, 53
 chemical safety in, 59–62
 chemicals for, 53–62
 fixer in, 56–58
 manual, 53
 washing in, 58–59
Film processors, quality control of, 69–81
 characteristic curve in, 77, 77b, 79f
 chemical activity in, 69–71
 cleaning procedures in, 71–72, 71b–72b
 for daylight systems, 77–78, 80f
 maintenance in, 72–73, 72b–73b
 monitoring in, 73–77
 troubleshooting in, 77, 80t

Film/screen contact
 in mammography, 240, 240f, 240b
 poor, 184
 resolution and, 49
Film/screen image receptors, 44–50
 intensifying screen speed in, 44–45, 44t
 in mammography, 198–199, 198f, 204
 screen condition in, 50, 50f, 50b
 screen resolution in, 46–50
 spectral matching in, 46
Film/screen radiography
 artifacts in, 181
  exposure, 183–184
  handling and storage, 184–186
  processing, 181–183
 computed radiography *vs.*, 143, 144f
 digital *vs.*, 138
 image quality in, 343
  contrast and, 345–348
  distortion and, 350
  optical density in, 343–345
  recorded detail and, 348–350
 mammographic systems for
 medical physicist responsibility in, 203–205, 206f–208f
 radiologic technologist responsibility in, 209–265, 234f–241f, 235b, 237b, 239b–240b
 repeat analysis worksheet for, 178–180, 180f
Film/screen spot film devices, 126, 126f
Film speed
 contrast and, 347, 347f
 optical density and, 344
 recorded detail and, 349
Film transfer systems, 38
Filtering, digital, 153, 350
Filters
 developer circulation system, 65–66
 safelight, 38–39
Filtration, 31
 emission spectrum and, 196, 196f
 by fluoroscopic equipment, 128b, 129t
 optical density and, 345
 by radiographic equipment, 98, 99b–100b
5 Whys of problem solving, 10
Fixer, 56–58. *see also* Chemicals. processing
 direct sale of used, 86–87
 ingredients of, 57–58
 mixing procedure, 58
 replenishment, 66
 silver accumulation in, 84
Fixing agent, 57, 57b
Flare, 133
Flat-fielding, 150
Flat-panel detector, of image intensifiers, 121
Flat-panel digital fluoroscopy systems, 153
Flat-panel or flat-plate imaging, 145
Flood replenishment, 66
Flowchart, 23, 23b, 24f
Flow meters, 70–71
Fluorescence, 44
Fluoroscopic equipment, 121–126. *see also* Digital fluoroscopy
 for cardiac catheterization and interventional procedures, 134, 134b

Fluoroscopic equipment (*Continued*)
 guidelines and protocols for, 121
 image intensifiers in, 121–124, 121f
 image monitoring systems in, 124–126
 quality control of, 120–136
  environmental inspection in, 128
  performance testing in, 128–134
  visual inspection in, 126–128
Fluoroscopic examinations, ALARA protocols for, 31–32
Fluoroscopic imaging, statistical phantom for, 191, 192f
Flux gain, 122
FMEA. *see* Failure Mode and Effects Analysis (FMEA)
Focal spot, 103
Focal spot blooming, 103, 105
Focal spot size
 for fluoroscopic equipment, 128b
 for mammography, 197, 203, 204t
 for radiographic equipment, 103–105, 104b, 105t
 recorded detail and, 348
Focal spot test tool, 104, 104f, 105t
Focus groups, 10, 12
FOCUS-PDCA, 15–16, 16f
Fog
 age, 185
 chemical, 181, 181f
 darkroom, 237–240, 239f
 light, 185
 optical density and, 344
 radiation, 185
 safelight, 38, 40f, 185
 subject contrast and, 346
Fog density, 345
Food and Drug Administration (FDA)
 mammography regulation by, 199, 201–202
 mammography requirements by, 4–5
 medical devices and, 4, 30
 MQSA inspection by, 263, 264b–265b
Foot-candles, 43b
Foot-lambert, 42b
Foreign objects, artifacts due to, 188–189, 189f
Foreshortening of image, 350
Fourier transformation, 48–49
"14 Points for Management," Deming's, 7–8, 8b
Frame averaging, 153
Frame rate, 156–157
Frequency, 20
Full-field digital mammography systems, 199
 medical physicist responsibility in, 205–209, 210f–233f
 radiologic technologist responsibility in, 241–263, 242f–262f
Full-wave rectified generator, 91–92, 92f, 101
Full width-half maximum (FWHM), 48

G

Gamma camera
 scintillation, 320–322, 320f–321f, 322t, 322b
 SPECT, 322b, 328, 329f, 331f
Gas-filled detectors
 chamber, for performance testing, 96
 quality control of, 333–334

Darkroom (*Continued*)
 environment of, 36–41
 film and chemical storage, 41
 function of, 36
 light and leakage testing in, 39–41, 40f,
   237, 239b
Darkroom disease, 37
Data collection and organization, 12
Data Form for Daily CT Equipment Quality
   Control, 277, 278f
Data set, 20
Daylight systems, 80f
 quality control of, 77–78
Dead time, 323–324
Decompression, mammographic system,
   205
Deficit Reduction Act, 6
Deming, W. Edwards, 3, 7–9, 15–16
Densitometer, 343
Densitometry, bone, 173–175, 175f
 for safelight testing, 42b
 for processor monitoring, 74–75, 74f
Density control function, automatic
 exposure control, 112–113, 113b
Dependent variables, 20
Depth calibration accuracy, 308
Depth of visualization, 305
Design, in Cycle for Improving
   Performance, 13–14, 15f
Destructive or atrophic diseases, 344–345
Det Norske Veritas, 6–7
Det Norske Veritas Healthcare, 6–8
Detectability, in magnetic resonance
   imaging, 289, 289b
Detection number, 17
Detective quantum efficiency (DQE), 146–147
Detectors
 area, 339
 automatic exposure control, 110, 110f,
   112, 112b
 dose calibrator, 334–335, 334f
 gas-filled, 333–334
 gas-filled chamber, 96
 personal, 338–339
 scintillation, 335–336, 335f, 336f
 solid-state, 110
 X-ray output, 100–101, 101f
Developer, 53–56, see also Chemicals
 processing
 activity of, 55
 components of, 53–55
 mixing, 56
 replenishment, 66
Developing agents, 54
Development
 contrast and, 346
 optical density and, 344
Diagnostic imaging, 2, 138
Diagnostic performance measurement,
   189–191, 190f
Diagnostic range, for optical density, 75
Dichotomous variables, 21
Dichroic stain, 182
DICOM. *see* Digital Imaging and
 Communications in Medicine
   (DICOM)
Digital dosimeter, 96, 97f

Digital fluoroscopy (DF), 152–154
 digital subtraction angiography in,
   154–155, 154f
Digital image recorders, 126, 168–169, 169b
 quality control for, 155–156
Digital images, archiving and management
 networks for, 170–173, 173b
Digital imaging
 image distortion, 350
 optical density, 343–345
 recorded detail or spatial resolution with,
   349–350
Digital Imaging and Communications in
 Medicine (DICOM), 171
Digital kilovolt (peak) meter, 100f
Digital mammography systems, 199–201
 quality control for
 radiologic technologist responsibility
   in, 241–263, 242f–262f
Digital photospot imaging, 168–169
Digital radiographic imaging systems,
   138–156, 139f
 computed radiography, 140–145, 140f
 digital radiography, 145–147, 145f
 quality control for, 148–152, 149b, 152b
 secondary capture, 138–140, 139f–140f
Digital radiography (DR)
 artifacts in, 186–189
 computed *vs.*, 147
 equipment for, 145–147, 145f
 manufacturers for, 148
 quality control for, 149b, 152b
 repeat analysis worksheet for, 178–180, 180f
Digital subtraction angiography, 154–155,
   154f
Digital temporal filtering, 153
Digital thermometer, 70, 70f
Digital X-ray radiogrammetry, 175
Digital X-ray timer, 101–102, 101f
Direct-conversion digital radiography
 system, 146–147
Directional effect, 75b–76b
Direct-power units, X-ray generators, 117
Direct-to-digital radiographic systems
   (DDR), 145
Disease presence
 optical density and, 344–345
 subject contrast and, 346
Disintegrations per minute (DPM), 336
Displacement method, of silver recovery,
   84, 84f, 85b
Distance from radiation source, 33
Distance measurement accuracy, in
 ultrasound, 303, 308–309, 309f
Distortion
 display device, 159
 fluoroscopic image, 132
 radiographic image, 343, 350
 spatial, 307
D log E curve, 77, 346
Doppler ultrasound testing, 314–315
Dose area product (DAP), 31
Dose calibrator, 334–335, 334f
Dose creep, 30
Dosimeters, 96
Dosimetry, in mammography, 204, 204f

Double exposure, 184, 188, 188f
"Double read" method, 191
DR. *see* Digital radiography (DR)
Drain stoppage, 85
Drive motor, 64
Drive subsystem, 64, 64f
Dropped pixels, 189
Drying film, 53
Drying system, of film processor, 66, 67f
Dry laser printer film, 39
Dry laser printers, 166–168, 166f
 artifacts due to, 189
 in digital mammography, 200
 hard copy image quality control of,
   in digital mammography, 200
Dry-to-drop time, 67
Dual-energy subtraction, 155, 200
Dual-energy X-ray absorptiometry (DEXA),
   174, 174t
Dual focus multifield image intensifiers, 122
Dual-photon absorptiometry, 174
Dust filters, visual inspection of, 304
Dwell time, 87b

E

Echogenicity variation, in ultrasound, 313,
   313f
Edetate. *see* Ethylenediamine tetraacetic
 acid (EDTA)
Edge definition, monitor, 307
Edge enhancement, 141–142, 143f, 350
Edge packing, 324
Edge spread function, 48, 49f
Edison, Thomas, 44
Effective focal spot, 103, 348
Effectiveness of care, 12
Efficacy of care, 12
Efficiency of care, 12
Eight-penny (nine-penny) test, of light field-
 radiation field congruence, 105–106,
   106f, 107b
80/20 Rule, 8, 24–25
85/15 Rule, 8
Electrical system, of film processor, 66–67
Electrolysis, 85
Electrolytic silver recovery, 85–87, 85f–86f,
   86b–87b
Electronic display devices, 156–161, 157f
 quality control of, 158–161, 159f
Electronic probe tests, for ultrasound
 transducer, 315–317, 315f–316f
Electrostatic focusing lenses, in image
 intensifier, 121f, 122
Elon, 54
Elongation, of image, 350
Emission spectrum, 195–196, 196f–197f
Emulsion pickoff, 181
Energy resolution
 of nuclear imaging equipment, 322–323,
   323f
 of scintillation detector, 335–336
Energy subtraction, 142, 143f
Entrance rack, 63
Entrance roller marks, 182, 182f
Entrance rollers, 63, 63f
Environmental inspection
 in fluoroscopic equipment, 128
 of radiographic equipment, 95–96

Index **363**

Index

Spatial accuracy
  in computed radiography, 150
  in digital radiography, 149b, 150f
Spatial distortion, 307, 350
Spatial frequency, 47–48
Spatial linearity
  of gamma camera, 327
  in magnetic resonance imaging, 287, 287f
Spatial resolution, 138, 139f
  comparison of, 48t
  in computed radiography, 143
  in computed tomography, 271–272, 271b
  in digital imaging, 349–350
  in digital mammography, 200
  of display device, 159
  of gamma camera, 326, 326f–328f
  of image receptor, 349
  of intensifying screens, 47–50, 47f, 48b
  in magnetic resonance imaging, 287–289
  in tomographic imaging, 115, 115f
  in ultrasound, 309–310
Special procedures laboratory, 173
Specific absorption rate monitor, 293b
Specific gravity
  measurement of, 71, 71f
  of solution concentration, 55
Specificity, 178, 191
SPECT. see Single-photon emission computed tomography (SPECT)
Spectral matching, 46
Spectrum
  emission, 195–196, 196f–197f
  radionuclide, 323, 323f
  visible light, 38, 38f
Specular reflection, 160b–161b
Speed indicator, 75b–76b
Spinning top test, of timer accuracy, 101–102, 101f–102f
Spot film camera, 126
Spot images and spot image size, 32
Staff reports, 12
Standard deviation, 21–22
Standard entrance exposure rates, for fluoroscopic unit, 130–131, 131f
Standard precautions, 4
Standardized uptake value, 331, 332b
Standby replenishment, 66
Start-up effect, 21
Starter in developer, 55
State pollution laws, 83–84
Static artifacts, 185–186, 186f
Static electricity, 36
Statistical analysis
  terminology used in, 20–23
  tools for, 23–26
Statistical inference, 20
Statistical quality control (SQC), 7–8
Statistics, 20
Steel wool cartridge, for silver recovery, 84–85
Step tablet, 73–74, 74f
Stereotactic localization, in mammography, 201
Sterling silver, 83
Stop bath or water rinse, 53
Storage area network (SAN), 172
Storyboard, 13, 13f
Stratification, 65
Streaking, 65, 182, 183f
String test objects, for Doppler ultrasound, 314
Stub lines, 182
Subject contrast, 345–346
Sulfurization, 86
Superfund Amendments and Reauthorization Act (1986), 59–62
Supplier, 8–9
Surface area, in silver recovery, 87b
Surface coils performance, in magnetic resonance imaging, 293b, 296
SWOT analysis, 14–15, 15f
Synergism, 51
System, 8
System cleaner, 72
Systematic errors, 21

T

Table angulation and motion, in fluoroscopic unit, 128
Table locks, in fluoroscopic unit, 126
Tanning agent, in fixer, 58
Target angle, for mammography, 197
Target composition, 195–197, 196f
Target material, emission spectrum and, 196, 196f
Taylor, Frederick Winslow, 3
Technetium-99m, 322–323, 323f, 337
Technetium-99m pertechnetate, 337
Technology, advances in, 2
Teleradiology, 139
Television camera, 124–125
Television monitor, 125
Temperature
  ambient, 45
  chemical activity and, 70, 70f
  darkroom, 37
  developer activity and, 55
  film and chemical storage, 41
  silver recovery and, 87b
  solution, in developer, 55, 56f
Temperature control system, of film processor, 64–65
Temporal mask subtraction, 155, 155f
Temporal resolution, 134
10-Step monitoring and evaluation process, 11
Terminal electrolytic unit, 86
Test objects
  for computed tomography, 275, 275f
  for ultrasound, 310–314
Test patterns
  AAPM TG18-AD, 164f
  AAPM TG18-CT, 162f
  AAPM TG18-CX, 164f
  AAPM TG18-LN01, 162f
  AAPM TG18-LN08, 162f
  AAPM TG18-LN18, 162f
  AAPM TG18-MP, 163f
  AAPM TG18-PQC, 164f
  AAPM TG18-UNL10, 163f
  AAPM TG18-UNL80, 163f
  for display devices, 158–159, 159f
  for dry laser printer, 168f
  for film, 290

Test patterns *(Continued)*
  for fluoroscopic unit, 134, 134f–135f
  for gamma camera, 326, 326f–327f
  for multiformat camera, 165f
  picture archiving and communication system, 172f
  for ultrasound images, 306, 306f
The Joint Commission (TJC), 4, 6
  accreditation procedures of, 2
  continuous quality improvement and, 7–8
  Cycle for Improving Performance of, 13–14, 15f
  nuclear medicine program of, 320
  safety guidelines of, 28–29
  10-step monitoring and evaluation process of, 11
Thermoluminescent dosimeter (TLD), 338–339
Thermometer, 70, 70f
Thermostatically controlled system, of film processor, 64–65, 65f
Thin-film transistor (TFT), 145–146, 145f
Thought process map (TPM), 10–11
Three-phase generators, 92–93, 92f
  six-pulse, 92, 92f
  12-pulse, 92–93, 93f
Threshold of acceptability, 26
Thyroid uptake probe, 336, 336f
Time
  automatic exposure control, 111
  developer processing, 70, 70f
  of radiation exposure, 33
Timed replenishment, 66
Time-in-solution test tool, 70, 70f
Time-interval difference subtraction, 155, 155f
Timeliness of care, 12
Time-of-day variability, 75b–76b
Timer, in fluoroscopic unit, 127
Timer accuracy, of radiographic unit, 101–102, 102f
Tissue attenuation coefficients, 302, 303b
Tissue density
  fluoroscopic image brightness and, 123b
  optical density and, 344
  subject contrast and, 345–346
Tissue equalization, 200
Titus, Donald E., 66
TJC. see The Joint Commission (TJC)
TN fraction, 191
Tomographic angle, 113, 113f
Tomographic systems, conventional, 113–115
  quality control of, 113–115, 114f
  types of, 113
Tomography
  linear (rectilinear), 113, 113f
  pluridirectional, 113, 114f
  positron emission, 330–333
  quantitative computed, 174–175
  single-photon emission computed, 328
Tomosynthesis, 201
Total loss control. *see* Risk management
Total quality control (TQC). *see* Total quality management (TQM)
Total quality improvement (TQI). *see* Total quality management (TQM)
Total quality leadership (TQL). *see* Total quality management (TQM)

Index

Total quality management (TQM), 7–8
Total repeat rate, 180–181
Tower, in fluoroscopic unit, 126
TP fraction, 191
Transducers, ultrasound
 choice of, 304–305
 electronic probe tests for, 315–317, 315f–316f
 visual inspection of, 304
Transmission-based precautions, 4
Transmission densitometer. *see* Densitometer
Transmit gain, in magnetic resonance imaging equipment, 287
Transmitted light, 74, 74f
Transmitter setting, in magnetic resonance imaging, 293b
Transport rack subsystem, of film processor, 63–64
Transport rollers, 63, 63f
Transport system, of film processors, 63–64, 63f
Tree static, 185
Trend chart, 25–26, 26f
Trending, 25–26
Trifocus multifield image intensifiers, 122
Troubleshooting, processor, 77, 80t
Troy oz, 82
True negative (TN), 190–191
True positive (TP), 190–191
Tungsten, as target material, 196, 196f
Tungsten-rhenium alloy target, 195–196, 196f
Turnaround rack, 63, 63f

U

Ultrasound equipment
 basic quality control tests for, 304–309
 distance measurement accuracy in, 303, 308–309, 309f
 documentation for, 309, 310b–312b
 Doppler testing for, 314–315
 electronic probe tests for, 315
 preventive maintenance, 302
 quality assurance, 301–318
 components of, 302–304
 tasks of, 309
 quantitative, 175
 spatial resolution tests for, 309–310
 test objects and phantoms
  anechoic voids in, 310–313, 313f
  desiccation of, cautions about, 303–304, 304f
  design of, 302–303, 303f
  Doppler flow, 314–315, 314f
  spherical object, 313–314, 313f

Ultrasound equipment (*Continued*)
 string, 314
 tissue-mimicking, 302
 tissue properties represented in, 302
 with varying echogenicity, 313, 313f
Ultraviolet (UV) light, 41
Uniformity correction flood, 329, 329f
Uniformity in digital radiography, 150
Universal precautions, 340, 340f

V

Validity, 21–23
Variable-aperture collimator, 94, 105–106, 106f
Variance, 22
Variation, 22
Veiling glare, 122–123, 133
Velocity accuracy, in Doppler flow phantoms, 315
Ventilation, in darkroom, 37
Vertical distance measurements, in ultrasound, 308, 309f
Vertical or deep racks, 63, 63f
Video monitor performance, in fluoroscopic image, 134, 134b, 135f
Videotape and videodisc recorders, 168, 169b
Video waveform, in fluoroscopic unit, 133, 133f
Vidicon, 124
Viewbox illuminators, 41, 205
Viewbox quality control, 41, 42b
Viewing conditions, 205
Vignetting, 124
Visible light spectrum, 38, 38f
Visitor protection, 32
Visual checklist, 277, 280f
Visual inspection
 of fluoroscopic equipment, 126–128
 of magnetic resonance imaging equipment, 290
 of mammographic equipment, 235, 238f
 of radiographic equipment, 94–95
 of ultrasound equipment, 304
Voltage ripple, 93, 197, 197f
Voltage waveform
 emission spectrum and, 197, 197f
 of fluoroscopic equipment, 129
 optical density and, 345
 of X-ray generator, 100–101, 100f
Volume flow accuracy, in Doppler flow phantoms, 315
Volume of computed tomography dose index (CTDI$_{vol}$), 276
Volume replenishment, 66

W

Warm-water processor, 64, 65f
Washer or coin method, for beam alignment measurement, 109b
Washing film, 53

Water computed tomography number and standard deviation, 277, 280b
Water-controlled system, of film processor, 64, 65f
Water Pollution Control Act, 59–62, 83b
Water rinse or stop bath, 53
Water spots, 182, 183f
Weiner spectrum graph, 49, 49f
Wet laser printer quality control, 277, 281b
Wet-pressure sensitization, 182, 184f
Wetting agent, 53
Wheels and wheel locks, visual inspection of, 304
White light, 38
Wide area network (WAN), 171
Window level, 153
Window width, 153
Wipe test, 339
Wire mesh test, of film/screen contact, 49, 49b, 50f, 240, 240f, 240b
Wisconsin Test Cassette, 98–100, 99f
Workflow, in mammography, 200
Workstation, computed radiography, 141, 142f
Work teams, 10
World Health Organization (WHO), 174, 174t

X

X-ray beam-Bucky tray alignment, 108, 108f, 108b
X-ray field/light field/image receptor/ compression paddle alignment, in mammography, 204
X-ray generators, 91–93
 for fluoroscopy, 121
 for mammography, 195, 195f
 performance testing of, 73–74
 portable and mobile, 117–118
 power ratings of, 93
 quality control of, 90–119
 types of, 91
 voltage ripple of, 93
X-ray output detector, 100–101, 101f
X-ray tube accessories, 94
X-ray tube heat sensors
 for fluoroscopic unit, 129, 129b
 for radiographic unit, 109
X-ray tubes, 94
 angulation indicators for, 108
 for fluoroscopic unit, 121
 for mammography, 195–197, 196f–197f
X-ray tube window, for mammography, 195
X-Y scales, accuracy of, 107, 107b

Z

Zebra pattern artifact, 184, 185f